Too Much Medicine Not Enough Health

Too Much Medicine Not Enough Health

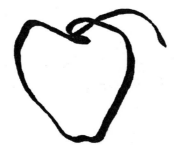

Jeffry Fawcett PhD

Layna Berman

From the Producers of

Your Own Health and Fitness

Published by 8½x11 Productions, PO Box 460, Camp Meeker, CA 95419, www.8x11p.com

Second printing.

Designed by Layna Berman

Text is set in Century Schoolbook and Futura.

Printed in the United States of America.

Library of Congress Control Number: 2009901990

ISBN13 978-0-9754237-0-7

Contents

𝒢

Contents

Prologue

This book is a collection of 48 articles from the quarterly *Progressive Health Observer: A News Commentary Alternative to Big Box Medicine* (PHO). The articles are organized into 15 sections, each introduced by an original essay.

PHO articles share a common structure. They open with a news item or event about a health, medical, or related issue. The news is often the report of research. The article then examines the actual research and discusses how the research fits with other research and how accurately the science was actually reported by the media. Typically, alternative resources are discussed and cited, enabling readers to learn more and make informed decisions.

The articles are always critical in the neutral sense of "critical thinking"—they are written to invite the reader to carefully consider the information presented in the news and in the research. However, the articles are also often critical in the negative sense of "finding fault." All too often, the journalism is weak, the meaning of research results is not supported by the evidence, researchers' conclusions are not supported by their own data, and the research design itself is flawed.

So the PHO is part media studies, part science education, and part health information.

The sections of *Too Much Medicine, Not Enough Health* are not organized as you might expect for a "health book." Our intention is to disrupt the ordinary, diagnosis-and-treatment mode of thought typical of books about health. We also intend to disrupt the false distinction between books about personal action (the self-help mode) and books about collective action (the public health/public policy mode).

The title *Too Much Medicine, Not Enough Health* means what it says: our failing health care system is too much about medical diagnosis and treatment and not nearly enough about actual health. In fact, we argue that this failure is at the very core of our health care crisis.

The inspiration for the book is the work of Layna Berman through her weekly radio show *Your Own Health And Fitness* and in her private practice as a health educator. It is her work that inspired and informs the *Progressive Health Observer* from which this book is constructed.

Although the PHO articles include references, they are not formally footnoted. Instead, references are placed at the end of the article. Conventional footnoting is used in the essays that introduce each section. We hope this does not interfere with the book's usefulness.

The information in this book is intended to complement your other health information sources. In particular, it is not a substitute for professional advice. Before acting on any health information, including the information in this book, you should weigh the benefits and risks, then decide using your own best judgment.

Health care is in crisis.

The great public debate on the crisis is principally about economics: who does and does not have access to health care, how to pay for it, who pays for it, and how to control health care costs. A secondary issue, connected to controlling costs, concerns the quality of care and the capacity of current health care institutions to deliver it.[1]

Some health care professionals argue that business interests— pharmaceutical companies and medical device manufacturers in particular—have completely warped the care people receive.[2] Still others argue further that the crisis has been caused by overdiagnosis and overtreatment in the practice of medicine, creating fertile ground in which business can plant the seeds for profit.[3]

What's missing from the debate is an acknowledgment that our health care system isn't about health. It's about medicine: being diagnosed and treated for a disease or injury. We have been conditioned to think of our health as the absence of disease.

That way of thinking is a mistake. Health is not the absence of disease. It's the capacity to thrive. Our institutional failure to grasp the difference is at the core of the health care crisis.

The problem is demonstrated no more clearly than in preventive medicine. Preventive medicine is central to many health care reform proposals. It is positioned to play a major role through its promise to reduce the incidence of disease and the cost of disease.[4] H. Gilbert Welch, MD is a vocal critic of this approach, going so far as to call it a myth.[5]

What the preventive medicine strategy for health care reform promotes is the idea that by actively attending to the factors that predict illness, the medical system can both keep people healthy longer and, by avoiding serious illness, reduce long-term health care costs. Dr. Welch argues that both assumptions are false.

Dr. Welch argues that the actual practice of preventive medicine is about turning healthy people into patients. The actual practice of preventive medicine consists of routine screening for risk factors in the absence of overt symptoms of illness. The result of tests and examinations are compared to standards for these risk factors. The standards, in turn, are set in order to ensure that patients are compliant with treatments. The treatments consist principally of prescription drugs, medical procedures, and the installation of medical devices.

Although it's supposed to be about keeping people healthy by avoiding illness, in the social dynamics of the doctor's office preventive medicine is about treating yet another disease. The person-as-patient understands quite clearly that she is sick. That's because it's the doctor's office and that's what doctor's do: they treat the sick.

For example, hypertension is just such a disease. We discuss what's wrong with this diagnosis in our article "Hypertension All Around" in this book's section on Illness. High blood pressure is a sign that the body is under stress. Instead of finding ways to reduce the stress, physicians typically prescribe a drug that forces the body to lower its blood pressure, leaving the underlying cause unexamined and unresolved. Frequently, the drug creates side effects, creating another illness that requires its own treatment.

Preventive medicine that turns healthy people into patients has pushed the envelope still further by putting "pre" in front of medical conditions. Some examples of these new diseases include pre-hypertension and pre-diabetes, created by lowering risk factor standards further so that more people are at risk and so treated earlier.

This strategy of preventive medicine as something delivered in the doctor's office has been in force for many decades. Dr. Welch's concern is that, despite the actual history of its failure, this kind of prevention is being sold to us as the cure for our health care system's ills.

One illustration of that failure is the billions of dollars that have been spent over many decades on heart disease and cancer. Yet these two conditions remain our major causes of death.[6]

Another illustration is, on the one hand, the increasing number of people taking prescription drugs and, on the other hand, the increasing incidence of death and injury from these drugs. During the 1990s, the number of adults taking at least one drug increased by 10% to almost half and the number of people taking three or more drugs almost doubled.[7] During the same period, the rate of deaths from prescription drugs almost doubled.[8]

Prescription drugs are not the only source of overtreatment. Medical procedures such as surgeries can have side effects that lead to additional procedures, additional pharmaceutical prescriptions, or both with equally dire consequences.

We believe that there is more than ample evidence that the real source of prevention is not in the doctor's office or in the medical system. Instead, it is in our communities and other social environments, where we health care civilians make our lives, that prevention has its proper place: social networks of family and friends, places of work, formal community and professional organizations, informal neighborhood gatherings, relationships created over common social or political interests, and, of course, governments. A vast body of research supports this idea. We discuss that research in many of the articles in this book.

The misconception of health shows up in another form in this book. Enabling health care civilians to make informed health and medical decisions requires that they be well informed and able to use their best judgment. Yet de facto, the health care system is the functional arbiter of what counts as valid health and medical information and sound judgment.

There is no viable alternative to the system of knowledge institutionalized in the health care system that is dominated by conventional medicine. The media is as close as it comes—and it is a very weak reed. As we describe in this book, the media are enraptured by this very system of experts.

In other words, medicine is the loadstone for our discourse on health. Even critical thinking on health care has medicine, disease, and healing as its center of gravity.[9] With no countervailing force, health has come to mean the absence of disease—essentially, you're pronounced healthy if a doctor can't find anything wrong with you.

With this book we want to contribute to another center of gravity for the discourse on health. The idea at the core of *Too Much Medicine, Not Enough Health* is that we health care civilians have been conditioned to think and act as though health is another medical condition. It's not. It's the biological capacity to to live a full, rich life.

It's important to dwell on this briefly before moving on.

In the existing health care system, the operational meaning of "health" is that it is a condition (or absence of one). It's something each person has—by luck or circumstance. So as a condition, health is something that happens to you—something that might even be your fault.

In contrast, the idea of health as a capacity is about what each person and their body are able to do. It's a capacity that develops in response to what each person wants from life. It's a capacity that develops based on what each person knows and learns. It's a capacity developed in response to the circumstances in which each person finds herself, the circumstances she seeks out, and the circumstances she creates, on her own and with others.

In other words, health is about power—the power not only to care for infirmities but the power to take action that purposefully makes life better.

This points us in a direction that's very different from the way the health care system is arranged. The central relationship in the health care system is between a health care provider and a patient in a clinical setting. The central relationship we want to promote is between each person and their circumstances, both physical and social..

We health care civilians have among us a wealth of capacities, resources, and knowledge that can enable us to thrive. What we have is the raw material for sustainable health—the capacity of people and their communities to thrive. That force needs to be mobilized.

This is a subversive concept. It runs against the winds of the culture of expertise that enshrouds the health care system.[10]

As we said earlier, the core relationship in the health care system is one-on-one—one health care practitioner engaged with one patient in a clinic. Communication of knowledge and calls to action in that relationship are in one direction: from practitioner to patient.

In contrast, it is our vision that well-informed people and their communities can create a foundation of knowledge of and support for health practices that meet their personal and cultural needs. Experts don't captain this ship, but instead provide support based on the demonstration of valued service rather than on the assumption of authority.

The three articles that follow develop these ideas.

"The Placebo Effect" challenges what counts as real in medical science and practice. It also offers an alternative perspective on where health and healing come from: instead of being the result of interventions by health professionals, health and healing first and foremost come from the body's capacity to sustain itself and heal when harmed.

"Health as a Commodity" discusses how choices in health become narrowed by the culture of expertise and the limitations of market capitalism in meeting health needs. The article describes the powerful social forces that prevent people from exercising their own best judgment in solving health problems.

"Social Medicine, Social Health" discusses how socially responsible medicine is not enough for health. Although a powerful force for correcting the corrosive health effects of socioeconomic inequality, it's still about disease and its absence. The article argues for the necessity of directly building the capacity of people to act on behalf of their own and their community's health using their own knowledge and resources.

Notes

[1] For example, Donald Barlett and James Steele (2004) *Critical Condition: How Health Care in America Became Big Business and Bad Medicine*. See

also the results of a survey conducted by the AFL-CIO in AFL-CIO (2008) *2008 Health Care for America Survey.*

[2] For example, John Abramson (2004) *Overdosed America: The Broken Promise of American Medicine,* Marcia Angell (2004) *The Truth About the Drug Companies: How They Deceive Us and What To Do About It.*

[3] H. Gilbert Welch, et al. (2007) "What's Making Us Sick Is An Epidemic of Diagnoses." See also H. Gilbert Welch (2004) *Should I Be Tested for Cancer? Maybe Not and Here's Why.*

[4] For example, see California's campaign for single payer health care Health Care for All http://www.healthcareforall.org. At the national level see Physicians for a National Health Program http://www.pnhp.org.

[5] H. Gilbert Welch has been one of the most vocal critics of preventive medicine as currently practiced. See his critique of the proposals by presidential campaigns in H . Gilbert Welch (2008) "Campaign Myth: Prevention as Cure-all."

[6] Steven Woloshin, et al. (2008) "The Risk of Death by Age, Sex, and Smoking Status in the United States: Putting Health Risks in Context." See also "Health Care Bankruptcy" on page 62.

[7] National Center for Health Statistics (2004) *Health, United States, 2004, with Chartbook on Trends in the Health of Americans* Table 86, p. 299-300.

[8] Centers for Disease Control and Prevention (2007) "Unintentional Poisoning Deaths - United States, 1999-2004" and Centers for Disease Control and Prevention (2005) "Increase in Poisoning Deaths Caused by Non-illicit Drugs - Utah, 1991-2003."

[9] Discussed more fully in "Social Medicine, Social Health" on page 22.

[10] See Frank Fischer (1990) *Technocracy and the Politics of Expertise.* See also Douglas Walton (1997) *Appeal to Expert Opinion: Arguments from Authority.*

THE PLACEBO EFFECT

There are many exceptions, but we generally expect a better product when we pay more for it. Our economy works that way; our culture works that way. Price means value.

The identity of price and value even works in medicine. A 2008 study by Rebecca Waber and her fellow marketing researchers demonstrated this with placebos. When people were told a placebo cost $2.50 per pill it was more effective in alleviating pain than when told it cost 10¢.

This is quite remarkable: price signaled more than market value; it signaled pain relief. What's even more remarkable is that both groups experienced significant pain relief: 85% of the $2.50 pill group reported pain relief while 61% of the 10¢ pill group reported relief. (A fairly consistent result in studies of the placebo effect is that at least one third of people respond positively to a placebo.)

No Cheaters Allowed

Newspapers had some fun with this. Their spin was that people's expectations were set by the price and those expectations affected the outcome. It almost seems like cheating.

Placebos have an aura: those who improve when they take them aren't playing fair. In fact, there's a characteristic of clinical trials called "placebo washout" that systematically identifies and excludes potential cheaters.

The purpose of placebo washout is to eliminate people who will respond positively to a placebo so it doesn't interfere with the results, which, of course, are intended to show the efficacy of a drug. In other words, built into the very methods of clinical trials is the assumption that it's about the efficacy of an "intervention" rather than the capacity of people to heal.

What a placebo does, in essence, is send a signal that "Help is here." Few researchers ask about that signal and how it works.

Help Is Here

The study and the news coverage frame the placebo effect in terms of expectations. In other words, a great deal of meaning was packed into the price difference. That meaning created expectations of relief.

"It's all about expectations" really begs the question. How exactly does the mental state of expectation affect the body? Or are expectations only part of the picture?

Another 2008 study points to an answer. It supports the idea that your body understands the signals it receives when you take a placebo or receive any other kind of care that says "Help is here." The study is by Henk Aarts and his colleagues and involved how performance of a task was affected by words delivered both subliminally and consciously.

The task was to squeeze a handgrip when signaled. The subliminal words flashed to participants were about physical exertion, words such as "vigorous." The consciously visible words were about encouragement and consisted of positive adjectives such as "good."

Those who experienced only the subliminal words gripped more forcefully than the control group, in an extensively studied process that's called *priming*. In other words, meaning was communicated directly to the body without conscious thought.

Those who experienced both subliminal exertion words and consciously visible encouraging words had still greater grip strength. Note that this isn't about expectations because there were no rewards for better performance and the task itself had no intrinsic value. The participant's bodies were getting positive signals—some conscious, some unconscious.

Autonomous Healing

The Aarts experiment wasn't about expectations, it was about how meaning affects the body. Meaningful acts are not restricted to words. Taking time to listen, sharing a meal, or giving a pill that's not supposed to do anything can all mean that "Help is here." All support the body's capacity to heal.

The signal by a placebo or other meaningful act, whether received consciously or unconsciously, depends on cultural context. For example, a placebo pill administered to someone who has no understanding of a drug delivered in this way won't respond. The pill has no meaning.

The literature on the placebo effect alludes to this connection between meaning and health effect. In this literature the placebo effect is seen as a middle ground between the body's innate capacity to sustain and heal itself (called *autonomous healing*) and the intervention of a priestly healer (whether MD or shaman) with substances and technologies to do what the body cannot.

The remarkable thing is that what priestly healers do most of the time is enable the body to heal itself. If you break a bone, what does the doctor do? Immobilize it so it can mend. What's a doctor doing when she vaccinates you? She's prompting your immune system to create an antibody that will do the work of protecting you. What are doctors doing when they treat someone for cancer? They're pushing back a process until the body is able to control that process, not to mention clean up the mess left behind.

In other words, our body's capacity to heal is at the core of virtually every kind of medical intervention, whether conventional, alternative, or traditional.

Support for Protection and Healing

Viewing placebos as a middle ground is limiting. It's part of the continuum of support for the body in protecting, sustaining, healing, and recovering. Placebos, along with other meaningful, caring acts, are one kind of support. Medical interventions are another.

Don't forget that medical interventions are meaningful acts in their own right. The meaning of healer-patient interactions can be more powerful than the substances and technologies the priestly healers use.

Unfortunately, the aura of "It's all in your head" remains. Do animals experience placebo effects? If so, that would argue strongly against "It's all in your head." Just such evidence exists, although not framed as experiments in placebo effects.

Bernard Weiss and David Bellinger cite animal studies in which social environments affect sensitivity to environmental toxins. For example, mice who have a rich social life are more resistant to toxins than mice that have limited contact with other mice. As another example, mice who receive more nurturing as pups are more resistant than less nurtured mice.

A robust social environment and nurturing have meaning for mice, even without benefit of language (and likely without expectations). That meaning affects their health and their capacity to heal. It is meaning that has direct biological effects akin to the placebo effect.

It's obvious why the placebo effect doesn't get more research attention: it's a financial washout for drug companies, medical device manufacturers, and the medical organizations that protect the interests of priestly healers. For reasons of both cost and humanity, healing should start with what the body is already capable of doing. Start by supporting that capacity and then move on to sending signals that tell the body "Help is here." Only as a last resort should someonemove on to the priestly healers—who take a lot of credit for what the body knows how to do on its own.

The News
Carey, Benedict. 2008. More Expensive Placebos Bring More Relief. *New York Times.* March 5, 2008.

The Research
Aarts, Henk et al. 2008. Preparing and Motivating Behavior Outside of Awareness. *Science.* March 21, 2008 (319):1639.

Waber, Rebecca L. et al. 2008. Commercial Features of Placebo And Therapeutic Efficacy. *JAMA.* March 5, 2008 (299:9):1016-7.

Welch, John S. 2003. Ritual in Western Medicine and Its Role in Placebo Healing. *Journal of Religion and Health.* Spring 2003 (42:1):21-33.

Weiss, Bernard and David C. Bellinger. 2006. Social Ecology of Children's Vulnerability to Environmental Pollutants. *Environmental Health Perspectives.* October 2006(114:10):1479-85.

Resources
Your Own Health And Fitness. Resources on Alternative Healing. Access at http://www.yourownhealthandfitness.org/topicsAlternative.php.

❦

HEALTH AS A COMMODITY

We're all understandably worried about climate change. Information is churning away in our infosphere about what it means and what we can do: reduce our carbon footprint, purchase carbon offsets, and support legislation that forces manufacturers to offer low greenhouse gas alternatives.

Without these actions, scientists such as those who sit on the Nobel Prize winning UN Intergovernmental Panel on Climate Change predict significant public health effects such as increased incidence of infectious disease.

Although sensible, this is a biased perspective of the problem that reflects an equally biased perspective on health generally. It takes some effort to see this as a perspective at all instead of simply as the way things work. Purchasing products to lower our carbon footprint and regulatory actions that lower greenhouse gas emissions leaves unchanged the social processes that actually make those choices seem natural.

The Cost of Doing Business

A study in the *Proceedings of the National Academy of Sciences* (PNAS) looked at who benefits and who suffers from ecological damage, including climate change. In economics, this type of damage is an externality: a cost or benefit from producing or consuming that isn't accounted for in a product's price.

For example, the loss of forests increases damage from flooding. The timber company buys the land, cuts the trees, and is paid for the lumber. Rain that falls can't be held and destruction happens downstream. The cost of the destruction isn't included in the price of the lumber; it has to come from the people who suffer, their insurance companies, or their government. Or they simply have to walk away.

You should not be surprised to learn that nations such as Bangladesh with a low per capita income bear the burden of damage and little of the benefit while high income per capita nations such as the United States reap most of the benefit and little of the damage. This story of unequal exchange is an old one, much older than our current era of globalization. It really starts with the rise of European imperialism centuries ago.

For example, 500 years ago the Spanish began to strip the land of the Mixteca in Oaxaca, Mexico, of its trees. The Spanish also destroyed the indigenous water conservation system. An estimated 15 feet of top soil has eroded since then. The damage is now being reversed by a group of farmers who, over the past 25 years, have planted trees, restored the old water system, and reintroduced indigenous crops.

Climate change is only one of the six so-called drivers of ecological damage that the PNAS researchers examine: agricultural expansion and intensification, ozone depletion, deforestation, overfishing, and mangrove forest destruction. Ecologically, it's easy to see how climate change is linked to these other drivers of damage.

Migration

Ecological damage makes a place uninhabitable or at least increasingly difficult to inhabit. Ecological damage then damages health in the most profound sense. As areas become uninhabitable, people will die, adapt, or migrate. Some will migrate to areas nearby, some to the city, and some, with or without permission, from one nation to another.

While activists, political leaders, and even some corporate leaders exhort personal choices and government standards that reduce our carbon footprint, few societies are preparing for the onslaught of mass migrations that is likely over the coming decades. Nor are they preparing for ways to enable itinerant migrants to adapt to or recover from ecological damage so they can remain in their homes.

No doubt activists, artists, and some politicians will put on spectacular events to raise money for those who suffer. It's not likely that events will be scheduled to alleviate the social inequities that are at the root of these migrations.

To do so would question the sanctity of market capitalism as a way to provide people with the things they need. It's that sanctity that makes it difficult for us to look beyond personal decisions about what we buy—both literally and figuratively—as solutions to what are clearly social and global problems.

To be clear: these personal choices are far from irrelevant. But they are only half the picture. The other half is what we do together as communities that determines the alternatives from which we get to choose.

The sanctity of the market and its operations creates a world for us, a world of consumption, that makes it look like what we buy brings health, that commodities give us our health, that even health itself is a commodity—something for us to purchase.

Natural and Organic

In a study conducted in 2008, the Organic Consumers Association found that 46 of 100 personal care products labeled either "natural" or "organic" contain a known carcinogen (1,4-dioxane). The substance was not an ingredient but a byproduct of the production process. Happily, none of the products certified as "Organic" by the Department of Agriculture contained the substance. Unhappily, many of the manufacturers of tainted products had no idea it was present.

One reason for this problem is that the FDA has no standards for labeling personal care products "natural" or "organic." The USDA label only guarantees that product ingredients are grown according to certain standards. However, that doesn't guarantee an organic product is any better for your health than one with ingredients cooked up in the lab.

It's organizations such as the Organic Consumers Association and the Environmental Working Group's Skin Deep program that are providing consumers with information about personal care products. As for the market, it's essentially late 19th Century capitalism: buyer beware.

The same is true for the rapidly growing carbon offsets industry. Businesses are appealing to consumer concerns by offering a wide variety of ways to offset the climate changing effect of the products they purchase. Yet there are no standards here either. The Federal Trade Commission is looking into it. That's it.

Is the problem that regulatory agencies are failing their mission to protect consumers?

There's another story here. As Andrew Szasz argues, we have created a culture in which we protect ourselves with an inverted quarantine. A standard public health quarantine consists of isolating an environmental threat from the population. In an inverted quarantine we isolate ourselves from an environmental threat through individual consumption.

This strategy makes sense when we think the only thing we can control is our personal consumption decisions. However, as Szasz shows, it's a strategy that fails because the environmental threat and the forces that created it are unaffected.

Paying attention to the health effects of personal decisions is critical for protection and prevention. Paying attention to the human ecology in which we make those decisions is equally important. We can control our human ecology. But making changes to it is something we have to do together. Resources include the website for the documentary *Unnatural Causes* and the Local Chapters Program of the Sustainable Health Institute.

The News
Shin, Annys. 2008. Toxin Found in 'Natural,' 'Organic' Items. *New York Times.* January 9, 2008.

Singer, Natasha. 2007. Natural, Organic Beauty. *New York Times*. November 1, 2007.

Story, Louise. 2008. FTC Asks if Carbon-Offset Money Is Well Spent. *New York Times*. January 9, 2008.

The Research

Hunter, Lori M.. 2007. Climate Change, Rural Vulnerabilities, and Migration. *Population Reference Bureau*. June 2007. Access at http://www.prb.org/Articles/2007/ClimateChangeinRuralAreas.aspx.

Srinivasan, U. Thara et al. 2008. The debt of nations and the distribution of ecological impacts from human activities. *Proceedings of the National Academy of Science*. February 5, 2008 (105:5): 1768-73.

Resources

California Newsreel. 2008. *Unnatural Causes: Is Inequality Making Us Sick?* Access at http://www.unnaturalcauses.org/.

Environmental Working Group, Skin Deep Cosmetic Safety Database. Access at http://www.cosmeticsdatabase.com/.

Fine, Ben. 2002. *The world of consumption: The material and the cultural revisited*. New York: Routledge.

Organic Consumers Association, Coming Clean Campaign. Access at http://www.organicconsumers.org/bodycare/index.cfm.

Sustainable Health Institute, Local Chapters Program. Access at http://www.sustainablehealthinstitute.org/.

Szasz, Andrew. 2008. Shopping Our Way to Safety. *Your Own Health And Fitness*. Broadcast April 8, 2008.

Szasz, Andrew. 2007. Shopping Our Way to Safety: How We Changed from Protecting the Environment to Protecting Ourselves. Minneapolis: University of Minnesota Press.

SOCIAL MEDICINE, SOCIAL HEALTH

Disease prevention has fallen on hard times. This according to a New York Times article titled "What's a Pound of Prevention Really Worth?"

The article opens with a description of Dr. Arthur Agatston's practice. Although he is most famous as a diet doctor for writing *The South Beach Diet*, he's a practicing cardiologist—like Robert Atkins, whose diet also originated with a concern for preventing heart attacks. In fact, the South Beach Diet bears more than a passing resemblance to the Atkins diet, but that's another story.

Dr. Agatston claims that last year only 3 out of his 2,800 patients had heart attacks. He attributes his success to the time and attention he and his staff take with each of his patients to change their diet, exercise, and other aspects of their life (such as how to stop smoking). The regimen also includes doses of statins and other drugs, with time and attention devoted to dealing with the side effects.

What's the problem?

There's No Money in It

Dr. Agatston summarizes the situation this way: "The time we spend with patients—we get rewarded almost zilch." He is able to do it because he has the South Beach Diet empire as an independent source of income. Other doctors who are not so blessed avoid preventive care because it doesn't turn a buck.

Boo-hoo.

And so the article blathers on about what looks like an intractable problem: prevention is good but money can't be made by the doctors who deliver it.

But wait.

Why are doctors responsible for prevention in the first place? A piece of the answer is in a series of articles published in 2006 in the Public Library of Science (*PLoS Medicine*) on the topic of social medicine.

The strategy that Dr. Agatston uses is intended to change individual behavior, one patient at a time. The strategy of social medicine is to change the environment for medical care—including both treatment and prevention.

Social Medicine and Prevention

Instead of working one-on-one to persuade, coax, or bully someone to adapt to a prescribed diet, social medicine works to change the patient's food environment: access, affordability, and so on. Some advocates of social medicine go so far as to suggest that a redistribution of income and wealth by itself would improve medical care outcomes.

Fancy that.

Treatment as advocated by social medicine has a different slant as well. It is concerned not just with what happens within the clinic's walls but with how best to get people to the clinic—for example, by making access to transportation part of medical care. They even work on how to deliver medical care to people outside the clinic—for example, by transporting health professionals trained to deliver culturally appropriate care to people who might not otherwise travel to a clinic.

This socialized approach to medical care is more prevalent in Europe than in the United States because of a stronger tradition of socialized medicine and a strong, independent public health movement. In the United States, public health was first eclipsed and then colonized by the medical profession.

Despite an ongoing interest in social medicine by public health researchers and officials, a complex of institutional, political, and financial factors have forced the practice of public health to become an extension of individualized medical care. "Prevention" means vaccination, but not day care. That's changing, although slowly.

It's Still Medicine

Yet even if social medicine were to gain strength, it's still medicine. Prevention is still medicine, even the socialized prevention described by the authors in the PLoS Medicine series. It's about prescribing environmental change so that people will avoid being diagnosed and treated in the first place. Even alternative medicine (for example, that found in the essay collection *Ecological Medicine*) is still medicine, it's still about receiving or avoiding diagnosis and treatment.

What happened to health?

The problem is that we're trapped by the notion that health is the absence of disease. That's a notion that both medical science and medical practice foster: medicine confers health by preventing and curing disease.

Who do you think has good health? Someone who is without disease? No. It is someone vibrant and full of life. That's because health is the capacity to thrive.

In one respect, health is like illness: it comes from how your unique biology responds to your environment, both social and ecological.

Maintaining and improving your health isn't simply or even mostly about medical care, whether for prevention or treatment. In fact, your health might actually be better served by avoiding medical care. Your health is very much affected by your circumstances: the toxins to which you're exposed, the socioeconomic stress you experience, the personal relationships you enjoy, the pleasures available to you, and much more. These are the characteristics of the communities of which you are a member.

It is in this respect that, like social medicine, social health is about communities. Only it is not about how communities deliver medical care. It's about how communities create and sustain the social and ecological environments that enable people to live life fully, to thrive.

You won't find health in the doctor's office or in the hospital. You'll find it in your kitchen and the farmer's market, on the streets and paths you walk, with your loved ones, among the people with whom you work to make your community a better place to live.

The News
Leonhardt, David. 2007. What's a Pound of Prevention Really Worth? *New York Times*. January 24, 2007.

The Research
Murray, Christopher et al. 2006. Eight Americas: Investigating Mortality Disparities across Race, Counties, and Race-Counties in the United States. *PLoS Medicine*. September 2006 (3:9): e260. DOI: 10.1371/journal.pmed.0030357.

Pappas, Gregory. 2006. Geographic Data on Health Inequities. *PLoS Medicine*. September 2006 (3:9): e357. DOI: 10.1371/journal.pmed.0030260.

Resources
Ausubel, Kenny ed. 2004. *Ecological Medicine: Healing the Earth, Healing Ourselves*. San Francisco: Sierra Club Books.

Farmer, Paul et al. 2006. Structural Violence and Clinical Medicine. *PLoS Medicine*. October 2006 (3:10): e449. DOI:10.1371/journal.pmed.0030449.

Holtz, Timothy et al. 2006. Health Is Still Social. *PLoS Medicine*. October 2006 (3:10): e419. DOI: 10.1371/journal.pmed.0030419.

Navarro, Vicente et al. 2006. Politics and health outcomes. *The Lancet*. Online September 14, 2006. DOI: 10.1016/50140-6736(06)69341-0.

Unique Biology

Some people catch colds and flus easily. Some do not.

For some people, cows milk in any form is poison. Others can't get enough.

Each person has a unique biology. Health and illness come from how that biology responds to its environment, whether it's exposure to a virus, a particular food, a chemical in a consumer product, or waste from the production of that product.

The science that informs our understanding of "good health," the science that is the basis for medical care, loses sight of this simple fact. In the health care system, good health and good medicine are standardized.

Standardization has two aspects relevant to your unique biology.

First, standards are set by experts. These experts do not fall from heaven with an "Expert" label attached. They're selected to set standards by a government agency or professional organization. This means that politics and with it economics are deeply involved with who makes decisions about health and medical standards.[1]

Second, the concept of a standard assumes that its uniform application is the best approach to health. A standard, however qualified and nuanced, creates a one-size-fits-all plan of action for everyone. It places uniformity at the center of attention. Instead, we believe that each person's health should be based on his specific needs, circumstances, and biological history.

As an example, the USDA promotes the Food Pyramid[2] and the underlying *Dietary Guidelines for Americans*[3] as the standard for nutrition. The *Guidelines* are the result of an examination of science by a panel of experts with the stated purpose to "speak with one voice on nutrition and health."[4]

That food manufacturers are active participants in establishing these standards should be no surprise. A great deal is at stake for them.[5] In addition, a good deal of science that contradicts the *Guidelines* is ignored. The tawdry tale of how the most recent *Guidelines* were cooked is examined in greater detail in "Bureaucratic Food" on page 75.

What concerns us here is the science itself. Very broadly, the science that supports health policy and standards of care in medical practice are of two kinds.

The first kind is clinical trials, also referred to as provocation studies. In these studies, a group of subjects (whether human or lab animal) is divided into two (sometimes more) subgroups. One group receives a drug or other treatment intended to provoke a response— in other words, the provocation is intended to prevent illness or promote recovery. The other group is a control group that often receives a placebo—a drug or treatment that is not biologically active and is intended to provoke nothing. This group is a "control" because its members' illness or recovery is used to measure the effectiveness of the treatment being studied.

An emerging trend in clinical trials is to compare a new treatment to another treatment already in use. So instead of placebo control, the experiment is one of *active control*. Nevertheless, the principle is the same: does the new treatment work better than nothing at all (placebo control) or better than an existing treatment (active control).

The second kind of science comes from epidemiological studies, also referred to as observation studies. In these studies, there's no provocation. Instead, one or more characteristics of the experimental subjects are compared to the incidence of illness or speed of recovery among them. Often, a control group is identified for the same purpose as in clinical trials: to compare the effect of one or more characteristics on illness and recovery. For example, studying a group of people for the effect of smoking, the study would include non-smokers as a control group.

The differences between these two kinds of science are important but not relevant for showing how each person's unique biology is at the very heart of the science used to set health and medical standards.

Both types of science, clinical trials and epidemiological studies, base their conclusions on statistical analysis of measurements taken by researchers. For example, the *Guidelines* recommend that someone who consumes 2,000 calories per day should include 7 or 8 servings of grains as part of that diet. That's equivalent to 8 slices of bread or 4 cups of rice.

One of the studies upon which this recommendation is based comes from the *American Journal of Clinical Nutrition*.[6] The research team was based at Harvard's School of Public Health. Walter Willet, a leading expert in the relationship between nutrition and illness, served as the study's lead researcher. The researchers concluded that increased consumption of whole grains decreased the risk of cardiovascular heart disease—essentially the risk of having a heart attack or stroke.

The study uses five subgroups of people identified by the amount of whole grains each person ate during the study period, from least to most consumption. During the study, the researchers recorded the number of heart attacks in each subgroup. Then, using the group that ate the least as the control, the researchers compared each group regarding the relationship between whole grain consumption and the risk of heart attacks.

The statistic the researchers used for the comparison is called *relative risk*, expressed as a percentage. This is a common statistic reported in both clinical trials and observational studies.

For example, the relative risk of having a heart attack for people who ate the *most* whole grains was 79% compared to those who ate the *least*. That is, of the people who had heart attacks, those who ate the most whole grains were 79% as likely to have a heart attack as those who ate the least. Expressed another way, for every 100 people who ate little in the way of whole grains and had a heart attack, only 79 of the people who at lots of whole grains had a heart attack—that is, according to this study 21 people of every 100 people were spared because of their high consumption of whole grains.

The first thing to notice is that despite eating lots of whole grains, a high proportion (79%) of these people still had a heart attack. Any number of things could explain why people had heart attacks—even with whole grains prominent in their diet. It could be some factor the researchers didn't take into consideration, even though they took into account (statistically speaking) a wide range of factors such as smoking, age, and weight.

Certainly part of this unexplained variation comes from the differing biology of the people in the study. The biology of some grain eaters (21 out of 100) spared them from a heart attack. The biology of the rest (79 out of 100) did not.

Another number puts these estimates into perspective. So far, we've only discussed relative risk among the people who had heart attacks. This is commonly what's reported in the media. Virtually never is the *absolute risk* reported—either in the media or in the published research itself.

Absolute risk is taken from the perspective of the entire population of people in the study, not just those who had a heart attack. So this is something like the way somone would think about whether doing something decreases his risk. For the whole population of the study, the absolute risk reduction for whole grain eaters was 0.05%—out of 10,000 avid whole grain eaters, an additional five people would be spared a heart attack compared to 10,000 whole grain consuming slackers.

Yet another way to look at these numbers is using a statistic named *number needed to treat*. This statistic shows how many people would need to have a diet high in whole grains in order for 1 to be spared a heart attack. The number in this case is 2,183—that is, 2,183 people would have to eat lots of whole grains in order to spare one additional person of a heart attack; the remaining 2,182 would have heart attacks despite the whole grains in their diet.[7]

Not very impressive.

In addition to the estimated effect on risk reduction, the study reported the *confidence interval* of the estimate. The name suggests what this statistic means: the degree of confidence (statistically speaking) someone can have in the relative risk percentage that's been calculated.

When the study says that the relative risk for whole grain eaters is 79% compared to people who are not at all keen on whole grains, it means that it's what is most likely based on this particular study with this particular group of people. But lots of things could make that estimate high or low with regard to what's really going on. So when researchers calculate relative risk, they also calculate a likely range in which the actual relative risk might occur. In this case, the confidence interval was between 62% and 101%—which means that the actual number of people spared per 100 for eating whole grains could be as many as 38 fewer people spared from heart attacks or, embarrassingly, one additional person lost to a heart attack.

This uncertainty is the result of what's called in statistics *random variation*—that is, the estimate of 79% could be different from the actual risk because of unknown factors. The factors could be environmental or biological. Another factor is each person's unique biology.

For example, as we discuss in "Bureacratic Food," grains are a very problematic food. Grains are allergic in degrees from difficult digestion to anaphylaxis. Grains, as starches, contribute to metabolic and hormonal disruption as we discuss in "The Hormonal Consequences of Starch and Stress" on page 41, again an effect that manifests in degrees from no effect to extreme sensitivity.

Yet instead of advising people on the variable (and frankly not very impressive) result of whole grain consumption, the *Dietary Guidelines for America 2005* simply states that everyone should eat lots of whole grains.

Unfortunately, the way health and medical science is communicated and put into practice turns our attention away from our sense of and knowledge about our unique biology. This slight-of-hand makes it difficult to hold onto the tether that connects our own knowledge to what we receive in the form of medical diagnosis and treatment.

One phenomenon in our informational universe that has muddied these waters further is the rise of genetics as a causal explanation for disease and genetic testing as way to evaluate health risks. The reason is simple: we have been conditioned to believe that our genes are what confer our biological uniqueness.

The first article in this section, "Genetic Magic," reveals that belief to be far too narrow as a guide to health and healing. It also discusses how genetic testing is far from reliable in predicting health and medical conditions.

The second article, "Epigenetic and Proteomics," describes what we do and do not know about how our genes affect our biology and, more importantly, how our environment and biology affect our genes. It brings home the idea that our unique biology is the consequence of our unique biological history—genes responding to our biology responding to our environment through time.

Notes

[1] For a scathing review of the culture of expertise, see Sheldon Rampton and John Stauber (2001) *Trust Us, We're Experts! How Industry Manipulates Science and Gambles with Your Future.* See also the previously cited Frank Fischer (1990) *Technocracy and the Politics of Expertise.*

[2] MyPyramid.gov website.

[3] USDA and US Department of Health and Human Services (2005) *Dietary Guidelines for Americans, 2005.*

[4] The "experts" come from government, academia, and industry and are selected by the Secretary of the Department of Agriculture and the Secretary of the Department of Health and Human Services. The science that supports their recommendations is in Dietary Guidelines Advisory Committee (2005) *The Report of the Dietary Guidelines Advisory Committee on Dietary Guidelines for Americans, 2005.* The quote is from page 12.

[5] For example, see Marion Nestle (2002) *Food Politics: How the Food Industry Influences Nutrition and Health.*

[6] Simin Liu, et al. (1999) "Whole-grain Consumption and Risk of Coronary Heart Disease: Results from the Nurses' Health Study."

[7] These are estimates that have statistically (supposedly) accounted for all the other things that could increase the risk of a heart attack: whether someone smoked and how much fat, fiber, folate, vitamin B6, and vitamin E they ate. So we're supposedly only seeing the effect of how much grain each person ate.

GENETIC MAGIC

Genetic magic is in the air. Researchers have found that variants of two bits of DNA on chromosome 9 are associated with heart disease. What this means is made clear in a *New York Times* article: scientists will develop a test for these variants and if you have them you'll be treated to "early interventions such as cholesterol-lowering statins and methods to reduce blood pressure."

You take a test. It tells you that you've got the genetic variant for heart disease. Early intervention prevents you from having a heart attack. Doesn't that sound great?

But if you dig into the actual research, there's much less to this discovery than the news suggests.

Empty Promises

First, genetic scientists have yet to identify what this stretch of DNA actually does, which means they have no idea what biochemistry the two bits of DNA affect.

Second, these two bits of DNA aren't associated with any of the standard risk factors for heart disease. So if you have them you're a candidate for medication regardless of your levels of cholesterol or C-reactive protein or blood pressure or what have you.

The implication of these first two points is that rushing you into conventional treatments makes absolutely no sense.

On the other hand, we've been critical of those standard risk factors (for example, see our article "What Causes a Heart Attack"). Could it be that this DNA variant is pointing to the real cause of heart attacks, a cause that has nothing to do with cholesterol lowering and all the other conventional treatments?

Third, the two DNA variants are virtually absent in Africans. And while they're present in African-Americans, there's no association with heart attacks. That is, these DNA variants are risk factors for European-Americans only, not for African-Americans. So in contrast to the last point, could it be that this DNA variant is pointing to some utterly superficial relationship to heart attacks?

Fourth, the risks involved are not dramatic. Each chromosome has two strands of DNA. If only one strand has the variants, the risk goes up by about 20%. If both DNA strands have the variant, your risk goes up by 40%.

To put this in perspective, out of 1,000 people who *don't* have the two genetic variants, about 125 will have heart attacks. Out of 1,000 people who *do have* the two genetic variants on both strands of DNA (the worst case), 175 will have heart attacks. That's 50 additional people out of 1,000 or 5%.

However, of critical importance is the fact that most people with the DNA variants on both strands (825 to be exact) will not have heart disease. In other words, having the variants is far from a death sentence.

Basic Genetics

Let's review some basic genetics. A gene does its work in response to a biochemical signal. Ultimately, that signal comes from your environment: the nutrients and toxins in your food, water, and the air you breathe; the kind and quality of physical activity you have; the positive and negative stress you experience; the physical and emotional trauma you experience; the pollutants (including electrosmog) to which you're exposed.

Each of those exposures creates a biochemical cascade that starts on your surface—your skin, sinuses, lungs, mouth, stomach, and intestines are all where the outside meets your inside. The outside also gets inside through your senses: if you see a threat, your nervous system carries the message to your body.

What's called gene expression (how a gene does its work in response to a biochemical signal) starts at the cells on your surface and works its way in.

Simply put, the signal to your genes comes from an exposure in your physical or social environment. No exposure, no biochemical cascade, no signal, no gene expression.

Splashy news about gene magic typically leaps over that chain of events. Instead, the story you're told is that you have the genetic variation so you're at risk so it's off to the pharmacy for you.

It's a safe bet that you want to stay out of harms way. That's why the promise of this kind of story about genetic science as magic is so seductive. But in fact, it's completely unhelpful. It threatens to steer increasing numbers of people into the same old tired routines. Genetic magic simply adds a new way for you to suffer from overdiagnosis and overtreatment.

News such as this diverts your attention from what you can actually do to protect yourself: change your exposure to the things that send the wrong signal to your DNA.

Gene Testing

Avoiding exposures that send the wrong signal seems to beg the question of precisely what exposures to avoid. The answer is that epidemiological studies of humans and clinical studies of animals already point to risky exposures.

For example, studies indicate that people who live in smoggier areas are more likely to have heart attacks. The provocation seems to be through reactive oxygen species that cause mischief with your heart (and other organs).

But this is information about an entire population of people. It doesn't say anything about your specific risk. Wouldn't it be great to know whether smog puts you at risk of a heart attack?

This is the seductive quality of genetic research such as that concerning the two gene variants on chromosome 9. It is the source of a burgeoning field of genetic testing. These tests promise to pinpoint genetic weaknesses that might make you vulnerable to a wide variety of diseases.

Despite their popularity, the accuracy of these tests is in serious doubt. Little science supports the associations genetic testing vendors claim between genetic variants and risk of disease. The associations are also woefully uninformative as to the extent of the risk. Finally, the current model of the relationship between genes and functional states of your body are being called into question.

An international research consortium headquartered at the University of California, Santa Cruz has been laboring over how exactly genes work. In 2007, the program, named ENCODE (a labored acronym for Encyclopedia of DNA Elements), published its findings in analyzing 1% of the human genome.

Until now, the basic assumption behind the application of genetic research, including testing and therapy, has been that each gene produces a single protein that performs a particular function. That singular gene-function relationship is at the bottom of therapies based on the presence of genetic variants and the testing for those variants. The chromosome 9 variants and their association with heart attacks are an example. Others include gene variants associated with obesity, diabetes, cancer, and other chronic diseases.

What the ENCODE researchers reported is that the assumption of one-gene-one-function is wrong. Genes seem to work in complex, resilient, and adaptive relationships.

What this means is that researchers are a very long way from associating DNA variations with specific medical conditions. Practically speaking, simply avoiding risky exposures based on what you already know about your family history of illness is more likely to preserve your health than a genetic test of dubious accuracy.

The News

Caruso, Denise. 2007. A Challenge to Gene Theory, a Tougher Look at Biotech. *New York Times.* July 1, 2007.

Coghlan, Andy. 2007. Genetic Testing: Informed Choice or Waste of Money? *New Scientist.* October 3, 2007.

Wade, Nicholas. 2007. Gene Identified as Risk Factor for Heart Ills. *New York Times.* May 4, 2007.

The Research

McPherson, Ruth. 2007. A Common Allele on Chromosome 9 Associated with Coronary Heart Disease. *Sciencexpress.* May 3, 2007. DOI:10.1126/science.1142447.

ENCODE Project Consortium. 2007. Identification and Analysis of Functional Elements in 1% of the Human Genome by the ENCODE Pilot Project. *Nature.* June 14, 2007 (447): 799-816. DOI:10.1038/nature05874.

Resources

Your Own Health And Fitness. Resources on Cardiovascular and Heart Health. Access at http://www.yourownhealthandfitness.org/topicsHeart.php.

EPIGENETICS AND PROTEOMICS

A blueprint is not a house. We frequently see news about the discovery of the gene that controls this or that. For example, in 2005 the *New York Times* carried an article with the title "Study pinpoints gene controlling fear: Discovery could help humans with disabling anxiety."

The human genome is like a blueprint. The promise implied by the headlines and accompanying articles is that knowing what lurks behind our genetic closet doors will empower us to promote what's good and prevent what's bad. It's an idea that's one step away from "genetics is destiny."

How Genes Work

Let's step back a moment and remember how genes work. DNA makes up our genes, stored in each cell's nucleus and mitochondria. A chemical signal causes a segment of DNA to unwind. Using the chemical bits that make up the DNA segment as a blueprint, a protein is built. The protein launches a whole biochemical process that can have a long chemical path with many biological effects.

The chemical signal that starts it all can also be at the end of its own long biochemical path. What distinguishes one tissue—that is, one cell type—from another is whether a segment unwinds in response to a signal. The genes of your liver cells unwind to chemical signals that your brain cell genes do not.

This is a roundabout way of saying that genes express themselves in response to their environment, that the path from the environment to the gene and back out to the environment is not a simple one, and that genes in specific tissues respond according to what they're built to do.

Because each of your cells has the same DNA and therefore the same set of genes, which genes are "on" and which are "off" determine a cell's identity and behavior. When a gene that's supposed to be "on" is turned off or vice versa, the cell will not act according to its blueprint.

If the gene in question is a variant that can cause illness, switching it "off" is a good thing. If the gene is one that prevents illness, switching it "off" is trouble.

Express Yourself

The principal means by which genes are turned "off" is through a process called *methylation*. When *methyl* groups (a chemical consisting of one carbon atom and three hydrogen atoms) attach to certain parts of DNA that make up a gene, the DNA ignores the chemical signal that normally causes it to unwind and *express* the gene—that is, start a cascade of specific proteins.

Epigenetics is the study of how our bodies control which genes are expressed and which are not. Some of this pattern is just the normal function of cells as they develop and mature. But some is a result of what happens in our environment.

One of the most important discoveries is that an epigenetic pattern can be inherited. For example, a multi-generational study of men in England found that men who smoked before puberty were more likely to have sons and grandsons with metabolic syndrome.

Geneticists have proposed a Human Epigenome Project that would map the relationship between epigenetic patterns to health and disease. Unfortunately, as with the Human Genome Project, pharmaceutical companies hunger to dominate research in order to develop drugs customized to each person's epigenetics.

Genes and Proteins

The 22,000 genes identified by the Human Genome Project were far fewer than expected. It turns out that, genomically speaking, we're virtually indistinguishable from chimpanzees. What distinguishes us from chimps is our pattern of DNA methylation that causes a different pattern of gene expression.

On the other hand, we have somewhere between 400,000 to 1 million unique proteins. No reliable study has actually pinned down the number, which is why there is now a Human Proteome Project in the making—*proteome* meaning the complete map of all the proteins made by the human body.

Many of our most profound biological responses to our environment are built from this nexus of proteins, not from our DNA. It's a field parallel to, but vastly more complex than, genomics or epigenomics.

Does knowing which gene "causes" fear help us live a better life? Not by itself. But knowing the protein cascade that originates with the gene could help.

Research with mice looked at how nutrients can alter how genes respond to a signal. Mice that are well-nurtured are less prone to stress (and its health consequences) than mice that aren't nurtured. The researchers discovered the gene that was expressed by nurturing. Using a nutrient, they were able to turn off that gene and turn well-adjusted mice into stressed-out mice. Another experiment showed that the stress effect from lack of nurturing can be reversed by putting the mice in an environment where they are well-nurtured. In other words, nutrients and emotional environment affect gene expression.

Nutrigenomics

These are only discoveries along the way to better understanding how to support our health and well-being. They are not occasions for fawning over the control we think we have over our biology because we have looked at the blueprints and know where the closet door for fear or stress is located.

A field of study that is now emerging from proteomics and epigenetics is called *nutrigenomics*—captured by Jack Challem in the title of his book *Feed Your Genes Right*.

One of the major focuses of nutrigenomics is how to support the methylation process, both adding and removing methyl groups from DNA. The principal focus of attention is on antioxidants and B vitamins.

Antioxidants such as coenzyme Q10, lipoic acid, vitamin C, vitamin E, and glutathione protect against reactive oxygen species (*ROS*). ROS is a natural byproduct of your energy metabolism. Unless neutralized, ROS causes damage to DNA and disrupt the methylation process.

Folic acid, vitamin B6, and vitamin B12 are nutrients required to make the methylation process work. A deficiency in one or all of these B vitamins is common and commonly unrecognized.

From a blueprint, you can build a house of horrors or a palace of delight. Particularly if you feed your genes right. Not only are your genes not your destiny, they're not even most of who and what you are. In addition to nutrients, you need good nurturing.

Resources

Challem, Jack. 2005. *Feed Your Genes Right*. Hoboken, NJ: Wiley & Sons.

Challem, Jack. 2005. Feed Your Genes Right. *Your Own Health And Fitness*. Broadcast March 15, 2005.

Gilbert, Scott F. 2005. Mechanisms for the Environmental Regulation of Gene Expression: Ecological Aspects of Animal Development. *Journal of Bioscience*. February 2005; 30(1): 65-74.

Hooper, Rowan. 2006. Men Inherit Hidden Cost of Dad's Vices. *New Scientist*. January 7, 2006: 10.

Weaver, Ian CG et al. 2004. Epigenetic Programming by Maternal Behavior. *Nature Neuroscience*. 7: 847-54. DOI:10.1038–/nn1276.

Yasko, Amy and Garry Gordon. 2006. Nutrigenomic Testing and the Methylation Pathway. *Townsend Letter for Doctors and Patients*. January 2006: 69-73.

The Body as an Ecology

Bodies work like ecologies: each part and action supports or balances some other part or action. Ecologies are not worlds of intervention and opposition, but of exchange and adaptation. This is not to say that ecologies always adapt to change in a desirable way. Adaptation for an ecology might mean loss of habitat and with it loss of species.

Thinking of the body as an ecology is quite different from much of conventional medical and health science, which is based on interventions that oppose disease processes. Even so, interventions such as vaccination actually depend for their effectiveness on the ecology of the body's immune system: samples of a flu virus are presented to the immune system which adapts by producing antibodies, which is an adaptation that defends the body when it's infected by unknown organisms.

It's important to pause and grasp this idea: it's not the vaccine that's doing the work, it's the body's ecology.

This kind of misunderstanding causes mischief for people looking for health and healing. The story we step into when we seek health and healing through conventional health care institutions is one of intervention and opposition. The real story is often something quite different.

The Laws of Ecology, as Barry Commoner stated them in the seminal *The Closing Circle*,[1] serve us well as a guide to the body as an ecology. There are four.

1. Everything is connected to everything else.
2. Everything has to go somewhere.
3. There's no such thing as a free lunch.
4. Nature bats last.

Human contributions to global warming are an example. Our highly integrated global economy depends on transportation which depends on burning fossil fuels. The global transportation system and its infrastructure have wide ranging effects on ecosystem and human health. Everything is connected to everything else.

Fossil fuels and the engines they feed have allowed humans to break through the constraints of the solar economy:[2] we operate outside the global carbon cycle. Instead, burning fuels adds carbon to the atmosphere. Everything has to go somewhere.

The atmospheric chemistry that results from the additional carbon (not to mention the other products of fossil fuel combustion) does not disappear. Instead, they follow their own energetic path and, to a large extent because of Law #1, a chemical balance is struck that results in, for example, increased acidity in the oceans that ultimately depletes fish populations. There's no such thing as a free lunch.

One of those energetic paths traps heat in our atmosphere and contributes to its warming. In response to the resulting climate change, ecosystems adapt. Those ecosystem adaptations in turn cause humans to adapt. Nature bats last.

How the body responds to stress is a good example of how it acts as an ecology in adapting to change. We have come to think of stress as a bad thing. In some circumstances it is. But in others it is not.

1. Everything is Connected to Everything Else

The metabolic, hormonal, and neurological changes that take place when we're exposed to a stressor prepare us to fight, flee, or freeze—obviously handy for surviving a threat. But those changes also help us to learn and to focus on a task. Robert Sapolsky's *Why Zebras Don't Get Ulcers*[3] and Bruce McEwen's *The End of Stress as We Know It*[4] describe the operation of this elegant system.

The autonomic nervous system, the lymphatic system, and the adrenal glands and hypothalamus are directly connected. The autonomic nervous system regulates body functions (such as heartbeat) outside conscious thought. The lymphatic system is a key element to immunity. The hypothalamus and adrenal glands are part of the endocrine system: the hypothalamus releases hormones that control metabolic activity; the adrenal glands release stress hormones.[5]

So anything that causes a reaction in any one of these systems immediately causes a reaction in the other two. This is why, so far as your body is concerned, seeing a predator, having an infection, and being exposed to an endocrine disrupting pesticide are the same kind of event: a stress.[6]

2. Everything Has To Go Somewhere

The immediate effect of exposure to a stressor is to put the body on alert: heart rate increases, blood pressure goes up, blood sugar goes up, immune function goes up, digestion slows down, and sex hormones drop. These responses make very good sense for survival. It's time to focus all resources on fighting off the threat, running away from it, or hiding from it. It's not a time to have a nice meal or make babies.

This response is what you feel when you have to slam on your brakes or when you're confronted at work. After the immediate physical reaction, you're likely to feel fear or anger. From threat to nervous system to endocrine and immune systems to muscle and gut then back to the nervous system for emotional awareness and conscious action.

3. There's No Such Thing as a Free Lunch

But this reaction isn't meant to be permanent. Your body doesn't want to be in a permanent state of stress. Instead, the acute stress response brings with it a counter-balancing effect when the threat is no longer imminent.

What the body wants is rest and recovery following stress. Getting worked up to respond to a threat is metabolically very expensive. The body needs time to replenish itself.

4. Nature Bats Last

We live in a culture saturated with stressors. We also live in a culture that promotes constant engagement and devalues rest. Many people actively pursue a life of constant engagement. That life is integrated with and served by, for example, the food we eat and the stimulants we take. The body doesn't care. When stressed, it demands recovery. If it doesn't get it, it will compensate as best it can—often in unpleasant ways.[7]

The first article in this section, "The Hormonal Consequences of Starch and Stress," illustrates the four laws of ecology at work in the body from the standpoint of diet, stress response, hormonal disruption, and the consequences for health.

The second article, "Metabolic Syndrome Coming At You," describes how conventional medical science has recognized the body as an ecology in a distorted way. It has turned metabolic imbalance into a diagnosis that in practice only serves to promote early treatment of individual aspects of the imbalance such as high blood pressure rather than search for remedies for the imbalance itself.

The third article, "Intestinal Ecology," describes the complex ecology of our digestive system. In this case "the body as an ecology" is not a metaphor—we literally live in community and interdependency with a vast array of other organisms. When out of balance, our health suffers.

The last article, "Depression and Suicide," introduces the idea that our emotional life is integrated with our physiological life. The target of the article is the over-prescription of anti-depressants that increase the risk of suicide. We discuss how depression is the emotional consequence of, for example, nutrient or hormonal imbalance.

Notes

[1] Barry Commoner (1971) *The Closing Circle: Nature, Man, and Technology.*

[2] Robert Marks (2002) *The Origins of the Modern World: A Global and Ecological Narrative.*

[3] Robert M. Sapolsky (1994) *Why Zebra's Don't Get Ulcers: A Guide to Stress, Stress-related Diseases, and Coping.* See also Robert M. Sapolsky (2001) "The Biological Consequences of Stress."

[4] Bruce McEwen and Elizabeth Norton Lasley (2002) *The End of Stress as We Know It.* See also Bruce McEwen (2004) "Understanding Stress" and Bruce McEwen (2008) "Central Effects of Stress Hormones in Health and Disease: Understanding the Protective and Damaging Effects of Stress and Stress Mediators."

[5] Ronald Glaser and Janet Kiecolt-Glaser (2005) "Stress-induced Immune Dysfunction: Implications for Health."

[6] For a similar, ecological view from the perspective of how hormones and the endocrine system's signaling also follow the four laws of ecology, see Layna Berman (2005) "Hormone Intersect."

[7] For a discussion at greater length of the issues raised here, see Layna Berman and Jeffry Fawcett (2007) "Stress Related Illness."

THE HORMONAL CONSEQUENCES OF STARCH AND STRESS

The word *stress* has negative connotations. But stress is how we learn and adapt. The use of "stress" to refer to psychological and physiological states was borrowed from metal work where forces predict a metal's tempering into something useful. Without stress and its hormones we can't learn.

Instead of fearing stress we might respect its place in our development and adaptation. Stress becomes corrosive when our human brain seizes upon a disturbing thought and runs a long and frightening simulation.

Just One Thought

Neurobiologist, Stanford University professor, and author Robert Sapolsky, PhD points out in his groundbreaking book *Why Zebras Don't Get Ulcers* that humans are the only animals that stress themselves out with a single thought. Why did humans evolve to do that?

We do it because we want to protect ourselves. But the human body hasn't evolved to understand the difference between mental and physical stress and so it responds to both by preparing us to run or fight...for our lives. There's a big difference between quick or acute stressors such as an argument, and chronic stress states such as trauma or illness. Learning to recover from stress is the key to good health.

No Stress Without Hormones

Starting with the first hot rush of adrenaline followed by a chaser of cortisol, these stress hormones have a symbiotic relationship with your other hormones. This includes insulin, thyroid, and all your sex hormones.

Since stress is about adaptation, a healthy response occurs in a wave. Cortisol (made by the adrenal cortex) facilitates the movement of energy molecules to your big muscles, allowing you to run or fight. At the highest point in a stress response, cortisol levels are high, energy is high, and inflammation is low.

Because too much cortisol has a damaging effect on the body, the adrenal glands will slowly cut back production as you move into a recovery or rest phase. When cortisol levels are lower, you feel tired and it's easier to rest. And this is exactly what you should do.

Going Chronic

When you don't rest and recover you move from an acute situation into a chronic one. This may cause you to get stuck in either a high cortisol state or a low one.

Chronically high cortisol can cause anxiety, loss of muscle and bone, weight gain in the belly, insomnia, and can contribute to cancer promotion. Chronically low cortisol contributes to exhaustion, depression, low immunity, body-wide inflammation, and pain. Either way, cortisol levels affect hormone signaling and priming—that is, it starts the synthesis of other hormones. This in turn can lead to a lack of response by your tissues and a functional hormone imbalance or deficiency.

Diabetes is a perfect example of how chronic stress causes illness by interfering with normal hormone balance. High cortisol raises insulin and blocks thyroid and sex hormones. Too much insulin blunts a tissue's sensitivity to taking up blood sugar and other metabolic processes. Although weight gain, high blood sugars, and vascular problems are side effects of diabetes, chronic stress and too much cortisol might be the cause of these symptoms or of diabetes itself.

Low testosterone in men and low progesterone in women is caused by cortisol contesting the sex hormone's protective effects. For men, low testosterone causes vitality, libido, and muscle mass to decrease. It increases blood clotting and vascular anomalies.

In women, high cortisol and insulin decrease ovarian production of progesterone and increase production of testosterone. This in turn contributes to infertility, menstrual problems, acne, and even polycystic ovarian syndrome. All these conditions are associated with metabolic syndrome.

Did Someone Say Metabolism?

Nobody does metabolism such as your thyroid. Thyroid hormones drive your metabolism. Since thyroid priming is also affected by cortisol, stress can prevent the conversion of the thyroid hormone T4 into the active form T3.

T3 is involved in mood states. When T3 is too low, you'll feel fatigued and depressed. Diabetics, among other stressed out sick people, often have a corresponding thyroid deficiency.

Without healthy thyroid hormones you will be cold, constipated, your skin and hair will be dry, you'll be prone to psychiatric symptoms and, of course, all your other hormones won't work well since thyroid also effects hormone signaling and tissue sensitivity.

Come Here Often?

As you can see, chronic stress affects all your hormones, especially your sex hormones. Chronic stress lowers your production of sex hormones and their signaling—reproduction isn't a good idea when you're running or fighting to save your life. This decreases your vitality, mood, libido, and bone mass.

For both genders, testosterone is the main bone preserving hormone. In women, estrogen and progesterone play a bone-building role too. Stress is a catabolic state: your body cannibalizes itself for nutrients and minerals. Bones are made of minerals.

Take Two of These and Call Me in the AM

Scaring ourselves almost to death isn't the only way we make ourselves sick with stress. Humans also attempt to get away from these uncomfortable states of mind by ingesting a variety of medicating substances from pizza to Prozac. These habits can make the stress response more damaging in the long run.

Eating sugar and starch to comfort yourself isn't crazy. Studies confirm that these comfort foods lower the stress hormone cortisol, but only in the short term. Unfortunately, comfort foods that raise your blood sugar change your hormonal milieu in a way that ultimately results in more stress.

One More Dance and Then I Must Go!

Eating sugar and other so-called caloric sweeteners such as high fructose corn syrup as well as starchy foods causes your blood sugar to rise. In response, insulin goes up too. Along with its role in moving blood sugar in the form of glucose into tissues for fuel, insulin prompts your liver to store glucose for use later and to convert glucose to fatty acids for storage in your fat cells. In the process, your blood sugars are lowered.

When insulin stays too high because of frequent dietary sugar and starch spikes several things happen. Because insulin is a hormone, in excess it pushes back on your sex hormones. In men, it tends to couple with cortisol to contest and lower testosterone.

In women, excess insulin stimulates the follicles in the ovaries to overproduce testosterone instead of producing progesterone. Without progesterone, eggs can't mature and they become painful cysts that can burst. The result is irregular periods and infertility.

This condition is called polycystic ovary syndrome or PCO. It is considered to be an early consequence of metabolic syndrome and can lead to diabetes. Women with this disruption tend to put on weight in the waist and belly and have acne and oily hair. So for both genders, too much insulin from too much starch and sugar can lead to sexual dysfunction.

Heart Breaking

If sexual dysfunction isn't enough of a deterrent to medicating yourself with comfort foods, consider that insulin in excess is also cardio-toxic: it damages the heart muscle, as does too much sugar.

Additionally, the digestive system is affected by too much sweet stuff. Polypeptides in the gut are disrupted, more acid is produced, and gut flora are overrun with opportunistic organisms such as *Candida*.

Joint structures are also affected by sugar and caloric sweeteners. Arthritis is worse in people who indulge.

Finally, cancer cells love sugar—so much so that they have many more insulin receptors than normal cells. High sugar and insulin levels contribute to cancer cell growth.

Next Time You Buy Candy for Your Sweetheart

Sugar is very addictive. Our ancestry never prepared us for the large amounts of sweets in our modern diet. After an initial period of about two weeks without sugar, addictive cravings will back off. To avoid cravings eat more protein in servings sizes of less than 8 ounces at a time with plenty of vegetables. Snack on nuts or cheese and fresh, not dried fruits. You may find yourself feeling...well, sexier!

Resources

Berman, Layna. 2004. The Hunter-Gatherer Diet. *Your Own Health And Fitness*. Broadcast March 2, 2004.

Berman, Layna. 2004. The Hormonal Consequences of Starch and Stress. *Your Own Health And Fitness*. Broadcast February 3, 2004.

McEwen, Bruce. 2004. Understanding Stress. *Your Own Health And Fitness*. Broadcast January 20, 2004.

McEwen, Bruce. 2002. *The End of Stress As We Know It*. New York: National Academies Press.

Sapolsky, Robert. 2001. The Biological Consequences of Stress. *Your Own Health And Fitness*. Broadcast September 25, 2001.

Sapolsky, Robert M. 1994. *Why Zebra's Don't Get Ulcers: A Guide to Stress, Stress-Related Diseases, and Coping*. New York, WH Freeman and Company.

METABOLIC SYNDROME
COMING AT YOU

*R*isk factor is one of the most important concepts ever introduced into medical research and practice. It is also one that has led to the current medical practice of overdiagnosis and overtreatment.

The risk factor concept gained currency after World War II with the famous Framingham Heart Study. This ongoing research project, based in Framingham, Massachusetts, began in 1948. The study recorded how people live (for example, smoking) and how metabolic conditions (for example, blood pressure) related to who had heart attacks and who didn't.

The wedding of high cholesterol to increased risk of heart attacks was an early result of the Framingham Study. Today, people are diagnosed and treated for a wide variety diseases that they don't have. Instead, they are treated for the risk factors associated with disease and dysfunction: high cholesterol, high triglycerides, high blood sugar, high blood pressure, too much body fat.

The utility of the risk factor concept is that it enables people to take actions that prevent them from becoming ill. This is a good idea. Problems arise, however, in what gets counted as a risk factor and what actions are actually available to reduce risks.

Origins

In 1988, Gerald Reaven, MD of Stanford University introduced the concept Syndrome X. Reaven found that people with insulin resistance also had a greater likelihood of developing cardiovascular disease. In other words, when your body can't metabolize blood sugar properly and produces excess insulin in response, you're more likely to have a heart attack somewhere down the road.

What was remarkable about Reaven's finding was that it connected events from one system (hormone and energy metabolism) to another (cardiovascular). Also remarkable was that Reaven's prescription for reducing insulin resistance and with it the risk of heart attack consisted of abandoning the official low-fat, high-carb "heart healthy" diet and promoting an Atkins-like, low-carbohydrate diet in its place.

Perhaps because of this, many within health officialdom picked up the idea, but turned it into something more consistent with the dominant cholesterol-heart orthodoxy. Both the name and the risk factors changed. It was no longer Syndrome X, but The Metabolic

Syndrome. Insulin resistance was no longer the risk factor. Instead, a complex of risk factors was used that included cholesterol, triglycerides, body fat, and blood pressure in addition to insulin resistance.

What It Is

There is a growing consensus among official health researchers and practitioners that people with metabolic syndrome are at greater risk of not only heart attacks but also strokes, type 2 diabetes, polycystic ovaries, liver and kidney failure, and some cancers. What distinguishes metabolic syndrome is the complexity of its definition.

First, each individual criteria for insulin resistance, cholesterol, triglycerides, body fat, and blood pressure are subclinical. That is, taken alone, a test result would not get you diagnosed as having cardiovascular disease or diabetes or hypertension. But if two or three of the five factors test within a specified range, you'll get a diagnosis of metabolic syndrome.

One of the confusions in all this is that there are competing definitions of what those criteria ranges ought to be. There are three principal standards: from the World Health Organization (WHO), the National Institutes of Health's National Cholesterol Education Program Adult Treatment Panel (NCEP ATP), and the American Association of Clinical Endocrinology (AACE). These are summarized in the table below.

You will note that the criteria are not uniform across these standards, which creates problems for research. Some research finds connections with illness when using one standard, but no connection when using another.

Standards for diagnosis of metabolic syndrome

Criteria	WHO 3 or more	NCEP ATP 3 or more	AACE 2 or more
Fasting glucose	110-125 mg/dL	110-125 mg/dL	110-125 mg/dL
HDL cholesterol	<35 mg/dL Men <39 mg/dL Women	<40 mg/dL Men <50 mg/dL Women	<40 mg/dL Men <50 mg/dL Women
Triglycerides	>150 mg/dL	>150 mg/dL	>150 mg/dL
Blood pressure	>140/90 mm Hg	>130/85 mm Hg	>130/85 mm Hg
Body fat	BMI >30 and Waist-to-hip ratio >0.9 Men >0.85 Women	Waist circumference >102 cm Men >88 cm Women	

The AACE standard is of particular interest: it does not use body fat distribution as a criterion. This is because they take the position that excess body fat is a consequence of the already-measured insulin resistance.

Surprisingly, no measure of insulin itself is included in any of these major standards. Some clinicians and researchers, however, do include *hyperinsulinemia* (high blood levels of insulin) as a criterion. For insulin resistance, this makes better sense than blood glucose levels alone: when you're insulin resistant, your cells are insensitive to the insulin you produce and so your body produces more insulin to force the issue. Reavens' original concept was that hyperinsulinemia, not high blood glucose by itself, indicates insulin resistance.

Essentially, these standards are not the same but close. What ties them together is a welding of Reaven's insight about insulin resistance to the cholesterol-heart orthodoxy—with obesity orthodoxy thrown in for good measure; see our critique of this orthodoxy in "Fat and Death" on page 274.

What to Worry About

Singly, none of the metabolic syndrome criteria is enough to get you diagnosed with anything. However, if you test out with three (with the AACE you only need two), you get yourself a diagnosis and with that diagnosis you get treatment—which typically means drugs.

Several research projects have been well-publicized to raise a warning about the increasing incidence of metabolic syndrome. In one study, Earl Ford and his colleagues estimated that metabolic syndrome increased by 13% between 1990 and 2000. The biggest increase was among women (27%), especially young women between 20 and 40 years old (78% increase).

Ford estimated that in 2000 the prevalence of metabolic syndrome was 29% for the entire adult population, 28% for men, 30% for all women, and 18% for young women. In other words, well over one quarter of Americans have metabolic syndrome.

In Europe, the prevalence of metabolic syndrome is somewhat less—about a fifth of the adult population has it. In addition, the prevalence among men tends to be greater than among women.

These and other estimates of the prevalence and growth of metabolic syndrome were all population-based epidemiological studies. In a more novel approach, prescription drug management company Medco estimated that 15% of the people they manage had metabolic syndrome. The way they estimated this number was by counting up the number of people taking drugs for the various criteria conditions: glucose lowering drugs, cholesterol lowering drugs, and blood pressure drugs.

The surprise in the study was that $4 out of every $10 spent on drugs is being spent on metabolic syndrome, whether that's the diagnosis or not. And Medco claims that the prevalence of metabolic syndrome as measured by drug prescriptions increased by over a third between 2002 and 2004.

In other words, the Medco estimate of how many people have metabolic syndrome is about half of what population-based research indicates is out there, waiting to be diagnosed—and treated—with drugs.

Fitness as Prevention

In their press release, Medco describes how dramatically cardiorespiratory fitness improves metabolic syndrome. A significant body of research backs up that claim. The way to avoid the drug treatment is to avoid the diagnosis. And the way to avoid the diagnosis is to get and stay physically fit.

Although cardiorespiratory fitness works to keep metabolic syndrome away, an obvious question cries out for an answer: if this is a metabolic syndrome, what causes the metabolic disruptions that cause it? The thinking, if not the conclusions about metabolic syndrome, gives us a clue.

Metabolic syndrome looks beyond a single cause to a multiplicity of causes. Insulin resistance and the rest are *symptoms* of metabolic disruption. What we should be looking at are the exposures that derange your metabolism. The real risk factors underlying metabolic syndrome include

- inflammation and immune response from physiological stressors and infectious agents,
- oxidative stress from pollutants,
- psychosocial stress from inequity and other social conditions,
- nutrient deficiency from lack of access to nutrient-rich foods. and
- toxins that disrupt our endocrine and other metabolic systems.

In addition to protecting yourself from these real risk factors, you'll also have to protect yourself from the diagnosis. In concert with an epidemiological interest in metabolic syndrome, public health and medical association officials have started a campaign. In this campaign, physicians are encouraged to be ever-vigilant for the telltale signs of metabolic syndrome. This campaign targets children and teenagers as well as adults.

Some critics argue that metabolic syndrome is a made-up diagnosis intended to turn people into patients. It's true. The vast majority of health researchers, practitioners, and officials see no alternative when it comes to prevention. It's an infernal logic.

- It is their mission to prevent illness.

- To prevent illness, people must be treated for the factors that put them at risk.
- To treat someone to prevent illness, they must have a diagnosis—and the sooner, the better.

You'd be well advised to take cautionary prevention into your own hands and avoid the diagnosis. Some of the preventive actions you can take are

- rest and sleep,
- routine physical activity,
- antioxidants in your diet,
- a diet without starch and sugar,
- sex hormone balance,
- thyroid health,
- avoid exposures to chemicals and pollutants, and
- make deliberate choices to reduce stress.

Resources

Berman, Layna. 2005. Another Thyroid Show. *Your Own Health And Fitness*. Broadcast May 31, 2005.

Berman, Layna. 2005. Indoor Air Pollution. *Your Own Health And Fitness*. Broadcast March 1, 2005.

Berman, Layna. 2005. Designing a Sane Individualized Diet Plan. *Your Own Health And Fitness*. Broadcast January 4, 2005.

Duncan, Glen E, et al. 2004. Prevalence and Trends of a Metabolic Phenotype Among US Adolescents, 1999-2000. *Diabetes Care*. October, 2004 (27:10): 2438-43.

Ford, Earl S, et al. 2004. Increasing Prevalence of the Metabolic Syndrome Among US Adults. *Diabetes Care*. October, 2004 (27:10): 2444-9.

Hu, Gang, et al. 2004. Prevalence of the Metabolic Syndrome and Its Relation to All-Cause and Cardiovascular Mortality in Nondiabetic European Men and Women. *Archives of Internal Medicine*. May 24, 2004 (164): 1066-76.

Katzmarzyk, Peter T, et al. 2005. Metabolic Syndrome, Obesity, and Mortality: Impact of Cardiorespiratory Fitness. *Diabetes Care*. February, 2005 (28:2): 391-7.

Laaksonen, David E, et al. 2005. Physical Activity in the Prevention of Type 2 Diabetes. *Diabetes*. January, 2004 (51): 158-65.

Lee, SoJung, et al. 2005. Cardiorespiratory Fitness Attenuates Metabolic Syndrome Risk Independent of Abdominal Subcutaneous and Visceral Fat in Men. *Diabetes Care*. April, 2005 (28:4): 895-91.

Lunder, Sonya. 2004. Toxic Cosmetics. Your Own Health And Fitness. Broadcast August 17, 2004.

McEwen, Bruce. 2004. Understanding Stress. *Your Own Health And Fitness*. Broadcast January 20, 2004.

Scuteri, Angelo, et al. 2005. The Metabolic Syndrome in Older Individuals. *Diabetes Care*. April 2005 (28:4): 882-8.

Slater, Arthur. 2005. Controlling Pests without Toxins. *Your Own Health And Fitness*. Broadcast May 3, 2005.

INTESTINAL ECOLOGY

Testing water for intestinal bacteria is a cornerstone of public health. The tests are for benign bacteria that can be grown easily. The principle is that if a water supply is contaminated with benign bacteria from the human gut, then *pathogens* (disease-causing bacteria) might also be present.

Until a few decades ago, the control of pathogens was the focus of attention on the gut. Then researchers began to look at how bacteria and other microorganisms (*microbes*) play a role in digestion and immunity and their disruption. But until recently, scientists were unable to accurately describe the microbial ecology of the gut.

There are two reasons why it has been difficult to study what all those microbes are doing in your intestines.

First, stool samples were the only non-invasive way to collect intestinal microbes. This would be like studying the ecology of a watershed by taking water samples only at the mouth of the river.

The second limitation is that intestinal microbes are difficult to grow outside the intestine. It would be like trying to grow a rainforest in a lab to study rainforest ecology. And this is the area in which the greatest advances have been made.

5 Pounds of Microbes

Gut microbes make up about 5 pounds of your body's weight. Because the microbes are 100 times smaller than your cells, that 5 pounds contains 10 times the number of cells in your entire body.

The most significant discovery is that the five pounds of microbes consists of between 500 and 1,000 different species. This is about the same number cell types in the human body. What's different is that, for any individual human body, each cell type has the same genome. But for intestinal microbes, each species has its own genome giving that five pound mass 100 times the number of genes in the host's body.

What is that complex ecology of microbes doing? Apparently much more than previously thought.

One of the most prevalent species of bacteria produces enzymes that break down indigestible fiber into carbohydrates that we can absorb. And this bacteria does a better job because it produces 240 different enzymes compared to our body producing only 98 different enzymes for carbohydrate digestion.

This is a so-called *commensal* relationship: two or more species benefit each other by living together.

Experiments with mice have shown how the presence of commensal microbes might affect our ability to gain weight—specifically to store fat. Mice born and raised in a completely clean environment have no gut microbes. These mice could not gain weight.

But when the mice were taken out of the sterile environment and the gut became populated with microbes, they were able to gain weight. The popular press latched onto this as a new diet plan, a spin that is not only superficial but missed the true significance of the research.

Storing fat is essential to your health. This research tells us that your fat metabolism doesn't work without commensal gut microbes. Disruptions to gut ecology disrupt your basic energy metabolism.

Immunity

When pathogens and allergens reach your gut, commensal microbes form your first line of defense. Before bad guys get into your blood stream and your immune system kicks in, commensal microbes attack them and signal your immune system that something wicked this way comes.

This is a tricky business. Your gut microbes, just like your immune system, have to distinguish friend from foe. Conditions such as Crohn's disease occur when the gut's immune system mistakes normal commensal microbes for pathogens.

In a healthy gut, commensal microbes communicate with the cells that line the gut and the immune cells close by. The conversation helps maintain the integrity of the cell lining as well as help control inflammation in response to foreign substances that are not harmful—for example, substances that are food for you or food for your intestinal ecology.

Inflammation is the first response of your body to an invader. Inflammation signals your immune system to send in the troops. While commensal microbes are taking care of foreigners, they're also telling your gut to not get inflamed.

An immune system on alert from almost any source can increase the risk of inflammation. And with inflammation your intestinal ecology can become imbalanced, a condition called *dysbiosis*.

Healthy Gut

You know when your gut isn't working right. The best guide for navigating these waters is Liz Lipski's *Digestive Wellness* where dysbiosis is described.

Stress is a common instigator of gut problems. Stress shuts down your digestion so that all your resources can be used to fight or flee. In the short term, a good thing. But with chronic stress, your digestion is permanently affected. And that affects your commensal microbes, which can, in turn, affect your gut.

Antibiotics have a profound effect on your intestinal ecology. Antibiotics don't distinguish between commensals and pathogens. So use antibiotics prudently and sparingly. Your gut will need to recover from an antibiotic treatment. Probiotics (see below) can help repopulate your gut.

Allergies are a less obvious contributor to gut problems. Food allergies are proinflammatory and cause dysbiosis. Celiac disease is a well-known and extreme version of gluten allergies. So a place to start for a troubled gut is an allergy elimination diet that cuts out common allergic foods.

Mold allergies are another cause of gut problems. Molds are pervasive. Our allergic response to them is common—and commonly unrecognized.

Molds like dark, moist places such as behind furniture. Molds will also get into rugs and carpets.

In addition to keeping areas well-lit and dry, you can treat areas that are mold havens. Use a natural mycocide (mold-killer): mix equal parts tea tree oil and grapefruit seed extract in water. Or you can use hydrogen peroxide—but be careful because it bleaches where the tea tree-grapefruit seed mixture doesn't.

An air purifier (that doesn't produce ozone) also helps by precipitating mold spores out of the air so you can vacuum them up. To support your immune response and relieve symptoms, use homeopathic remedies for mold.

Sauerkraut is Good for You

Supporting your commensal microbes is as easy as eating sauerkraut or yoghurt. These and other cultured foods contain many of the beneficial species that populate your gut.

These *probiotic* organisms are also available as supplements. Probiotics has become a mainstay of the natural foods industry. But you need to take care when using probiotic supplements to make sure of their quality.

More recently, supplementation with *prebiotics* has received much attention. Prebiotics are food for commensal microbes. Prebiotics are complex carbohydrates that you can't digest but which your commensals can. More importantly, prebiotics (members of a class of carbohydrates called *oligosaccharides*) selectively nourish beneficial microbes.

Although prebiotics are available as supplements, the best source is a diet rich in vegetables. Supplements are sold that supposedly consist of specific oligosaccharides that benefit specific microbes. But the science in isolating which prebiotics benefit which microbes is still developing. The promise of prebiotics has become a marketing ploy for some supplement manufacturers that have charted a course in nutriceuticals—specially formulated supplements that claim astounding health and medicinal effects.

A common strategy for some supplement manufacturers has been to package probiotics with prebiotics and sell the mix as *synbiotics*. Too often, this *causes* rather than cures gut problems. The reason is that some oligosaccharides can't be digested by either you or your commensals and are instead gut irritants. So evaluate prebiotic supplements carefully.

Sauerkraut, on the other hand, is near perfect: probiotics and prebiotics you can create yourself. Stuff some shredded cabbage into a few canning jars, add 2 teaspoons of salt, cover with water, and put on the lids firmly (rub the threads of the lid with a little olive oil so it will open easily). Place the jars in a warm place (such as the top of the refrigerator) and in 3 or 4 days, you'll have a whole new food group to enjoy!

Resources
Bäckhed, Fredrik et al. 2005. Host-Bacterial Mutualism in the Human Intestine. *Science*. March 25, 2005 (307): 1915-20. DOI: 10.1126/science.1104816.

Badman, Michael and Jeffrey Flier. 2005. The Gut and Energy Balance: Visceral Allies in the Obesity Wars. *Science*. March 25, 2005 (307): 1909-14. DOI: 10.1126/science.1109951.

Eckburg, Paul et al. 2005. Diversity of the Human Intestinal Microbial Flora. *Science*. June 10, 2005 (308): 1635-8. DOI: 10.1126/science.1110591.

Ley, Ruth et al. 2005. Obesity Alters Gut Microbial Ecology. *Proceedings of the National Academy of Science*. August 2, 2005; 102(31): 11070-5. DOI:10.1073/pnas.0504978102.

Lipski, Elizabeth. 2004. *Digestive Wellness*. New York: McGraw-Hill.

MacDonald, Thomas and Giovanni Monteleone. 2005. Immunity, Inflammation, and Allergy in the Gut. *Science*. March 25, 2005 (307): 1920-5. DOI: 10.1126/science.1106442.

Macpherson, Andrew et al. 2005. Immune Responses that Adapt the Intestinal Mucosa to Commensal Intestinal Bacteria. *Immunology*. 115: 153-62. DOI:10.1111/j.1365-2567.2005.02159.x.

❦

DEPRESSION AND SUICIDE

In our first issue of PHO, we reported on the dangers of SSRI antidepressants when given to children ("What If They Gave An Antidepressant and No One Came?"). One study suggests that adults who take not only SSRI antidepressants but *any* antidepressant are at greater risk of suicide.

SSRIs (selective serotonin reuptake inhibitors) are the most widely prescribed medications for depression. These drugs work by disrupting your body's process of absorbing the neurotransmitter serotonin. By preventing reabsorption, SSRIs increase the concentration of serotonin circulating in your blood. Serotonin is a "happy" neurotransmitter that calms your troubled mind and helps you sleep.

Low levels of serotonin are associated with depression. Since your body recycles serotonin rapidly, drug makers invented SSRIs to prevent recycling and increase the amount of circulating serotonin.

But SSRIs do much more, including increase the risk of suicide.

Increased Risk of Suicide

In an article published in the *British Journal of Medicine*, Dean Fergusson, PhD and his colleagues reported on their review of over 700 studies comparing SSRIs to placebos, tricyclics (the class of drugs that SSRIs replaced), and other antidepressant drugs.

In comparing SSRIs to placebos, Fergusson and his colleagues found that the incidence of suicide and suicide attempts doubled. But when compared to tricyclics and other drugs, there was no difference in suicides and suicide attempts. In other words, both old and new antidepressants carry an increased risk of suicide.

After the furor over SSRIs and their suicide risk for children, the FDA applied a so-called black label on these drugs. Prescriptions for children declined significantly, although they're still being used. It's possible that the same might happen with adults.

The responses that accompanied the Fergusson article in the *BMJ* were revealing.

There was the usual cry from the official psychiatric community that the "risks have to be weighed against the benefits." The American Psychiatric Association has historically defended to the death (yours, not theirs) the virtues of throwing drugs at psychological problems.

But one such critic made an important point: while the risk was double, the actual impact was small. If the number of suicides doubles from 1 to 2 in a population of 100 people, that's a big deal. But in a population of 100,000 (the scale of the Fergusson study) the absolute risk doesn't seem so significant. Except, of course, to the parties involved.

As we noted in our PHO #1 article, suicide is only one of the many problems created by SSRIs, for which see Peter Breggin's *Antidepressant Fact Book*.

Yet another reviewer made an even more startling observation. This flap around SSRIs is really beside the point. Most of these drugs will be off patent soon—that is, the formula will no longer be protected by law and available for anyone to manufacture. So drug companies will be replacing them in their line-up with new, improved antidepressants that "solve" all the problems of SSRIs. In other words, who cares about SSRIs? They're going away soon. And with them, presumably the risk of suicide.

Remember that there's no difference in suicide risk between SSRIs, tricyclics, and other antidepressants? Is there any reason to believe that, drug company marketing campaigns aside, new antidepressants will be safer?

Vioxx and the other COX-2 inhibitors used for pain were supposed to be easier on the stomach than other, older non-steroidal anti-inflammatory drugs such as aspirin. In fact, they were only slightly easier on the stomach. But they did command a higher price.

Increased Depression

Between 1987 and 2000, the rate at which people were treated for depression doubled, from 4,373 cases per 100,000 people (4.4%) to 8,575 cases per 100,000 (8.6%). Between 1995 and 2001, the number of drugs prescribed for patients diagnosed with depression almost doubled from 138 per 1,000 patients to 238 per 1,000 (a 75% increase).

In other words, your risk of being diagnosed with depression doubled in 15 years. And, if you were diagnosed with depression, your risk of being treated with an SSRI almost doubled in 6 years.

As to suicide, death rates from suicide for adults is about 15 per 100,000 people. In the Fergusson study, suicide deaths were about 5 times that rate for people taking antidepressants, but only 2.5 times that rate for people who didn't take drugs.

This shouldn't surprise us. All the people in the Fergusson study were being treated for depression. In other words, people suffering from depression are at greater risk of committing suicide. Which begs an important question: the Fergusson study only compares SSRIs to other drugs, not other forms of treating depression, such as psychotherapy, nutrient therapy, or hormone replacement therapy.

Where Depression Comes From

1. <u>Hormone Imbalance</u> Thyroid imbalance affects your mood: too little thyroid promotes depression, while too much promotes anxiety. Sex hormone imbalance in either gender at any age can promote depression. Chronic stress creates its own hormonal imbalances that can promote depression. In addition to metabolic disruptions, endocrine disruptors from the environment can cause hormone imbalance.

2. <u>Food Allergies and Sensitivities</u> Foods common to our diet can be powerful allergens: grains, corn, soy, and dairy. Many of these are hidden ingredients in processed foods. Processed foods contain other provocative ingredients, such as MSG. Soy can be particularly provocative because it's not only a potential allergen, it can also inhibit your thyroid. Gut dysbiosis can also prompt an allergic response.

3. <u>Nutrient Imbalances</u> Deficiencies in essential fatty acids, amino acids, vitamins, and minerals can affect your mood. Some imbalances come from your diet, some come from hereditary factors, and some from metabolic disruptions such as gut dysbiosis, toxins, and allergens.

4. <u>Gut Dysbiosis</u> The balance of your gut flora not only affects digestion but your health generally, including your mental health. Dysbiosis (when your gut flora are out of balance) can lead to nutrients and byproducts leaking from your gut into your bloodstream. These become allergens that can affect your mood. In addition, gut dysbiosis leads to inadequate absorption of nutrients, which in turn affects depression.

5. <u>Toxins</u> A toxic reaction leading to depression can come from manufactured chemicals such as pesticides and heavy metals such as mercury.

6. <u>Pharmaceuticals and Recreational Drugs</u> Corticosteroids, antihistimines, anti-inflammatories, antihypertensives, cholesterol lowering drugs, birth control pills, tranquilizers, sedatives, and quinolone antibiotics have all been implicated in causing depression. In addition, mood-altering pharmaceuticals and recreational substances used to self-medicate (including comfort foods) make happy chemicals. Those exogenous happy chemicals overstimulate cell receptors and this down-regulates the production of your own, native happy chemical production (such as those released when you exercise).

7. <u>Health Status</u> People with diabetes, thyroid disorders, heart disease, lung disease, liver disease, cancer, multiple sclerosis, rheumatoid arthritis, lupus, Lyme disease, and chronic fatigue syndrome are at greater risk of depression.

8. Light Depression is often seasonal. Natural light affects your mood. More light, less depression.
9. Sleep and Rest Sleep deprivation and sleep debt caused by over-stimulation and hyperarousal from fatigue can cause depression.
10. Circumstances As Peter Breggin, MD notes, sometimes a person's circumstances really are depressing. However, "difficult" is not the same as "hopeless." When someone feels that there are no alternatives to difficult circumstances, they might develop a sense of helplessness—a feeling that is one of the most toxic forms of stress.
11. Exercise Endorphins are happy chemicals released when you exercise. More exercise, more happy chemicals. However, you will experience a stress response if you over-exercise and under-rest: exercise is a stressor; your body responds and adapts during sleep and rest.

Covert Depression in Men

For people in treatment for depression, antidepressants are prescribed half as often for men as for women: 15 prescriptions per 100 men treated versus 32 prescriptions per 100 women.

Women are treated for depression 50% more often than men: 7% of men are treated for depression, while 11% of women are treated.

Men commit suicide 4 times more often than women: 18 suicide deaths per 100,000 men versus 4 suicide deaths per 100,000 women.

Over the last 50 years, suicide rates have declined slightly, from 13 per 100,000 in 1950 to 11 per 100,000 in 2002. The exception is young men 15 to 24 years old. Suicide among young men has almost tripled: from 6.5 per 100,000 in 1950 to 16.5 per 100,000 in 2002.

In *I Don't Want to Talk About It*, Terrence Real refers to depression that is pervasive among men as *covert depression*. "Covert" because it is not recognized by the sufferer or anyone else as depression.

Real describes the lack of self-esteem at the core of depression as an attack by the self on the self for being less than it should. When the pain of that attack is felt as worthlessness, hopelessness, and shame, the sufferer's actions are what we commonly recognize as *overt depression*.

When the pain of depression's self-attacks-self is deflected and not felt, the feelings are externalized in actions that "prove" one's worth in status or material goods, addictions, and anger and violence.

Because women are better socialized to accept feeling the pains of depression, they are able to recognize the self-attacks-self and act positively on it. Men are not well socialized to acknowledge those feelings, but instead are trained to resist them with accomplishments and chemicals.

For Real, enabling men to experience overt depression would be an improvement. Writing from the context of "talk therapy," Real's book documents what hard work that can be.

It's a big emotional leap from covert to overt depression. Perhaps it starts by honestly recognizing that something doesn't feel right.

Resources

Breggin, Peter. 2004. Depressing News about Antidepressants. *Your Own Health and Fitness.* Broadcast May 25, 2004.

Breggin, Peter. 2001. *The Antidepressant Fact Book.* Cambridge, MA: Perseus Publishing.

Fergusson, Dean et al. 2005. Association between Suicide Attempts and Selective Serotonin Reuptake Inhibitors: Systematic Review of Randomized Controlled Trials. *British Medical Journal.* February 19, 2005 (330):396-403.

Marohn, Stephanie. 2003. *The Natural Medicine Guide to Depression.* Charlottesville, VA: Hampton Roads Publishing Company.

Real, Terrence. 1998. *I Don't Want to Talk About It.* New York: Fireside.

Real, Terrence. 1997. Male Depression. *Your Own Health and Fitness.* Broadcast July 15, 1997.

Walsh, William. 2005. Reducing Violent Behavior and Depression with Nutrients. *Your Own Health and Fitness.* Broadcast January 11, 2005.

In *Gut Feelings*, psychologist Gerd Gigerenzer tells a horrifying story of medical treatment gone wrong. A twenty-one month old boy was brought to a leading pediatric hospital with "nearly everything.. wrong with him."[1] The boy was withdrawn, underweight, refused to eat, and suffered persistent infections. The boy's family was dysfunctional—he received virtually no nurturing.

When the young doctor who took the boy's case took a blood sample to find out what might be going on, the boy withdrew and his condition worsened. So the doctor nurtured the boy and minimized invasive procedures. The boy began to eat and he improved.

The young doctor's superiors took him off the case and proceeded to assault the boy with a battery of diagnostic tests. The team assigned to the case was determined to find a diagnosis. Instead, the boy languished and died.

Our previous discussion in "The Placebo Effect" provides a window into why the young doctor's instincts helped: nurturing can have a profound effect on healing. For example, children who experience maltreatment are more strongly affected by environmental pollutants[2] and as adults are more likely to have a compromised immune system and suffer from diseases of inflammation such as diabetes.[3] In fact, such a simple thing as nurturing can lead to a better outcome than advanced technology. But as the story also illustrates, applying these simple things isn't always easy.

Diabetics have always been encouraged to eat carefully and get some exercise. But the primary treatment has always been the prescription of medications. Yet in a clinical trial that compared the efficacy of medication to so-called "lifestyle interventions" that encouraged diet and exercise, it was diet and exercise that were superior.[4]

During a radio interview of an expert on diabetes, a caller pointed out this superiority. The expert, an MD, agreed but argued that while she could prescribe drugs for her patients, she could not "make" them eat and exercise properly.

There are two lessons here.

The first lesson is that health practitioners are limited by their training, temperament, institutional constraints, and one-to-one relationship with patients.[5] Physicians are not trained to motivate people. They're trained to diagnose and treat. Temperamentally, they're prone to cures rather than the ongoing management of a condition.

Institutionally, how much time they can spend with a patient and the kind of treatment they can provide are constrained by the medical system. These constraints are imposed principally by insurance companies, government agencies such as Medicare, and government and professional regulatory organizations that establish and enforce standards of care.[6]

The second lesson is that prescribing changes in diet and exercise is the same as prescribing a new life. Food and physical activity are woven into each person's life. Without any support in overcoming the barriers to change, following orders to take a medication is typically easier for someone than changing her "lifestyle." It's easier for both the doctor and the patient.

But, at least in the case of diabetics, medication is neither simpler nor better.

It's not simpler because the medication has side effects, a fact we discuss elsewhere in this book. It's also not simpler because it exposes the body to what is in essence a toxin designed to oppose an adaptive balance the body has struck. The balance is not the desired, normal balance, but nevertheless is the body's attempt to adapt to an incapacity to metabolize blood sugar. Remember the four laws of ecology, especially that nature bats last.

On the other hand, there's common agreement that diet and exercise are better at treating diabetes. They're also simpler from the body's perspective. Nutrients and physical activity are not only known to the body but are craved by it. What diet and exercise are doing is working with the body to restore a normal balance using the body's own capacity to adapt.

What's missing from the picture is a prescription that enables diabetics to overcome the barriers to adopting these simple solutions. The health care system is not equipped at all to provide that kind of support.

This is true for a wide variety of diagnoses and medical conditions. The first article in this section, "Health Care Bankruptcy," describes how simple solutions are the obvious answer to the most common and costly medical conditions.

The second article in this section, "Life, Death, and Vegetables," discusses how simple solutions increase life expectancy. It helps us shift from thinking about how to treat medical conditions using the simplest things first to sustaining health using the simplest things first.

As with diagnoses and medical conditions, health generally is supported by doing the simplest thing first. The capacity to do those simple things has two sides.

On one side is knowing what those simple things are in the first place. The content of this book and its references provide some of that information. As important, the articles in this book provide examples of how to think through various issues of health and healing from a critical perspective.

The other side consists of finding and creating environments that make doing the simplest thing the easiest thing as well. The articles in this book are about overcoming those barriers.

The capacity to heal is a natural part of sustainable health. Thinking through problems of how to heal are cut from the same cloth as thinking through problems of how to sustain health.

For example, getting lots of rest when you're sick is a good idea. Often, the body communicates quite clearly its need for you to stop so it can heal. So it makes sense that resting is an important part of sustaining health too.[7]

Notes

[1] Gerd Gigerenzer (2007) *Gut Feelings: The Intelligence of the Unconscious* pp. 20-1.

[2] Bernard Weiss and David C. Bellinger (2006) "Social Ecology of Children's Vulnerability to Environmental Pollutants."

[3] Andrea Danese, et al. (2007) "Childhood Maltreatment Predicts Adult Inflammation in a Life-course Study."

[4] Diabetes Prevention Program Research Group (2002) "Reduction in the Incidence of Type 2 Diabetes with Lifestyle Intervention or Metformin." See also the review by a leading Finnish researcher in Jaakko Tuomilehto (2007) "Counterpoint: Evidence-based Prevention of Type 2 Diabetes: The Power of Lifestyle Management."

[5] For a description of what constrains the actions of physicians, see Oleg Reznik (2005) *The Secrets of Medical Decision Making: How to Avoid Becoming a Victim of the Health Care Machine.*

[6] See the description of one instance in David Leonhardt (2007) "What's a Pound of Prevention Really Worth?"

[7] For more on the practical application of doing the simplest things first, see Layna Berman and Jeffry Fawcett (2008) "Doing the Simplest Things First."

HEALTH CARE BANKRUPTCY

Health insurance is a crap shoot. Insurance companies bet that we will pay them more in premiums than they will have to pay us in benefits.

Insurance companies work from actuarial tables that describe the frequency with which people need medical care based on each person's characteristics (age, sex, etc.). Based on the characteristics of a group (for example, the people working at a business), an insurance company tries to figure out how many people in that group will need medical treatment and what treatments they will need. The company then sets premiums so that they will take in more money than they expect to spend.

You might think that insurance companies have a powerful financial incentive to reward prevention. You'd think they would reward people who take care of themselves. But they don't. All they know is what's in the actuarial tables, which tells them the chances that, given your age, etc., you'll have a heart attack or get cancer or break a leg. They're rolling the dice. And you're the dice.

Health Maintenance Organizations (HMOs) have an incentive to promote prevention because they are both the insurer and the provider. Unfortunately, HMO prevention is confined to the doctor's office (they couldn't get mercury out of your tuna even if they wanted to). And financially, their incentive is to keep you away from expensive treatments, not to support your health.

Medical insurance is a business. They know that the people they insure will get sick and injured. What they worry about is how much they will have to spend.

What we spend as a nation on medical care is the fastest growing portion of our national income. What we spend individually on medical care takes an increasing chunk out of our personal income.

The Top 15 Medical Care Costs

An article in *Health Affairs*, "Which Medical Conditions Account for the Rise in Health Care Spending?" looks at medical spending in 1987 compared to 2000.

Between 1987 and 2000 medical-care spending doubled before adjusting for inflation. After adjusting for inflation, so-called real dollar spending increased 46%, about 3.5% per year. Fifteen medical conditions accounted for over half of all medical spending increases. There are two parts to spending increases: the number of people treated for a medical condition and the cost of treating a person with that condition.

The 15 medical conditions that contributed the most to medical care spending, 1987 compared to 2000

Medical Condition	Percent change 1987 to 2000	
	Cost per case treated	Treatment prevalence
Mental disorders	+11.3%	+96.1%
Lung conditions	+31.5%	+49.4%
Hypertension	+57.2%	+16.9%
Heart disease	+16.5%	+0.6%
Stroke	+17.0%	+108.3%
Arthritis	+18.3%	+27.1%
Cancer	-1.1%	+17.0%
Skin disorders	+34.9%	+18.3%
Diabetes	-7.6%	+43.9%
Infectious disease	+91.2%	-11.3%
Pneumonia	+64.2%	-10.9%
Back problems	-7.9%	49.8%
Endocrine disorders	-7.2%	32.8%
Kidney disease	-22.6%	34.5%
Trauma	41.3%	-30.9%

When we think of medical cost increases, we often think of ever-more expensive treatments, especially the cost of pharmaceuticals and advanced technologies. However, the number of people treated has been an equally powerful cause of cost increases.

The number of people treated increases because there are more people *and* because a greater percentage of them get treated (treatment prevalence increases).

As an example, suppose the total population grew from 200 million in 1987 to 250 million in 2000. If the number of people treated for diabetes increased from 10 million people to 12.5 million, the treatment prevalence would remain the same at 5%. But if the number of people treated for diabetes increased to 15 million, both the number *and* the prevalence increase, the prevalence from 5% to 6%.

If the prevalence increases, something is affecting people more. It might be more actual sickness or it might be that doctors are paying more attention and finding people they would not have noticed before.

The table on the left shows the top 15 conditions along with both the change in per-treatment spending and the change in treatment prevalence. The conditions are listed by how much inflation-adjusted spending changed, from highest to lowest.

For example, spending on mental disorders increased the most (by $26 billion) between 1987 and 2000. While treatment costs increased by 11.3% (from $1,301 to $1,448), the prevalence of treated cases almost doubled (96.1% from 4.4% of the population to 8.6%). That is, people were suffering twice as many mental disorders or doctors were recognizing mental disorders more readily or some combination of the two.

Prevalence and Prevention

The most startling thing about the conditions listed in the table is that for all but three, their prevalence has increased: more people are getting sick or more doctors are noticing, diagnosing, and treating. Some increases have been dramatic—stroke and mental disorders in particular, followed by lung conditions, diabetes, and back problems.

In light of increased per-treatment costs, it would make financial sense to promote environmental changes that prevent these conditions. Unfortunately, our current health care is dominated by the medical model. Medical care requires a diagnosis. For something to happen, you have to enter the medical care system. Once in the system and diagnosed, you will be treated with drugs and technology.

This contrasts with a prevention-oriented health care system dominated by public health that eliminates our exposure to toxic social and physical environments that prevent disease before it starts.

Each of the 15 medical conditions listed is the result of your body's response to its environment. Most are affected directly by nutrition and physical activity: heart disease, stroke, arthritis, diabetes, hypertension, asthma, kidney disease, endocrine disorders, depression, and cancer. The other conditions are affected indirectly by the capacity of a well-nourished and well-conditioned body to withstand physical, chemical, and biological assaults.

For example, even conventional science recognizes that diet and exercise are better than drugs for preventing diabetes. Some research has shown that walking reduces the risk of Alzheimer's disease. And although hunter-gatherer diets such as the Atkins and South Beach Diet are sold as weight loss programs, both were developed to reduce the risk of heart attacks and strokes.

While we should work as citizens to reduce treatment costs and the availability of medical care, you don't have to wait. You can cre-

ate your own prevention program with
- whole, nutrient-dense foods supplemented by vitamins and minerals; and
- regular exercise that includes both aerobics (such as walking or swimming) and weight resistance (such as weight lifting or pilates).

The insurance industry won't reduce your premiums, but taking these preventive actions will help you avoid the medical-care horrors described in books such as *Critical Condition: How Health Care in America Became Big Business—and Bad Medicine* by Donald Barlett and James Steele.

Resources

Barlett, Donald and James Steele. 2004. Critical Condition: How Health Care in America Became Big Business and Bad Medicine. New York, Doubleday.

Berman, Layna. 2004. The Hunter-Gatherer Diet. *Your Own Health And Fitness*. Broadcast March 2, 2004.

Berman, Layna. 2003. Exercise How-To. *Your Own Health And Fitness*. Broadcast November 18, 2003.

Berman, Layna. 2002. The Science of Weight Training. *Your Own Health And Fitness*. Broadcast September 3, 2002.

LIFE, DEATH, AND VEGETABLES

How would you like to live 14 years longer? All you have to do is four simple things: don't smoke, don't drink more than an ounce of alcohol each day, engage in a moderate amount of daily physical activity, and eat at least 5 servings of fruits and vegetables each day.

Those are the conclusions the media drew from a study conducted in the English county of Norfolk as part of an ongoing health study with the grand acronym of EPIC (European Prospective Investigation into Cancer and Nutrition). This happens to be one of those studies that, despite its flaws, reinforces common sense.

Yet the study, by Kay-Tee Khaw and her colleagues and published in *PLoS Medicine*, does have limitations and flaws that are quite helpful in better understanding the result.

Healthy Lifestyle Score

The Khaw study began keeping track of people in 1993-1997 and followed up in 2006, an average of about 11 years. During that time the study looked at who died and who had the 4 healthy lifestyle characteristics.

The classification of each person in the study was quite simple: he or she scored 1 point for each of their lifestyle factors. More people with low scores died during the study than people with higher scores. The comparative death rate between those who scored 0 (no "healthy habits") and those who scored 4 (all of the "healthy habits") was equivalent to an average of 14 additional years.

Getting a point was not difficult.

Smoking   People who currently do not smoke got a point. The line could have been drawn more strictly so only people who never smoked scored the point.

Physical Activity Only people who were inactive failed to get a point. Four categories were used: active, moderately active, moderately inactive, and inactive. These categories combined routine physical activity at work and away from work. For example, someone classified as "active" might have a sedentary job but gets in more than an hour of exercise each day away from work or they might be whose job involves heavy manual labor regardless of outside activity. Someone who is classified as "inactive" has a sedentary job and gets no exercise outside work.

Alcohol   Those who consumed 4 ounces (112 grams) or less of alcohol per week got a point. That's equivalent to a pint of beer, an 8 ounce glass of wine, or a shot of distilled spirits per day.

Vitamin C   Those with a blood serum level of vitamin C of 8.8 micrograms per liter or greater got a point. From this level it is inferred that the person eats the recommended 5 servings of fruits and vegetables per day.

When the Khaw researchers stirred the statistical pot, they looked at how scores (0 through 4) were associated with who died and what from. Of the 2057 participants, 597 died during the 11 years of the study (the average age at the start was 58). That's about 28 out of every 100 participants who died. Of those 28, 13 died from cardiovascular causes (almost half), 11 died from cancer (about 40%), and the remaining 3 died from other causes (a little over 10%).

Using those who scored 4 as the standard, those who scored 0 were almost 4 times more likely to die from cardiovascular causes, 2½ times more likely to die from cancer, and 7 times more likely to die from other causes. As scores improved, so did the chances of surviving.

Fruits and Vegetables

No one argues with eating fresh fruit and vegetables as a way to sustain health. However, this study advertised fruit and vegetables as the health-promoting factor based on the level of vitamin C in participant's blood—an indirect link. The link is supported by research, but it points to another factor: stress.

Psychosocial stress creates oxidative stress through the immune system. We often think of oxidative stress as coming from exposure to environmental pollutants. But it also comes from the inflammatory response to stress that prepares your body to repair injuries.

Vitamin C is a master antioxidant called upon to combat oxidative stress. One study by Debbie Lawlor and her colleagues showed that the beneficial effect of vitamin C could be accounted for by the social status of study participants: the more difficult someone's social status, the more oxidative stress they suffered, resulting in lower blood levels of vitamin C, and, as a consequence, poorer health. Unfortunately, Lawlor drew the wrong conclusion: that vitamin C does not confer health protection. The obvious conclusion is that vitamin C depletion is the biological consequence of psychosocial stress. It's not one or the other.

Humans do not produce their own vitamin C and so must get it from food, particularly fresh fruit and vegetables. This is how the Khaw study was able to make the link between the amount of vitamin C someone has in their blood to the servings of fruits and vegetables they eat.

Like all antioxidants, vitamin C does not work alone. It's part of what's called the antioxidant network. The most basic antioxidants in addition to vitamin C are vitamin E, alpha lipoic acid, glutathione, and coenzyme Q10. The implication of low vitamin C is that the entire antioxidant network is weak because of oxidative stress.

Unlike the Lawlor study, the Khaw study found a benefit to vitamin C levels even after accounting for social status. In other words, regardless of social status, vitamin C (and by implication the entire antioxidant network) has a positive health effect.

One of the major flaws in the Khaw study is that it implies that vitamin C levels are simply the result of individuals choosing whether to eat the recommended level of fruits and vegetables. It does not point to the social and physical environments that promote or hinder consumption of fruits and vegetables.

Behaviors and Environments

The Khaw study's fundamental limitation is that it frames health issues strictly in terms of behavior. It restricts our understanding of what people choose and excludes understanding the alternatives that are available to them. For solutions, it points to changing your preferences but not to changing the environments in which your preferences are shaped and acted out.

In other words, someone's desire to smoke or drink or exercise or eat fruits and vegetables is affected by his or her ability to fulfill that desire. And the strength of the desire itself is affected by a wide range of factors in his or her personal and social environment—for example, what do friends and family do and what will they tolerate?

Each of the four health factors studied has this other, environmental dimension.

Smoking is an easy target. Everyone knows it's bad for health, even smokers. And it's addictive. Yet it's sold on the open market. Although fewer young people take a first puff these days, those who do are more likely to get hooked. Cigarette manufacturers are not unmindful of this fact. At the same time as laws become increasingly strict about second hand smoke, smoking is sanctioned in art and entertainment, especially the movies. It's a powerful drug in a social environment that doesn't provide enough support for prevention and recovery.

A study of Chicago neighborhoods by Ming Wen and her colleagues found that people in well-off neighborhoods are more likely to engage in physical activity than poor neighborhoods. In fact, they found that neighborhood socioeconomic status (measured by such things as the number of families living below the official poverty line) is the most powerful predictor of physical activity. They found that what increased physical activity is the degree of community connectedness.

Alcohol is a drug like tobacco. Like tobacco, taking alcohol can be a form of self-medication. And it can be addictive. However, the social environments that support the consumption of alcohol are more complex than those where tobacco is used. Alcohol is a natural part of eating, leisure, and celebrations. It is socially acceptable in a way that smoking is not.

Some people prefer not to eat fruits and vegetables or at least fewer than the 5 servings per day recommended. But for some, access to fresh fruits and vegetables is limited. In poor neighborhoods, supermarkets of any kind are scarce, let alone supermarkets with organic fruits and vegetables. This compounds the disadvantage because organic fruits and vegetables have antioxidant and overall nutrient density that's higher than industrial produce.

In disadvantaged neighborhoods, food takes a larger relative bite out of household income compared to well-off neighborhoods. In addition, it's more costly for people in poor neighborhoods to get to a store where they can purchase their 5 servings per day.

The message we need to hear is not only that people should stop smoking; and drinking too much alcohol; and that they should get some exercise; and eat 5 servings of fruits and vegetables each day. People also need to hear that they're capable of creating the social and physical environments that support achieving those goals. These environmental changes can be large and public (bringing a farmers market to your neighborhood) or small and personal (gardening for 15 minutes each day).

The News

Bakalar, Nicholas. 2008. Outcomes: Heeding Familiar Advice May Add Years to Your Life. *New York Times*. January 22, 2008.

Cheng, Maria. 2008. Healthy Habits Can Mean 14 Extra Years. *San Francisco Chronicle*. January 8, 2008.

The Research

Khaw, Kay-Tee et al. 2008. Combined Impact of Health Behaviours and Mortality in Men and Women. *PLoS Medicine*. January 2008(5:1):e12.

Lawlor, Debbie A. et al. 2004. Those Confounded Vitamins. *The Lancet*. May 22, 2004(363):1724-7.

Wen, Ming et al. 2007. Neighbourhood Deprivation, Social Capital and Regular Exercise during Adulthood: A Multilevel Study in Chicago. *Urban Studies*. December 2007(44:13):2651-71.

Resources

Fawcett, Jeffry. 2005. Nicotine Addiction. *Progressive Health Observer*. December 2004/January 2005 (4):4ff.

Glanz, Stanton. 2006. Smoking: The Truth. *Your Own Health And Fitness*. Broadcast February 21, 2006.

Linus Pauling Institute, Micronutrient Information Center. Access at http://lpi.oregonstate.edu/infocenter/.

McEwen, Bruce. 2004. Understanding Stress. *Your Own Health And Fitness*. Broadcast January 20, 2004.

McEwen, Bruce. 2002. *The End of Stress as We Know It*. Washington, DC: Joseph Henry Press.

Packer, Lester and Carol Colman. 1999. *The Antioxidant Miracle*. New York: John Wiley & Sons.

Your Own Health And Fitness. Resources on Aging. Access at http://www.yourownhealthandfitness.org/topicsAging.php.

Your Own Health And Fitness. Resources on Food, Nutrition, and Diet. Access at http://www.yourownhealthandfitness.org/topicsFood.php.

Your Own Health And Fitness. Resources on Exercise and Musculoskeletal Health. Access at http://www.yourownhealthandfitness.org/topicsExercise.php.

Y ou did something amazing with food today: you ate a meal. Amazing and very complex. What you ate, where you ate it, how you ate it, when you ate it, with whom you ate it, and why you ate it have explanations that range from the deeply personal to the deeply political.

The "what" of food takes up the majority of media space. In particular, book publishers frequently try to turn any book on health into either a cookbook or a weight loss plan. The thinking seems to be that what sells are directions on what to do rather than information that supports actions that meet individual needs.

Not here. Although the last article in this section, "Cooking for the Contemporary Hunter-Gatherer," covers the cookbook territory, it's presented as an example. It is not a sacred text.

There are competing views on what to eat, especially for people who want to eat for good health in a way that is socially and environmentally responsible. These range from the vegetarian[1] to the omnivorous[2] with many variations.[3]

The 500 pound gorilla in the kitchen is the United States Department of Agriculture (USDA) and its food guidelines, captured in the food pyramid. The first article in this section, "Bureaucratic Food," examines the faults of these guidelines, both scientific and political.

The second article, "Sweeteners: Not So Sweet," examines the particularly toxic sweetener food group from a similar perspective. Sweeteners are an example of empty calories: there's no nutrient value in them; they serve only as fuel. That extends beyond sweeteners to starchy foods generally that lack significant nutrient heft—foods such as baked goods made from refined grains.

The category of sweeteners highlights the fact that our food is a delivery system for nutrients and anti-nutrients. Nutrients are chemicals your body needs to sustain itself. Anti-nutrients are chemicals that interfere with your body's capacity to use nutrients. Artificial sweeteners are anti-nutrients as are refined sugars, especially the high fructose corn syrup that has become a ubiquitous ingredient in manufactured foods.

Food is also a delivery system for toxins such as pesticides. A study found elevated levels of metabolites of pesticides in children who ate conventional produce as compared to organic produce.[4] These are pesticides that have been shown to increase the risk of learning disabilities[5] and chronic disease later in life.[6] So deciding what to eat means more than nutrient density. It means understanding what your food is delivering to you. It also means understanding what nutrients you need that you're not getting from food.

This is a controversial topic. Some people believe that food should be the sole source of nutrients. Others believe that nutrient supplementation to meet individual health needs is absolutely required. We believe nutrient supplementation is needed because pollution and psychosocial and socioeconomic stress deplete nutrients and create nutrient imbalances. However, the caveat is to meet individual health needs. One nutrient supplement plan does not fit all.

Our third article, "Nutrient Supplements Are Good for You," looks at this issue by examining the bias in conventional research against the benefits of supplements.

Food is not only a delivery system for nutrients, it's also a delivery system for meaning. Food, first and foremost, satisfies desire, whether it's hunger, taste, identify, comfort, or self-medication. Food manufacturers have become very skilled at identifying each of these desires and selling to them.[7]

Meaning is also delivered through food traditions. Some restaurants serve breakfast, lunch, and dinner all day long. Some have a separate menu for each. The menu stands as a guide to what's appropriate to eat at particular times of the day. And even within this cultural structure, what is served depends on what is customary for the culture from which the restaurant's food originates.

Commercial food services and restaurants are only a small window into variations in eating. The meaning of food expands dramatically when considering each person's culture of origin, where he's traveled, what he's learned and where, and how he incorporates eating into his daily activities.[8] And then there is the meaning of food as psychotherapeutic.[9]

These microcosms of meaning are supported by a network of social structures that have been called by one researcher *food systems of provision*.[10] Food doesn't come to us all through a single, consistent process from growth of animals and plants to our mouths. Someone might grow some of his food, get some products from farmers markets, other products from local markets known for socially and environmentally responsible products, and yet other products from big box discount stores. Or someone else might eat at restaurants all the time, never preparing a meal for himself. Each type of food has its own path to that person's stomach. Each has both a unique political economy and a culture.

This incredibly complex process starts with what each person thinks he should eat for good health—and whether he thinks about it at all. That journey starts with the three principles we've discussed in the preceding three sections.

Unique Biology

The starting point is each person's unique nutrient needs.[11] Most simply, it begins with that person paying attention to how he feels and how his capacity to resist and recover from illness is affected. Many people we know who wanted desperately to be vegetarians felt so horrible and had so many health problems that they felt compelled to introduce animal protein into their diet. On the other hand, we know some people who do very well on a vegetarian diet.

The Body as an Ecology

The body needs more than energy. Any eating regime can lead to imbalances. One of the most common and least examined is the effect of nutrient imbalance on hormones.[12] The effect of anti-nutrients on hormones is equally important.

Do the Simplest Things First

Improving what's eaten might come most simply by changing where someone gets his food. If he eats at restaurants constantly, he might simply need to learn how to prepare simple meals for himself. If he already prepares his meals, he might simply look for better sources of food—if he currently shops principally at a big box discount store, he could try joining a community supported agriculture organization (CSA) to increase the fresh produce he gets from local farmers.[13] Often, CSAs make delivery part of their service—an instance where simpler can be easier.

Notes

[1] For example, Dean Ornish (2007) *The Spectrum: A Scientifically Proven Program to Feel Better, Live Longer, Lose Weight, and Gain Health,* John Robbins (2007) *Healthy at 100,* and the lesser known T. Colin Campbell and Thomas M. Campbell (2004) *The China Study.*

[2] For example, see the Weston A. Price Foundation website, Sally Fallon and Mary Enig (1999) *Nourishing Traditions: The Cookbook that Challenges Politically Correct Nutrition and the Diet Dictocrats,* Jessica Prentice (2006) *Full Moon Feast: Food and the Hunger for Connection,* and more commercially Robert Atkins (2002) *Dr. Atkins' New Diet Revolution.*

[3] As will be plain from the articles in this section and others, we fall squarely in the omnivorous camp. Nevertheless, as will also be made plain, we are not dedicated to spreading a true faith. We're primarily concerned with providing information and analysis that enables each person to make informed food decisions. See our webpage Resources on Food, Diet, and

Nutrition. Access at http://www.yourownhealthandfitness.org/topicsFood. php.

4 Chensheng Lu, et al. (2008) "Dietary Intake and Its Contribution to Longitudinal Organophosphorus Pesticide Exposure in Urban/suburban Children."

5 Duk-Hee Lee, et al. (2007a) "Association of Serum Concentrations of Persistent Organic Pollutants with the Prevalence of Learning Disability and Attention Deficit Disorder."

6 Duk-Hee Lee, et al. (2007b) "Association between Serum Concentrations of Persistent Organic Pollutants and Insulin Resistance among Nondiabetic Adults," Duk-Hee Lee, et al. (2007c) "Extended Analyses of the Association between Serum Concentrations of Persistent Organic Pollutions and Diabetes."

7 For example, the description of flavor science in Eric Schlosser (2001) *Fast Food Nation: The Dark Side of the All-American Meal.*

8 For example, Felipe Fernández-Armesto (2002) *Near a Thousand Tables: A History of Food.*

9 For example, Frances Kuffel (2004b) *Passing for Thin: Losing Half My Weight and Finding My Self* and Frances Kuffel (2004a) "Passing for Thin." But also see Ben Fine's analysis of eating disorders in Ben Fine (1998) *The Political Economy of Diet, Health and Food Policy* Chapter 3, The Political Economy of Eating Disorders.

10 For example, see Ben Fine (1998) *The Political Economy Of Diet, Health and Food Policy* and Peter Jackson, et al. (2006) "Mobilising the commodity chain concept in the Politics of Food and Farming."

11 For example, Richard Kunin (2006) "Nutrient Basics."

12 See the discussion in "The Hormonal Consequences of Starch and Stress" on page 41.

13 Community Supported Agriculture website. Access at http://www.nal. usda.gov/afsic/pubs/csa/csa.shtml.

BUREAUCRATIC FOOD

Every 5 years, the USDA's Dietary Guidelines Advisory Committee performs a checkup on *Dietary Guidelines for Americans.* In August, 2005, the Advisory Committee released a draft of the latest Guidelines. Four issues made the news:
* the health effects of sugar are buried in the details;
* exercise is highlighted, even though it's technically outside the Committee's mandate;
* attention is paid to the benefits of dietary fiber; and
* the iconic Food Pyramid survived as a tool for communicating what constitutes a "healthy diet."

Although they didn't make headlines, three other issues received attention from the Committee:
* the effect of environmental factors on what we eat;
* how nutrition affects chronic illness; and
* how nutrition affects health disparities by race and class.

It's a mixed bag, but the song remains the same.

The Guidelines still call for a carbohydrate-dominant diet, with 45% to 65% of energy from carbs. Saturated fats continue to be villainized. And while the Guidelines rightfully condemn *trans* fats, they tar saturated fats and *trans* fats with the same brush.

Since you're reading this book, chances are good that you think independently and do not follow the USDA's Guidelines slavishly. So why worry?

Where the Food Pyramid Lands

In *The Political Economy of Diet, Health and Food Policy*, Ben Fine refers to the standards such as those contained in the *Dietary Guidelines for Americans* as Current Human Nutritional Thinking (CHNT). "In effect, CHNT trickles down from scientists and ultimately ends up, symbolically speaking, in our stomachs."

Federal food programs and programs that receive federal funds must conform to the Guidelines. The most important are the National School Lunch Program, Head Start, and WIC (Special Supplemental Nutrition Program for Women, Infants, and Children). More generally, the Dietary Guidelines Advisory Committee tells us that "using the Dietary Guidelines helps policymakers, educators, clinicians, and others to speak with one voice on nutrition and health."

This chorus's captive audience include children at school, mothers receiving food support, and people who follow the dietary guidelines of organizations such as the American Heart Association and American Diabetes Association.

And let us not forget journalists who report on nutrition and health. For them, "healthy diet" means the Guidelines. In the course of reporting on an issue, journalists cite only experts who hew to the Guidelines' standards.

For example, last October, the Associated Press reported on research that compared the Atkins diet to the American Heart Association diet. The results showed that the Atkins diet not only worked better for losing weight and keeping it off, but that Atkins dieters could eat more and still lose more weight, just as Atkins predicted.

The experts consulted by the journalist (including the principal researcher in the study) were completely flummoxed. One expert said the results defied the laws of thermodynamics. Yet no experts from the Atkins organization were even asked for their explanation.

Then there are the scientists who study nutrition and health. For example, in 2002 the Diabetes Prevention Program (in the Centers for Disease Control and Prevention or CDC) released the results of their 5-year study. It showed that diet and exercise beat pharmaceuticals hands down in preventing diabetes.

Great news.

The bad news is that the diet used in the study was the American Diabetes Association's low-fat, high-carbohydrate diet. As a consequence, we'll never know from this study how well low carbohydrate diets such as those described in *Dr. Bernstein's Diabetes Solutions* and in *Atkins Diabetes Revolution* compared to the conventional low-fat diet.

What's Wrong with the American Diet

In a 2002 USDA report on food consumption trends, researchers were alarmed to report that 70% of people ate whatever they wanted. In this apparent free-for-all, the researchers asked how people ate compared to the Guidelines.

Surprisingly, the proportions of energy sources (carbohydrates, protein, and fats) recommended by the Guidelines closely match what people actually eat. The Guidelines recommend 45% to 65% of calories from carbohydrates, 10% to 30% from protein, and 20% to 35% from fat. What Americans actually eat is about 52% carbohydrates, 12% protein, and 36% fat.

In their *Comments on the Food Guidelines System*, Sally Fallon, Mary Enig, and Bill Sanda of the Weston A. Price Foundation note that the grain-based structure of the Guidelines looks suspiciously like the USDA guidelines for fattening livestock: 61% carbohydrates, 10% protein, and 29% fats.

Despite the 70% who eat with reckless disregard for the Guidelines, the proximity of actual eating to the Guidelines is not just a happy coincidence. It is the trickle-down effect of CHNT on everyday life.

As Marion Nestle describes in *Food Politics*, the corporate forces that dominate the American food system also dominate what ends up in the Dietary Guidelines. Industrial food companies, directly and through their trade organizations, are the Pharaohs of the Food Pyramid.

However, the real fuss comes from the quantity and quality of specific foods eaten. It is here that the Pharaohs have their way.

The Food Pyramid has seven components from which people are supposed to build meals. The table below compares the pyramid for a daily intake of 2200 calories (for the average adult) to actual, average consumption.

USDA Food Pyramid for a 2200 calorie diet compared to actual consumption in servings per person per day

Food Group	Pyramid	Consumed	Difference
Grains	9.0	10.6	+18%
Vegetables	4.0	3.8	-5%
Fruit	3.0	1.4	-53%
Dairy	2.2	1.6	-27%
Meat	6.0	6.2	+3%
Added fats	41.0	65.0	+59%
Added sugars	12.0	31.0	+158%

According to this, Americans eat about the right amount of vegetables and meat, not enough fruit and dairy, a little too much in grains, too much added fats, and way too much added sugars. However, the apparently optimal consumption of vegetables is an illusion: green and yellow vegetables are underconsumed, while potatoes and other starchy vegetables are quite dramatically overconsumed.

Added fats and sugars should rightfully be called hidden fats and sugars. The butter you put on vegetables and the honey you put in tea count in these categories. But most of the added fats and sugars come in manufactured foods: shortening in baked goods, oil in fried foods, and sweeteners added to a wide variety of food (see "Sweeteners: Not So Sweet" on page 81).

Most scientists worry about the overconsumption of added fats and sugars, as well they should. The calories from this excess alone are equal to the difference between the Food Pyramid's target of 2200 calories and the actual consumption of 2750.

During the first half of the 20th century, the calories consumed by Americans declined. Through the 1950s and 1960s, calories consumed leveled out. In 1970, calories consumed increased steadily from an average of 2300 per day in 1970 to 2750 calories in 2000 (a jump of almost 20% in 30 years).

How did Americans match their calories burned with the calories they ate without the Food Pyramid to guide them?

It's the Environment, Stupid

"[T]he Committee was struck by the critical and likely predominant role of environment in determining whether ... individuals consume excess calories, eat a healthful diet, and are physically active."

The environmental factors they cite did not fall from the sky. They are the often intended results of actions taken by commercial interests. For example, the Committee worried about the increased serving sizes provided at restaurants. As Greg Critser describes in *Fat Land*, "supersizing" was a very deliberate marketing strategy undertaken by fast food chains to increase profits.

But the Advisory Committee did not look very hard at "the environment," simply listing a collection of items such as food advertising. They fail to ask whether the foods themselves have caused us to overeat. For example, they didn't look at the differences between whole and processed foods or between organic and commercial foods.

Fat is Good for You

Journalists like to use the phrase "artery-clogging saturated fat." Colorful but untrue. Plaques in arteries are less than 25% saturated fat, less than body fat, which is 45% saturated fat.

Dr. Mary Enig, author of *Know Your Fats*, has long argued that *trans* fatty acids have been confused in research with saturated fats and that it is *trans* fats that are the bad players.

The Advisory Committee warns against *trans* fats. But, in a demonstration of how old ideas die hard, the warning lumps *trans* fats with saturated fats. Journalist now use "artery-clogging saturated and *trans* fats."

Trans fatty acids are associated with heart disease, cancer, diabetes, obesity, immune dysfunction, and bone loss. Saturated fats comprise 50% of your cell membranes, contribute to your bone health, protect your liver from toxins, support your immune system, and are your heart's, your liver's, and your muscles' preferred fuel.

Trans fats come from food manufacturing. They are produced when plant-based polyunsaturated oils (these days, that means soy, with canola a distant second) are hydrogenated to saturate them, conferring on foods the desirable properties of saturated fats.

Any manufactured food label that lists hydrogenated or partially hydrogenated vegetable oil contains *trans* fats.

Margarine. Shortening from vegetable oil. Oils used for commercial frying. All are loaded with *trans* fats.

Until 1940, Americans consumed an average of about 30 pounds each year of butter and lard. From 1940 to 1980, annual consumption fell to 10 pounds per year.

As for margarine, vegetable shortening, and cooking oils, consumption doubled from 10 to 20 pounds per year between 1910 and 1940. From 1940 to 2000, consumption tripled to 60 pounds, with most of that increase from cooking oils. The reason? Vegetable oils are cheaper than animal fats.

And Grains Are Not

Given the Guidelines' restriction on fats, how are we supposed to meet our calorie requirements? The Guidelines' answer: grains.

Consumption consists almost entirely of grains refined into flours and meals. Wheat dominates, with corn a distant second: 75% wheat to 15% corn. But overall consumption of grains declined by half from the beginning of the last century through the mid-1950s, when the decline slowed, bottomed out in the 1970s, then started a steady climb.

This recovery corresponds to the increased prevalence of manufactured foods (packaged and fast food) and the ascent of the low-fat orthodoxy.

As Fallon, Enig, and Sanda describe in their *Comments*, the refining process strips grains of vitamins and minerals. For example, refining removes B vitamins, without which your body can't break down the grain's carbohydrates. To compensate, flour manufacturers add B1 and B2, but not B6. Your body then has to draw upon other B6 sources.

Whole grains are often recommended as an alternative because their nutrients are preserved. But as Melissa Smith points out in *Going Against the Grain*, whole grains have their own problems.

For example, refining removes much of the lectins from grains, which is a good thing. Lectins are anti-nutrients. Most seriously, they can affect the permeability of your gut and enable proteins to enter your bloodstream which prompts inflammation and autoimmune reactions.

And refined grains, as Smith describes, are allergic and addictive. Which might have something to do with why Americans can't stop eating them.

None of this information, however, appears in the Dietary Guidelines for Americans. Yet.

Resources

Bernstein, Richard. 1997. *Dr. Bernstein's Diabetes Solution: A Complete Guide to Achieving Normal Blood Sugars*. New York, Little, Brown & Company.

Critser, Greg. 2003. *Fat Land: How Americans Became the Fattest People in the World*. New York, Houghton Mifflin.

Diabetes Prevention Program Research Group. 2002. Reduction in the Incidence of Type 2 Diabetes With Lifestyle Intervention or Metformin. *N Engl J Med*. February 7. 346(6): 393-403.

Dietary Guidelines Advisory Committee. 2005. *The Report of the Dietary Guidelines Advisory Committee on Dietary Guidelines for Americans, 2005*. Access at http://www.health.gov/DietaryGuidelines/dga2005/default.htm.

Enig, Mary. 2000. *Know Your Fats: The Complete Primer for Understanding the Nutrition of Fats, Oils, and Cholesterol*. Silver Spring, MD, Bethesda Press.

Fallon, Sally and Mary Enig. 2003. *Comments to the 2005 Dietary Guidelines Advisory Committee*. December 18, 2003.

Fine, Ben. 1998. *The Political Economy of Diet, Health and Food Policy*. New York, Routledge.

Nestle, Marion. 2002. *Food Politics: How the Food Industry Influences Nutrition and Health*. Berkeley, University of California Press.

Smith, Melissa Diane. 2002. *Going Against the Grain: How Reducing and Avoiding Grains Can Revitalize Your Health*. New York, Contemporary Books.

USDA and US Department of Health and Human Services. 2005. *Dietary Guidelines for Americans, 2005*. Access at http://www.health.gov/DietaryGuidelines/dga2005/document/.

SWEETENERS: NOT SO SWEET

$3 billion. That's what Coke and Pepsi spent last year on advertising. Their sugar-sweetened soft drinks and others like them account for most of the added sugars in the American diet.

The August 25, 2004 edition of the Journal of the American Medical Association (JAMA) reports on the health effects of soft drink and juice consumption. No surprise: sugared soft drinks and juices are associated with weight gain and type 2 diabetes.

The details hold some interesting information. The study is based on the Nurses' Health Study II, initiated in 1989. The women entering the study were between 24 and 44 years old. (We note with regret that in science "nurse" is synonymous with "woman.")

The JAMA study looked at data for more than 50,000 participants from 1991 to 1999. In doing so, they followed changes in a wide variety of factors in addition to soda and juice. At each stage in the study, women were grouped by their level of soda and juice consumption, from low to high: less than 1 serving per month (the control group), 1 to 4 servings per month, 2 to 6 per week, and 1 or more per day.

First, even the lowest consumption (1 to 4 servings per month) had an effect on weight gain compared to the control (less than 1 serving per month).

Second, the average weight of all the women in each group increased, although the details are worth noting.

- The greatest weight gain was for women who went from low to high consumption.
- The least weight gain was for women who went from high to low consumption.
- But women who were consistent low consumers gained about the same on average as the women who were consistent high consumers.

Third, type 2 diabetes increased with consumption for the two highest-consuming groups, even after accounting for weight gain and total calories.

Fourth, there was an increased risk of diabetes associated with diet soft drinks, although the relationship was weak.

Fifth, heavy juice and soda drinkers tended to smoke more, eat more calories over and above those from the sugared drinks, eat less protein, and were less physically active. Although we might be tempted to speculate about addictive personalities, we should probably first speculate about addiction-sensitive metabolisms.

High Fructose Corn Syrup

The USDA classifies sweeteners as caloric (such s table sugar and honey) and non-caloric (such as aspartame and stevia). As the name suggests, caloric sweeteners add calories. The most widely used caloric sweetener is high fructose corn syrup (HFCS). It long ago replaced sugar as the sweetener used in soda and sweetened juices because it is cheaper because of federal corn subsidies.

Per capita consumption of caloric sweeteners has doubled since 1966, principally delivered in soft drinks and manufactured foods. HFCS, which was first introduced in 1966, now accounts for half of all caloric sweeteners.

At one time, fructose was considered a safe alternative to table sugar, especially for diabetics. It enters your blood stream more slowly and has little effect on blood sugar and insulin levels. However, fructose is metabolized in your liver, which converts it into fatty acids faster than glucose (blood sugar). In fact, test animals fed lots of fructose develop the liver of an alcoholic.

Research suggests that fructose contributes to complications of diabetes through reactions with proteins and disruptions to mineral metabolism (specifically copper, magnesium, and chromium) that lead to problems with bones, connective tissue, heart, and blood sugar homeostasis.

Table sugar (sucrose) has been notorious much longer than fructose. Chemically, sucrose is made up of one molecule of glucose linked to one molecule of fructose. When it's digested, the molecules are separated. As a result, sucrose has a lower glycemic index than bread.

The glycemic index measures a food's effect on blood sugar—that is, glucose. The complex carbohydrates in bread and other starches are nothing more than strings of glucose molecules. When digested, all of it affects blood sugar. But, because only half of a sucrose molecule is glucose, only that half affects blood sugar.

Sucrose consumption is linked to kidney, liver, and heart disease; hyperactivity; and addictive behavior. Sucrose disrupts your blood's calcium-to-phosphorus equilibrium. It lowers phosphorus and raises calcium. With low phosphorus, calcium can't be metabolized and can even become toxic. Calcium rises because it is leached from bone and teeth, causing bone loss and tooth decay.

A Safe Alternative?

Aspartame (trade name Nutrisweet) is the most widely used non-caloric sweetener. Diet sodas are almost exclusively sweetened with aspartame. While diet sodas were not associated with weight gain and only weakly associated with diabetes in the JAMA study, aspartame is not a safe alternative to sugared drinks.

Aspartame breaks down into phenylalanine, aspartic acid, and methanol.

Phenylalanine can convert into a carcinogen when warm or in storage. The FDA warns against aspartame for pregnant and lactating women, people with a compromised liver, and people who have phenylketonuria (a condition that damages neurological function and development).

Both phenylalanine and aspartic acid are amino acids contained in foods. The trouble is that when they are consumed as isolated amino acids, as they are when aspartame is metabolized, they enter the nervous system in abnormally high concentrations. This can cause a variety of toxic effects and functional havoc in nerve tissue.

Methanol is a poison. Although fruit juice also contains methanol, the amount of aspartame in a diet soda delivers up to 100 times the methanol as an equivalent amount of fruit juice. The EPA says that up to 7 milligrams per day is safe. A liter of diet soda creates 56 milligrams of methanol. And methanol can convert to toxic formaldehyde.

Aspartame is associated with Parkinson's disease, Alzheimer's disease, and Gulf War Syndrome. It's also been linked to visual impairment, numbness, hypertension, pancreatitis, and birth defects.

Aspartame's Material Safety Data Sheet tells workers handling it to seal themselves off from contact: chemical goggles, protective gloves, a protective apron, and an air-purifying respirator.

Exposures

One of the ironies of the low-fat diet orthodoxy that dominates American eating is that it promotes the consumption of sweeteners. Caloric-sweetener consumption doubled in the last 35 years. Non-caloric sweeteners quadrupled between 1966 and 1991 (after which the manufacturers withheld the data).

When low-fat (particularly low saturated fat) became the standard, food manufacturers adapted. They replaced saturated fats with hydrogenated polyunsaturated fats. But a good deal of flavor was lost.

Humans seem to have a natural affinity for two tastes: sweet and salt. All others seem to be learned. So to make foods more palatable and therefore more desirable (that is, in order to sell as much as possible), food manufacturers load their products with the taste of sweet and salt.

Although soft drinks and sweetened fruit juices account for the bulk of added sugars in the American diet, caloric and non-caloric sweeteners are in a wide variety of unlikely products. Peanut butter. Pasta sauce. Ketchup.

The first step in protecting yourself from sweetener overload is to read the label of any packaged food. Sugar might not be listed, but corn syrup and dextrose might.

The second step is to remember that organic or natural sweeteners are still sucrose, fructose, or some other sweetener. And if you are prone to drinking fruit juices, remember that their sugar load is much greater than a piece of fruit: the juice doesn't have the pulp that slows digestion and portion sizes are deceptive (an 8-ounce glass of orange juice has the sugar of three oranges; you might easily drink an 8-ounce glass but be quite content with a single orange).

The third, and perhaps most difficult step is to de-sweeten your diet. After a time, you'll find that a whole apple is more than enough sweetness.

Resources

Fallon, Sally, Mary Enig, and Bill Sanda. 2004. *Comments on the Food Guideline System/Food Guide Pyramid.* August 26, 2004. Washington, DC: Weston A. Price Foundation.

Roberts, HJ. 1990. *Aspartame: Is It Safe?* Philadelphia: The Charles Press.

Schulze, Matthias B., et al. 2004. Sugar-Sweetened Beverages, Weight Gain, and Incidence of Type 2 Diabetes in Young and Middle-Aged Women. *JAMA*, 292(8), August 25, 2004, 927-34.

NUTRIENT SUPPLEMENTS ARE GOOD FOR YOU

The Enlightenment philosopher Baruch Spinoza argued that we can never know the whole truth. Because we are finite creatures, the best we can ever have is partial knowledge because we view the world from a unique perspective. Spinoza concluded that the right thing to do was understand that perspective so that we do not become its captive.

Over the last two decades a movement has taken hold within conventional medical science calling itself *evidence-based medicine.* Traditionally, standards of care—the rules for treatment that govern medical practice—had been set by panels of experts. Advocates of evidence-based medicine have argued that this system is prone to bias: the experts who populate the panels tend to be well-established, conservative, and self-selecting. As a consequence, emerging science might not be considered when standards are set because the established experts rely on what they know—which is likely out of date.

Evidence-based medicine was intended to break through the biases of expert panels. Medical standards and practice would be based on the results of the best science available.

And so with this sword of objectivity in hand, the Agency for Healthcare Research and Quality (AHRQ, which lives within the US Department of Health and Human Services) turned its attention to the use of multivitamins. The investigation was a large undertaking. It was requested by the National Institutes of Health (NIH), the US agency responsible for evaluating medical and health science. The NIH's objective for the investigation was intended to

- evaluate the effectiveness of multivitamins in preventing chronic disease and
- evaluate the safety of vitamins and minerals.

Protecting Consumers

The AHRQ study, led by Han-Yao Huang, PhD, formed the basis of the NIH's statement on multivitamins. The NIH statement is a de facto policy on multivitamins: although not an explicit standard, its word carries weight. And so its conclusions were picked up by the media and given wide coverage.

The take-home message of the NIH statement is that multivitamins don't seem to do much. The Los Angeles Times headline was "Benefits from Vitamins are Few" while the Washington Post's article managed to cast a somewhat brighter light with the headline "Panel Finds Conflicting Data on Multivitamin Benefit."

The NIH statement (as well as the AHRQ study) begins with the observation that "half of American adults take a dietary supplement, the majority of which are multivitamin/multimineral (MVM) supplements." With this in mind, the ostensible objective of the study and statement were to provide consumers with the best information available about the benefits and safety of multivitamins.

But the real bottom line is in the concluding section of the NIH statement.

> The current level of public assurance of the safety and quality of MVMs is inadequate, given the fact that manufacturers of these products are not required to report adverse events, and the FDA has no regulatory authority to require labeling changes or to help inform the public of these issues and concerns. It is important that the FDA's purview over these products be authorized and implemented.

In other words, increase regulation of nutrient supplements to protect consumers. As Robert Verkerk, PhD of the London-based Alliance for Natural Health discussed on an edition of Your Own Health And Fitness, the same reasoning is being used by the European Union to severely restrict access to supplements, herbs, and other natural health products. Many agencies and organizations in the US are pressing for similar restrictions, with the direct and indirect support of the pharmaceutical industry. In the US, Citizens for Health is a major activist organization resisting these efforts.

But do consumers need protection beyond the current labeling requirements for supplements?

State-of-the-Science

The AHRQ study was designed using the methods of evidence-based science.

- A wide variety of databases were searched for published articles in peer-reviewed journals on the relationship between vitamin supplements and chronic disease.
- A careful process was used to review each article for its suitability in addressing the issue of vitamin benefit and safety.
- The studies that passed were examined for their results.

When the study was complete, the NIH held a conference to evaluate it. A panel of experts presided over the conference at which invited experts discussed the AHRQ study. The NIH statement is the result of the conference. The panel's conclusions allegedly describe what is currently known and what further research needs to be conducted.

You will notice that this sounds very much like the old system where a panel of self-selected experts decides on a standard. In this case, however, the panel has draped itself with the cloth of evidence-based science in the form of the AHRQ report. Two things happened: the AHRQ report was quite selective in what counted as science and the NIH panel interpreted the report from a particular perspective.

The panel found little to support the idea that multivitamins were of benefit in preventing chronic disease. They also found little of merit in using the single vitamins they included in their study. Yet their own statement includes a description of the benefits of vitamin D on bone loss, vitamin E in certain cancers and cardiovascular disease, folic acid on birth defects, and selenium on cancer. And although the AHRQ study found only five multivitamin studies that met its requirements, they showed benefits such as reduced risk of cancer, cataracts, and macular degeneration.

When it got to the issue of safety, the panel became concerned. The NIH statement opens its discussion of safety by referring to the well-known harm done to smokers by beta-carotene in increasing lung cancer risk. But that was the only specific instance of demonstrated harm cited by the panel.

The extensive and biased AHRQ search found precious little that demonstrated harm from vitamins. Yet in a nice piece of twisted logic, the NIH panel worries mightily over the potential harm of vitamins because of this lack of evidence. If the FDA followed the NIH expert panel's logic, the pharmaceutical industry would come to a halt.

Biased by Design

The AHRQ study was biased in many respects. The following are just a few.

How Studies Were Selected

To evaluate benefits, only randomized controlled trials (RCTs) were allowed in. RCT is the so-called "gold standard" for evidence-based medicine because it allegedly shows only the effect of a multivitamin or other substance.

Yet when it came to evaluating safety, observational studies were allowed in addition to RCTs. Observational studies are allegedly of lesser value because they supposedly do not isolate the effect of a multivitamin as well as RCT.

In other words, when it came to the safety issue, the AHRQ went fishing for multivitamin harm. And didn't come up with much for their effort.

Where They Looked for Studies

The database search was supposedly comprehensive. But as the Orthomolecular Medicine News Service (OMNS) noted in responding to the AHRQ report, not one article from the Journal of Orthomolecular Medicine was considered.

The same is true of the Journal of Alternative and Complementary Medicine. Without trying very hard, we found several articles that were RCT studies of multivitamins, such as a study on autism. This is also the journal in which the work of Stephen Schoenthaler, PhD has appeared—RCTs of the beneficial effects of multivitamins on emotional and developmental disorders.

How They Judged Study Quality

The process used by the AHRQ study included an evaluation of each selected study's quality. However, this had a very limited meaning.

One of the common criticisms of vitamin studies is their use of small doses. While the AHRQ researchers noted dosing, they made no use of that information in evaluating results.

The AHRQ researchers also did not evaluate whether a study included drugs taken by the subjects: pharmaceuticals are notorious for depleting nutrients. In addition, the AHRQ researchers did not look at whether a study evaluated their subjects' nutrient status.

In other words, the AHRQ researchers didn't look at whether a study was well-designed from the standpoint of how nutrients work. They looked at the multivitamin studies as just some more drug trials.

Where Are the Bodies?

In its response to the NIH panel, the OMNS asked "Where are the bodies?" The system that reports incidents of poisoning in the US tracks reports of toxic responses in hospitals and other medical facilities. When a group of orthomolecular physicians looked at these statistics, the found thousands of poisonings deaths from prescriptions drugs but none from vitamins—with one exception.

Minerals in sufficient quantity can have a toxic effect. In 2003, 3 deaths from iron supplements were reported. These were children who ate iron and iron-containing supplements like candy because the supplements had a candy-like coating. No such deaths were reported in 2004.

Nutrient Status and Stress

Observational studies of vitamins tend to show benefits where RCTs tend to show no effect. Devotion to the "gold standard" aside, this might have been a reason why the AHRQ researchers excluded observational studies.

In an *RCT*, subjects are typically divided into two groups: one group receives an intervention such as a drug or in this case a multivitamin; the other group receives a placebo that contains nothing. It's why these are called provocation studies: they are designed to provoke a response by actively intervening in the experimental subject's life.

On the other hand, *observational studies* simply keep track of what people do. After a period of time, researchers look to see whether health outcomes are associated with what people were doing, such as taking a multivitamin.

Several years ago The Lancet published an article titled "Those confounded vitamins" by Debbie Lawlor, PhD and her colleagues. The Lawlor article examined why there was such a difference between vitamin RCTs and vitamin observational studies. The researchers compared vitamin C and vitamin E studies and their effect in preventing chronic disease.

The observational studies they looked at measured actual blood levels of vitamin C and E—that is, they were measuring people's actual nutrient status. The original studies found a strong association between these blood levels and the risk of chronic disease. However, when these researchers adjusted these outcomes for each person's social status, the association weakened or disappeared entirely. In other words, social status was associated with nutrient status.

Unfortunately the conclusion Lawlor and her colleagues came to was that it wasn't nutrient status that explained chronic disease risk, but social status. And thus RCTs were somehow preserved as the "gold standard."

We think the Lawlor study tells another story entirely.

Social status causes health effects through stress and limits on access to medical care. "Stress" in this context encompasses the psychosocial stress due to such factors as income security as well as physical stress from exposure to toxins.

The people who participate in RCTs are allegedly selected randomly. Yet social status is typically no part of the selection process. Nor does the analysis of health outcomes typically include the effect of social status. In an RCT, a body is just a body, it has a biology but no history.

Observational studies are more likely to capture social status as a factor. What the Lawlor study showed was that, in fact, the much maligned observational studies were the better studies because they revealed the pathway by which vitamins affect health: social status affects stress affects nutrient status affects health.

Although the take-home message of the NIH statement and the mainstream media was that multivitamins don't do much (and might even be dangerous), the take-home message we want to leave you with is that vitamin supplements most certainly do affect your health for the better.

However, the take-home message includes the understanding that the effectiveness of vitamin supplements is specific to your individual nutrient needs and your individual nutrient status. The resources we list below by Kunin, Higdon, and Balch are a good place to start.

The News

Gellene, Denice. 2006. Benefits From Vitamins Are Few. *Los Angeles Times.* May 18, 2006.

Squires, Sally. 2006. Panel Finds Conflicting Data on Multivitamin Benefit. *Washington Post.* May 18, 2006. A15.

The Research

Huang, Han-Yao et al. 2006. Multivitamin/Mineral Supplements and Prevention of Chronic Disease. Evidence Report/Technology Assessment No. 139. AHRQ Publication No. 06-E012. Rockville, MD: Agency for Healthcare Research and Quality. May 2006.

NIH State-of-the-Science Panel. 2006. Multivitamin/Mineral Supplements and Chronic Disease Prevention. *Annals of Internal Medicine.* 145(5).

Resources

Adams, James and Charles Holloway. 2004. Pilot Study of a Moderate Dose Multivitamin/Mineral Supplement for Children With Autistic Spectrum Disorder. *Journal of Alternative and Complementary Medicine.* 10(6): 1033-9.

Alliance for Natural Health. Access at http://www.anhcampaign.org/.

Balch, Phyllis. 2002. *Prescription for Nutritional Healing: A-To-Z Guide to Supplements, 2nd Edition.* Avery: New York.

Citizens for Health. Access at http://www.citizens.org/.

Higdon, Jane. 2003. *An Evidence-based Approach to Vitamins and Minerals: Health Benefits and Intake Recommendations.* Thieme: New York.

Independent Vitamin Safety Review Panel. 2006. Report of the Independent Vitamin Safety Review Panel. *Orthomolecular Medicine News Service.* May 23, 2006. Access at http://www.orthomolecular.org/resources/omns.

International Orthomolecular Medicine Society. Access at http://www.orthomed.org.

Kunin, Richard. 2006. Nutrient Basics. *Your Own Health And Fitness.* Broadcast January 31, 2006.

Lawlor, Debbie et al. 2004. Those Confounded Vitamins: What Can We Learn from the Difference between Observational versus Randomized Trial Evidence? *The Lancet.* 363 (May 22, 2004): 1724-7.

Schoenthaler, Steven et al. 2000. The Effect of Vitamin-mineral Supplementation on the Intelligence of American Schoolchildren: A Randomized, Double-blind Placebo-controlled Trial. *Journal of Alternative and Complementary Medicine.* 6(1): 19-29.

Verkerk, Robert. 2006. Protecting Access to Natural Products. *Your Own Health And Fitness.* Broadcast June 20, 2006.

COOKING FOR THE CONTEMPORARY HUNTER-GATHERER

This special edition of the *Progressive Health Observer* is far from a complete cookbook. Instead, it attempts to give you ideas and guidelines for the practical problem of following a style of eating we have found beneficial.

In our consultation practices, after we've discussed the risks of a high starch diet filled with empty calories, toxins, and allergens, we are often asked, "But what do I eat?" This special edition is the start of an answer.

Food habits develop from traditions, inattention, and addiction. Not for nothing are high starch foods called "comfort foods." Those starches turn into blood sugar that stimulate neurotransmitters that make us feel good. The tab that comes due on those foods is insulin resistance, polycystic ovaries, diabetes, heart disease, and much, much more.

Because you're not reading this by accident, you are no doubt aware of those health risks. Yet chances are good that your meals consist of something such as cold cereal and a cup of coffee for breakfast, a sandwich for lunch with fries on the side, and fish with rice for dinner with a glass or two of wine topped off with a chocolate chip cookie for dessert.

It's not our mission here to take apart what's wrong with this eating pattern. We use it to illustrate what people we work with report as their healthy diet.

Instead, we're going to give some recipes for meals that we eat ourselves. It isn't our intention to persuade you to eat what we eat. But we do intend to stimulate your thinking about how you nourish yourself.

We've organized this special edition into breakfast, lunch, and dinner because that is a common and familiar structure. However, you can eat any of the dishes we describe at any time. We do. Bacon and eggs for dinner is not uncommon. Chile verde over cauliflower rice is a favorite breakfast.

One of the things you'll notice is that every meal has protein and fat. These two types of nutrients are essential as raw material for your cells. So we believe your body works better when supplied throughout the day with them.

A fundamental principle in these dishes is what's not there—namely, common allergic foods. No soy. No grains, either on their own or processed into breads, pastas, and so forth. And except in a few dishes, no dairy. You'll also find that we don't use onions and garlic. For one, we've noticed that these tend to be overused in cooking to the detriment of the foods flavor. For another, they can cause digestive problems in some people.

We don't use polyunsaturated fats for cooking—we recommend butter or ghee (clarified butter from which the milk solids have been removed) or tropical oils high in saturated fat such as palm oil or coconut oil.

On the economic side, these dishes are relatively inexpensive. Of course, you'll pay more for organic produce and sustainable meat—which we strongly recommend. Also with regard to economics, many of these dishes are either fast to fix or freeze (and thaw) well so you can economize on time.

So give it a try. Follow your tastes. And eat well.

Layna Berman and Jeffry Fawcett, PhD

RECIPES

BREAKFAST

COOKING WITH EGGS

Eggs are a terrific food. They're a great source of protein, an essential macronutrient, found in the whites while the yokes contain important micronutrients such as phosphatidyl choline, a major constituent of cell membranes.

Eggs were wrongly maligned as a cause of high cholesterol—a mistaken notion itself, but that's another story. Research has since shown that the fats in eggs are very good for health and don't contribute to cholesterol imbalances. In addition, eggs contain lots of vitamin B12, which is especially important for vegetarians—and everyone else!

Eggs are also tricky business when cooking. It's easy to turn them into something that should be on your doorstep to wipe your feet rather than on your plate to eat. The three typical ways we cook eggs are to hard (or soft) boil them, scramble them, or (most elegant of all) wrap them around food as an omelette.

Boiled Eggs, Hard and Soft

A hard boiled egg might not seem that appealing, but it is one of the most portable, high nutrient foods around. It's also fast food—in a little over 10 minutes, it's ready to eat.

A soft boiled egg is not transportable, but it's still a great, simple food.

INGREDIENTS
2-3 fresh, cage free eggs   1 tsp vinegar

INSTRUCTIONS
1. Place the eggs in a pot and add water until the eggs are covered.
2. Add the vinegar—this helps make the shell easier to remove.
3. Leaving the pot uncovered, bring the water to a rolling boil over the highest heat.
4. Immediately turn off the heat. If you're using an electric stove, remove the pot to a burner that's cool.
5. Cover the pot and wait 10 minutes.
6. Pour off the now-warm water and pour in cold water—this stops the eggs from continuing to cook.

VARIATIONS
Soft Boiled For a soft boiled egg, just reduce the cooking time from 10 minutes, typically to 3 minutes.

Scrambled Eggs

There are two philosophies in scrambling eggs. One is the throw-it-together philosophy and the other is the care-in-preparation philosophy. Those in a hurry like the former. Those with a more leisurely attitude toward eggs like the latter.

INGREDIENTS

2-3 fresh, cage free eggs
1 tsp water (optional)

1 tsp butter or Ghee
Accompaniment (see below)

INSTRUCTIONS

1. Heat the butter/ghee in a frying pan over medium heat. The butter/ghee should be melted and bubbling slightly, not burnt.
2. Here's where the two philosophies diverge.
   - For those in a hurry, crack the eggs directly into the pan and stir them with a spatula.
   - For those of a leisurely disposition, crack the eggs in a bowl and whisk. If you want fluffier eggs, add the water. Now pour the mixture into the pan.
3. Turn the heat down to low.
4. Stir the eggs continuously.
5. While the eggs are still semi-solid, add the accompaniments.
   - However, the amount of liquid in what you add will affect the cooking: with more liquid you'll have to have a higher heat.
   - And when you add the accompaniment will affect how cooked and blended it is with the eggs. Typically, you should wait until the end to add tomatoes, but cheese you can add early.

ACCOMPANIMENTS

Salsa
Sautéed vegetables
Herbs
Peppers
Diced tomato and avocado
Olives and mushrooms
Sour cream (recipe below)

Cheese—the softer the cheese, the faster it melts and blends with the eggs
Cooked meat, cubed or ground, including salt cured, nitrate- and preservative-free bacon or ham

A Perfect Omelette

An omelette is a perfect little package of food. But if the eggs aren't cooked right, it can turn into a meal wrapped in paper. Luckily, there's a way to cook the eggs that requires little attention. But you do have to make sure the heat is controlled correctly.

INGREDIENTS

1 tsp butter or ghee

3 fresh, cage free eggs

1 tsp water (optional)

EQUIPMENT

A 9" omelette pan or frying   A mixing bowl
pan with curved sides   A small whisk

INSTRUCTIONS
1. Put the omelette pan over a medium flame.
   - "Medium flame" means that the flame just licks the bottom of the pan.
   - If you're using an electric stove, you'll have to experiment.
2. While the butter/ghee is melting, break the eggs into the bowl then whisk it.
   - Yes, you can use a fork, but a whisk is better.
   - For a fluffier omelette, add the water.
3. When the butter/ghee is thoroughly melted and bubbling, rotate the pan so it's spread uniformly over the bottom then add the whisked eggs.
   - This is a delicate step. You want the pan hot to immediately set the eggs, but not so hot as to burn them. If the butter/ghee has turned brown, the pan is too hot.
4. Check the depth of the egg around the pan. If it's deeper on one side, your omelette will be thicker on that side. But there's a solution described in step #6.
5. Immediately cover the pan and turn the flame to low.
   - "Low" means that the flame is well below the bottom of the pan. At this point, all you want is to maintain the heat that's already in the pan.
   - To warm your serving plate, use it to cover the pan.
6. If your stove isn't level, let the eggs cook for 30 seconds then rotate the pan so the handle is pointing in the opposite direction (180°) to distribute the egg that remains liquid to the "thin" side.
7. Cook until the eggs are set, typically a few minutes then turn off the flame.
8. Add fillings to one side, fold over, and slide it onto a plate.

VARIATIONS

Bacon and Tomato Omelette Slice two strips of salt cured, nitrate- and preservative-free bacon into 1" bits and fry them in the omelette pan, keeping the pan covered. While that's cooking, cube the tomato (usually, half a medium tomato is enough) and salt them to your taste. Prepare the eggs. When the bacon is done to your satisfaction, remove it from the pan, turn the heat to low, pour off all but a teaspoon of the bacon grease, return the pan to the heat, and add the eggs as in step #3 and continue.

Warm and Cool Fillings If you wait until the eggs are completely set, your filling will not heat much if its cold—and will cool down the omelette. So fillings should be at room temperature or warmed. Cold eggs are no fun. For cheese that you want melted, add it before the eggs are set. If you do try to warm the filling after the eggs are set, you'll end up burning the eggs on the bottom.

Cauliflower Brei

I came up with this idea because I was looking for a substitute for Matzo Brei, an old family favorite of matzo soaked in egg and scrambled. My Dad used to make it on Sunday mornings while listening to opera.

This version is grain free and has no starch. It's a good way to get cauliflower into people who think they don't like it. It also seems as though you're eating something starchy in your eggs without messing up your blood sugar and insulin levels or causing an allergic reaction, unless you have the misfortune to be allergic to eggs.

INGREDIENTS
2-3 fresh, cage free eggs
2 T butter or ghee

Brittany or sea salt to taste
¾ cup cauliflower, grated

EQUIPMENT
A 9" omelette pan or frying
pan with curved sides

A mixing bowl
A small whisk

INSTRUCTIONS
1. Melt 1 T butter/ghee in an omelette pan while whisking the eggs with a splash of water and salt.
2. Pan fry the grated cauliflower at a maximum heat until cooked, stirring frequently to avoid burning—about 5 minutes.
3. Add the other 1 T butter/ghee and stir until melted.
4. Add whisked eggs. They should make a hissing sound when they hit the pan.
5. Turn heat to low and cook slowly until you can lift an edge with a spatula.
6. Gently scramble the eggs and cauliflower together to your favorite consistency.
7. Put on a good performance of *La Bohème* and enjoy!

Fruit "Pie" Omelette

This recipe is for people who like something sweet in the morning but don't want sugar and starch. Use any fruit in season. I like to go out in the morning and collect blackberries in the yard. But you can use any fruit you like—even combinations. This recipe cooks up in about ten minutes or less.

INGREDIENTS

2-3 fresh, cage free eggs	2 T cinnamon or to taste
¼ tsp cardamom or mace	1 T butter or ghee
Brittany or sea salt to taste	¾ medium apple or pear or a cup of fresh berries

INSTRUCTIONS

1. If using apple or pear, start by slicing it thin and warming it in just enough water to avoid burning. Cook until it's soft then set aside.
2. Melt butter/ghee in a clean pan while whisking the eggs with a splash of water, salt, cinnamon and cardamom. Yes, it's brown!
3. Whisked eggs should make a hissing sound when they hit the pan.
4. Immediately turn heat to low or just above. Cook slowly until you can lift an edge with a spatula.
5. Gently but quickly turn the eggs.
6. Pile the fruit onto half the eggs and fold the other end to cover.
7. Turn off the heat and let sit while you get your tea or set your place.
8. Close your eyes and take a bite!

VARIATIONS

Frozen Berries Most frozen fruit isn't as healthful as fresh. Berries freeze best. The fruit sugar of other fruits tends to become more "refined" after freezing, so the sugar may cause more blood sugar spikes. This is true especially of frozen fruit juice.

Sour Cream Live it up and put a dollop of organic sour cream or crème fraîche on top (if you're not dairy sensitive). Homemade sour cream is easy and assures that you are getting organic.

Your Own Sour Cream

Sour cream is a fabulous source of probiotic cultures throughout all of Europe. Who needs a pill when you can have sour cream!

INGREDIENTS

1 T cultured sour cream for a starter—you'll be able to use your own after you've made your first batch
1 pint organic whipping cream

EQUIPMENT

A 1½-pint glass container with lid
A spot in the kitchen that's consistently warm—such as the top of the refrigerator

INSTRUCTIONS
1. Pour the organic cream into the glass container.
2. Whisk the cultured sour cream starter into the cream.
3. Cover the cream with a piece of waxed paper.
4. Set the container in a consistently warm spot.
5. Allow one week for the culture to mature, then put the lid on the container and refrigerate.

VARIATIONS

Raw Milk Instead of using pasteurized organic milk, try raw milk. It is a food that is loaded with nutrients destroyed by the pasteurization process.

Breakfast without Eggs

If you're allergic to eggs, all hope is not lost. Use any of the other recipes we describe for breakfast. We have it on good authority that it's legal.

For a warm breakfast, heat a slice of meatloaf (recipe below) and have it with some steamed green beans. For a cold breakfast, have a cooked chicken thigh out of the refrigerator with some homemade sauerkraut (recipes below).

LUNCH

SALADS

Yes, you can go to a salad bar and get lots of creative salads, but they're not hard to make at home. Then you just go to your frig when the taste for salad hits.

These salads get better as they marinate, with all the flavors playing off each other. They're great with cold chicken or turkey (recipes below).

Jicama-Carrot Slaw

This is a new spin on coleslaw. Instead of cabbage, I substitute jicama. Investing in an electric grater or a food processor is a good idea if this becomes a habit.

INGREDIENTS

½ medium jicama, skinned and grated
3 medium carrots, grated   ½ fresh orange
2-3 T mayonnaise   Brittany or sea salt

INSTRUCTIONS

1. Mix the jicama and carrot in a bowl.
2. Squeeze in the juice of the orange and add the mayonnaise.
3. Mix and salt to taste.

Celery Root and Daikon

This is another alter ego to coleslaw that tastes great as it marinates. It lasts at least a week refrigerated.

INGREDIENTS

1 celery root, peeled and grated   1 good sized daikon
2 T unrefined toasted sesame oil   Japanese radish, grated
Brittany or sea salt or gomasio   Rice vinegar
   (sesame salt) to taste   1 cup cucumber, grated (optional)

INSTRUCTIONS

1. Mix the grated celery root, daikon, and cucumber (if you decide to use it) in a bowl.
2. Add the sesame oil and rice vinegar to taste.
3. Mix and salt to taste.

Coleslaw Variations

These two recipes are variations on cabbage-based coleslaw. If you want regular coleslaw, follow the Jicama-Carrot Slaw recipe and substitute chopped or grated cabbage for the jicama. For added pizzazz, mix red and white cabbage.

VARIATION

To vary regular coleslaw, add grated raw cauliflower or zucchini to the raw grated cabbage. Use a dressing of mayo and toasted sesame oil with a splash of your favorite vinegar. or just use oil and vinegar. Try macadamia nut oil for a treat.

Cobb Salad

This is a classic. My first taste of a Cobb salad was at the legendary Brown Derby on Hollywood Boulevard where it was invented. Although there are numerous variations, this is close to the original. One of its most important features is that it's a chopped salad. You can make a Cobb for one, two, or many. Just scale up the ingredients.

INGREDIENTS

2 cups crisp lettuce (the original used a combination of head lettuce, romaine, watercress, and chicory)
2 strips of salt cured, nitrate- and preservative-free bacon, cooked crisp and crumbled
5 ounces of cooked chicken breast, cubed
1 small tomato, cubed
½ small avocado, cubed
1 hard boiled egg
¼ cup blue veined cheese (such as Roquefort or gorgonzola)
Dressing (see below)

EQUIPMENT

A large salad bowl   A food chopper

INSTRUCTIONS

1. Place everything except the dressing in the bowl and mix.
2. Chop and mix the salad.
3. Add the dressing and toss.

DRESSING

The simplest dressing is mayonnaise, especially if you make your own. Next simplest is oil and vinegar. Nut oils such as walnut and macadamia add to the richness of the salad. Avoid wine vinegars because of the allergens in the wine.

A dressing reminiscent of the original includes olive oil, vinegar, lemon juice, and a dash of dry mustard.

VARIATIONS

To save time, skip the chopping. However, it won't be the same.

YOUR OWN COLD CUTS

Nothing quenches hunger like some protein. So it's a good idea to have a roast chicken or turkey breast or thigh waiting for you in the refrigerator when you're stomach calls.

Having roast chicken or turkey in the frig also lends itself to healthy, whole fast foods. Of course, you don't have to wait for the chicken or turkey to cool in the refrigerator. Eat it hot with steamed vegetables.

Roast Chicken

The first step in roasting a chicken is selecting the chicken. There are two issues: size and feed.

The size affects the tenderness of the cooked meat: for a large chicken, make sure you roast it a long time. How long? Until the meat is falling off the bone. Otherwise, the meat will be tough. What's a large chicken? For roasting, anything over 4 pounds.

The feed affects the flavor of the meat. Most organic chickens are fed soy and so, at least to some tastes, it's less palatable than so-called free range chickens fed corn. We've found organic chickens fed a combination of soy and corn. The taste improvement is noticeable.

INGREDIENTS
   1 chicken   Brittany or sea salt

EQUIPMENT
   A flat pan   A poultry rack
   A meat thermometer   A roaster (optional)

INSTRUCTIONS
1. Pre-heat the roaster to 400°F.
2. Thoroughly wash the chicken.
3. Salt the chicken all over.
4. Place the poultry rack in the pan and the chicken in the rack breast down and then the whole contraption in the roaster.
   • Spread the wings and legs so the heat can get at the chicken.
5. Cook at 400°F until
   • the skin is golden and pulled back from the leg
   • the wing tips are crisp
   • when you test with the meat thermometer, liquid from the breast is clear and the temperature is 180°F
   • for a 4 pound chicken, that will take about 1½ hours; for a 5 pound chicken 2 hours or more

VARIATIONS
Roaster During the summer, you won't want to fire up the oven to roast a chicken. That's why this recipe calls for a roaster that you can put outside when it's hot.

Lemon-Rosemary Chicken You can add flavor by stuffing the body cavity with sliced lemon and fresh rosemary.

Roast Turkey Breast

It's easy to turn a turkey breast into something that gets stuck in your throat when you take a bite it's so dry. And that after chewing for days it's so tough. All because it cooked a little too long.

Tender roast turkey breast takes good timing—no doubt revenge on the part of the bird.

INGREDIENTS
1 half of a split turkey breast	Toasted sesame oil
Brittany or sea salt	

EQUIPMENT
A roasting pan with lid	A meat thermometer
A roaster (optional)	

INSTRUCTIONS
1. Pre-heat the cooker to 375°F.
2. Thoroughly rinse the turkey breast.
3. Apply the toasted sesame oil liberally to the turkey breast then salt it all over.
4. Place the turkey breast in the roasting pan, bone down, breast up. Put on the cover. Stick it in the roaster.
5. Cook at 375°F until
   • when you test with the meat thermometer, liquid from the breast is clear and the temperature is 140°F
   • a 3 pound breast takes about 1 hour.

VARIATIONS

Roaster As with roasting a chicken, a roaster allows you to roast when it's hot without heating up the house.

Leg and Thigh This recipe works for a leg and thigh too. The cooking time turns out to be about the same even though the leg and thigh weighs less than the breast. That's because they have more fat and bone. You'll have to worry less about the cooked meat being dry, but you will have to make sure that the meat next to the bone is fully cooked.

Homemade Sauerkraut

A friend from the local farmers market claims that homemade sauerkraut is its own food group. With a little effort and patience, you can find out for yourself.

Sauerkraut is a near perfect food for gut health. Because it's a food created by fermentation caused by Lactobacillus microbes, it's loaded with probiotics and prebiotics.

This recipe makes about 6 quarts of sauerkraut. It's less taxing to make sauerkraut in large batches because of the set-up and clean-up.

INGREDIENTS

3 large heads of white cabbage   Brittany or sea salt
Purified water

EQUIPMENT

6 1-quart glass canning jars with lids
A pounder
A food processor or slicer (optional)
A large enameled flat pan
A spot in the kitchen that's consistently warm—such as the top of the refrigerator

INSTRUCTIONS

1. Thoroughly wash the canning jars.
2. Shred the cabbage into thin strips.
   - You can do this by hand with a good kitchen knife, but you'll need to keep it sharp.
   - A mechanical device such as a food processor or slicer will make your life easier. So you know we're not asleep at the wheel, we are aware that food processors throw off electromagnetic fields when they're in operation.
3. Spread the shredded cabbage in the roasting pan.
4. Pound the cabbage thoroughly until it's glistening. Don't be gentle.
   - You can also just use a clean countertop. However, this step is messy, with cabbage bits flying about—depending on the vigor of your pounding.
   - What you've just done is release the Lactobacilus and mixed it with the nutrient rich liquid of the cabbage—its food for the fermentation process.
5. Press the shredded cabbage into the canning jars, leaving about 1½" of space at the top.
   - Do your best to thoroughly press the cabbage in.
6. Place 2 teaspoons of salt on the cabbage then pour in purified water until the top of the cabbage is just covered with water.
   - If you've done a good job of pressing in the cabbage, it will bubble and hiss a bit as the water fills the voids. You'll likely have to do 2 or 3 pourings.
   - You might need to press in the cabbage one last time.
7. Put the lids on the jars and tighten then place the jars in a warm place.

- You might want to set the jars in a pan in case the fermentation process causes the liquid to overflow.
8. Let the sauerkraut ferment for one week.
9. Refrigerate to stop the fermentation process.

VARIATIONS

If you're really committed, get a large ceramic crock built for making sauerkraut and put the whole batch in it. My father remembered going to his grandmother's and nipping sauerkraut from her crock, left in the root cellar where it was cool. The cold stops the fermentation process so the sauerkraut isn't unbearably sour.

Of course, most houses (let alone apartments) don't have cellars so you'll have to stow the crock in the refrigerator or transfer the sauerkraut to smaller containers. You can purchase a one gallon crock for less that $40, but make sure the glaze is lead-free.

DINNER

CAULIFLOWER RICE AND MASH

A friend over for dinner kept asking "This isn't rice?"

Nope. It was grated cauliflower, sautéed in ghee (clarified butter). We haven't had actual rice for years. But we miss the texture when eating. One day some synapses fired and we grated and sautéed some cauliflower.

In addition to being a low starch replacement for rice, grated cauliflower takes less time to cook. And depending on how much you dress it up (for example, with herbs and spices) your taste buds can't tell the difference.

Cauliflower Rice

This recipe makes 3 cups of cauliflower rice. Depending on how firm you want the dish, it will take from 5 to 8 minutes to cook. It refrigerates well, maintaining its texture when you warm it up later.

INGREDIENTS

4 cups cauliflower. grated   1 tsp Brittany or sea salt
2 T tropical oil (palm or coconut)

EQUIPMENT

A food processor or electric grater (optional)

INSTRUCTIONS

1. Wash and cut a head of cauliflower.
   - Use the florets, not the stalk.
   - Depending on the size of the head, you might have florets left over.
2. Grate 4 cups of raw cauliflower.
   - A food processor is handy, but not essential.
   - The 4 cups will cook down to 3 cups of finished cauliflower rice.
3. Heat a frying pan over a high flame and add the tropical oil.
   - We like palm oil. But care is required in selecting a brand: severe ecological damage is being caused by harvesting. So we use Spectrum's vegetable shortening because they pay attention to their source.
4. When the oil is melted, add the grated cauliflower and salt.
5. Turn the cauliflower to distribute the butter/ghee and salt evenly.
6. Cover the frying pan.
   - For brown, firm cauliflower rice, keep the flame high.
   - For white, soft cauliflower rice, turn the heat down to a medium flame.
7. Every minute or so, turn the cauliflower to make sure it cooks evenly.

VARIATIONS

This is a simple dish that invites infinite variations. As you learn how to control the firmness and whiteness of the dish, you can pull out any rice dish and use cauliflower rice as the base.

Cauliflower Mash

Miss mashed potatoes? Or just looking for a low starch alternative? This recipe makes about 2½ cups of cauliflower mash. It takes about 15 to 20 minutes to prepare.

INGREDIENTS

4 cups cauliflower florets	2 T butter or ghee
1 tsp Brittany or sea salt	

EQUIPMENT

A mixer, blender, or food processor

INSTRUCTIONS

1. Wash a head cauliflower and cut the florets.
   - For a creamier texture, use the tender heads and as little of the stems as possible.
2. Steam the florets until they are tender but firm.
   - You should get a little resistance when you test a floret with a fork or knife.
   - This takes about 10 minutes.
   - This is a critical step. The firmness to which you cook the cauliflower will determine whether the final product is creamy or runny.
3. Drain the cauliflower, but keep the liquid.
4. Put the cauliflower in the mixer's bowl or blender or food processor then add the butter/ghee and salt.
   - If you like, you can use a potato masher to pre-blend the ingredients. If you don't mind your mash lumpy, you can stop here.
5. Whip the cauliflower in the mixer, blender, or food processor.
   - Adjust the creaminess of the mash using the liquid from step #3.

Cauliflower Lore

A cup of mashed potatoes has 31 grams of carbohydrates and contributes 135 calories to a meal. A cup of mashed cauliflower has 5 grams of carbohydrates and contributes 28 calories to a meal. Cauliflower is loaded with vitamin K and vitamin C. It's also rich in B vitamins.

Like other cruciferous vegetables, cauliflower is loaded with compounds that support your liver's detoxification processes. High consumption of crucifers is associated with a lower risk of cancer.

One note: too much raw crucifer can inhibit thyroid function, although "too much" is far more than anyone ordinarily eats.

MEATLOAF

We continue our promotion of cauliflower by substituting it for bread crumbs traditionally used in meatloaf. We also pull some other tricks.

This recipe invites variation, which is how we got to this version. If you want your grandmother's meatloaf, start there and replace the bread crumbs with the cauliflower and egg.

Like all good meatloafs, this one is terrific cold. It's good served hot with steamed green beans or with cauliflower mash or both if you're up to it.

Crumbless Meatloaf

INGREDIENTS

2 pounds ground beef
   (fresh is best)
¾ cup cauliflower, grated
¼ small green pepper, grated
2 tablespoons melted ghee
   or butter

½ apple, grated
2 eggs
1 tsp cinnamon
1 tsp Brittany or sea salt
1 tablespoon Herbs de Provence
   (also called French herbs)

EQUIPMENT

A roaster
A roasting pan

A large mixing bowl
A food processor or electric
   grater (optional)

INSTRUCTIONS

1. Preheat the roaster to 350°F.
   • As with roasting chicken or turkey, a roaster enables you to heat the great outdoors instead of your kitchen during hot weather.
2. Cut and wash a fistful of cauliflower florets.
   • Use the stalks, it helps add bulk.
   • "Fistful" just means whatever grates up into ¾ cup.
3. Grate the raw cauliflower so you have ¾ cup and put it in the mixing bowl. Then grate the apple and green pepper in with the cauliflower.
4. Place the rest of the ingredients except the ground beef in the mixing bowl and mix thoroughly.
   • You're doing this to minimize the amount you have to work the ground beef, for reasons discussed in the next step.
5. Add the ground beef and combine the ingredients until it's a uniform mixture.
   • Use your hands to work the ingredients together. It's an opportunity to play with your food.
   • But don't play too much: the loaf tends to toughen as you work it.
6. Form a loaf and put it in the roasting pan. Leave it uncovered.

7. Cook uncovered for 1¼ to 1½ hours.
   - Check it at 1¼ hours by slicing in the middle.
   - You'll have goo in the bottom of the pan from the liquid in the loaf. Cats like the goo (they'd like the meatloaf too, but enough's enough).

Pork Loaf

This is a variation of the Crumbless Meatloaf recipe, with emphasis on "variation." There's more to it than substituting ground pork for ground beef.

INGREDIENTS
2 pounds ground pork
1 stalk celery, grated
½ bunch cilantro chopped
1 tsp Brittany or sea salt
2 eggs

¾ cup cauliflower, grated
¾ cup red bell pepper, chopped
1 tsp cumin seed, crushed
1½ T toasted sesame oil

EQUIPMENT
A roaster
A roasting pan
A mortar and pestle (optional)

A large mixing bowl
A food processor or electric
   grater (optional)

INSTRUCTIONS
1. Preheat the roaster to 350°F.
2. Wash the vegetables.
3. Grate cauliflower and celery into mixing bowl, add the rest of the ingredients except the ground pork, and mix well.
   - For best results, grind the cumin seed in a mortar.
4. Add the ground pork and massage all of the ingredients together until well mixed.
5. Form it into a loaf and place it in a roasting pan.
6. Cook uncovered for 1¼ hours.

EQUIPMENT
A roaster
A roasting pan

A large mixing bowl

SERVE
Served hot, this loaf is good with sautéed zucchini or broccoli. It's also good cold, either by itself, with vegetables, or in a salad.

VARIATIONS

Pork and Fat Ground pork is usually made from the butt so it tends to have a good deal of fat. However, this will cook off. If you choose a leaner cut of pork such as the loin, you might need to add a little fat to the mixture.

Cumin You can substitute ground cumin for crushed seeds. The cumin, red bell pepper, and cilantro are what give this loaf its flavor so you'll probably want to experiment to get it right.

Onion and Garlic We haven't tried onions or garlic and don't think the recipe wants it. But if you're so inclined, give it a try. The same is true for spicing it up with either hot peppers or hot sauce: we haven't tried it and don't think it wants it.

Soy-free Stir Fry

I love Chinese food but I'm allergic (as are many people) to soy. Hard to imagine stir fry without it? Read on. I believe I can get you out of "food jail!"

There are ample opportunities to experiment with this recipe by adding different vegetables and meats. This dish is really fast to make. From start to finish, probably 15 minutes—depending on how fast you chop!

This recipe makes a good sized single serving or two small ones.

INGREDIENTS

5 ounces of any meat, poultry or fish you like, cut in equal sized chunks
1 celery stalk, sliced
Equal size chunks of your favorite vegetables. Try broccoli, carrots, and shiitake mushrooms.
¾ cup of cooked cauliflower rice (see recipe on previous page)
2 T fresh cilantro, chopped
1 small clove garlic, chopped (if it works for you)
1 tsp fresh ginger, chopped
1 heaping T Ume Boshi paste
A splash of rice vinegar
1½ T tropical oil (palm or coconut)

INSTRUCTIONS

1. Heat the oil over a high flame.
2. Rinse the vegetables and the meat and let them dry on a clean cloth.
3. If you've not already made the cauliflower rice, stir fry the grated cauliflower first at a high heat, turning often until it's as brown as you want it.
4. With the pan still hot, add the cilantro, celery, garlic, and ginger until they are hot.
5. Now add the other vegetables, keeping the heat high and stirring often.
6. Put the Ume Boshi paste in a small mixing bowl, add a splash of rice vinegar, mix, then stir into eveything else with the meat.
7. Traditionally, stir fried vegetables are still crunchy, so your dish may be done unless you prefer softer vegetables. If so, cover and turn the heat down and cook until tender.

• Be careful not to overcook your meat since it will be more tender with less and faster cooking.

Stir in a whole egg at the end and scramble it in.

Chile Verde

Pigs were domesticated from wild boars about 9,000 years ago. Vikings believed that in heaven they would have an endless supply of pork from Sæhrímnir, the cosmic hog that regenerates itself overnight.

Pork from sustainably raised pigs, while not quite up to Sæhrímnir's virtuosity, provides a high quality, nutrient dense source of protein, fat, and micronutrients. And pound for pound, pork tends to be less expensive than beef or poultry.

This recipe uses the shoulder butt. This cut of meat can have a lot of fat. If you buy it as a roast, it will be rolled so you should take a careful look to make sure it doesn't have too much fat beyond what is marbled in the meat itself. Of course, you can always use leaner cuts such as the loin.

This recipe offers many opportunities for experimentation, but however you fix it you'll be able to cook a large batch. If you're not feeding Vikings, you can freeze some (or most) for later. This is the basic from which you can add or remove ingredients and change amounts.

INGREDIENTS

3 pounds pork shoulder butt	1½ pounds tomatillos
1 bunch cilantro	1 large clove garlic
2 tsp ground cumin	2 tsp Brittany or sea salt
2 limes	3 T tropical oil (palm or coconut)

EQUIPMENT

A pressure cooker or Dutch oven   A food processor or blender

INSTRUCTIONS

1. Rinse the vegetables and the meat.
2. Cut the meat into 1" cubes and set aside. If you bought a roast, this is where you might need to trim fat.
3. Heat the tropical oil in the pressure cooker or Dutch oven over a high flame with the lid off.
4. When the oil is melted, add the meat, salt it, and mix it to coat it with oil.
   • As you're fixing the vegetables, keep stirring the meat so each cube loses its color on all sides.
5. Put the tomatillos, cilantro, cumin, and garlic in the food proces-

sor or blender, squeeze in the juice of the limes, then liquefy the whole thing.

6. Pour the liquefied tomatillo mix into the pot and bring to a boil.
7. Put on the lid.
   - If you're using a pressure cooker, bring it to pressure and let it cook at pressure for 1 hour.
   - If you're using a Dutch oven, turn the heat to low and simmer for 3 hours, stirring occasionally so it won't burn.

SERVE

Make some cauliflower rice (recipe on page 105) and serve the chili verde over it in soup bowls.

VARIATIONS

<u>Chicken Chile Verde</u> Replace the pork with chicken. To get three pounds of meat, you'll have to bone 2 small chickens or one large one. You'll need to take care in browning the meat because it's leaner than pork. For the same reason, you might need to add some additional cooking oil for flavor. To avoid boning, stew the chicken in the tomatillo sauce then pull the meat off the bone and dice it.

<u>Tropical Oil</u> Tropical oils are high in saturated fat and that makes them cook well at high heat. Spectrum makes a nice product it calls Organic Shortening made from palm oil. Jungle Products makes a tasty coconut oil. If you can find clean lard, use that—although we haven't found a source so if you find one, let us know. You could use butter, but we've found that taste-wise the tropical oils work the best.

<u>Tartness</u> The addition of lime adds tartness to an already tart dish. If that's not to your taste, leave out the lime or keep the lime, add broth and reduce the amount of tomatillo.

<u>Soupiness</u> You can increase the soupiness of the final product in two ways. Adding more tomatillos will increase the tartness of the broth. Adding chicken or beef broth will sweeten up the broth a little.

<u>Heat</u> If you like your dishes spicy, you can add hot peppers or hot sauce to the tomatillo mix. Both, but especially the hot sauce, will affect the flavor. We recommend trying it once without the spice. Then you can liven it up to your heart's (and tongue's and stomach's) content.

Sustainable Pork

Buying sustainably raised pork is not difficult. You'll have to buy it from a butcher who knows their business. You might have to educate your butcher about what "sustainable pork" means.

Sustainable isn't the same as organic, although they're close. "Organic" refers to what the hogs eat. "Sustainable" refers to the hogs' overall living conditions and farm practices.

Sellers of sustainable meats such as Organic Prairie (www.organicprairie.com), BN Ranch (www.preferredmeats.com/BNranch_network.htm), and Humane Farm Animal Care (www.certifiedhumane.com) describe their practices on their websites. The Animal Welfare Institute's criteria for raising pigs (www.awionline.org) include

- freedom to roam, root, and play;
- year-round access to fields;
- rotation of fields fertilized by the hog's own manure;
- clean, dry bedding;
- housing that is roomy and promotes healthy social relationships; and
- piglets are not weaned prematurely.

Resources

These are two comprehensive cookbooks we find useful: Sally Fallon and Mary Enig (1999) *Nourishing Traditions* and Jessica Prentice (2006) *Full Moon Feast*. Both authors have been interviewed on *Your Own Health And Fitness*.

The basic principles behind our recipes are discussed on two shows: Berman (2005c) "Designing a Sane Individual Diet Plan" and Berman (2004c) "The Hunter-Gatherer Diet."

Exercise is good for you. Few people disagree. Yet exercise seems to be avoided more than sought.

A century ago most people were paid to exercise: most people worked at jobs that required physical exertion that was often arduous. It was a time when the majority of people were engaged as manual laborers in agricultural, construction, and manufacturing.

Today, dramatically fewer people work as manual laborers in these industries. Machines have replaced human muscle and endurance in many occupations. Jobs have shifted from manual labor to office work and service jobs. Although many of these jobs can be physically taxing, they do not involve the kind of exercise to which our forebears were subjected.[1]

Instead, we now pay to exercise. Several industries sell exercise products. These include the obvious health club membership as well as sporting goods, exercise clothing and footwear, exercise equipment, and exercise programs offered in a variety of media: books, videos, seminars, fitness clubs, personal trainers, and even electronically with the wireless Wii technology.

Paying to exercise reaches into the public sector with taxes spent on recreational parks and the design of public places that encourage physical activity.

Why is exercise good for you?

Your body is put together so it can move—to walk, run, lift, throw, and carry. All these are useful capacities for a hunter-gatherer.

But your body is also put together to conserve nutrients and energy. Some of what's behind that capacity is the physical need to balance the nutrients consumed with the nutrients used. Just as important, your body is put together so it will recover from the stress caused by the physical exertion of hunting and gathering.

Both nutrient conservation and recovery from stress are very adaptive for hunter-gatherers who had to literally catch a meal. As hunter-gatherers in a food environment that requires effort to obtain nutrients, a balance needs to be struck with the physical need for recovery. Those in turn need to be balanced with personal and social needs.

In 1966, the anthropologist Marshall Sahlins introduced the idea of hunter-gatherers as the original affluent society.[2] Based on then-current anthropological studies of modern day hunter-gatherer societies, Sahlins estimated that these peoples spent approximately 20 hours per week "working" at hunting and gathering. The remainder of their time was spent in domestic work (for example, preparing food) and personal and cultural activities (for example, playing games).

The workweek for modern day hunter-gatherers typically consists of 2 to 4 days hunting and 2 to 3 days gathering. There's a rhythm here of work (which is exercise) and rest. With this work (and exercise) schedule, modern-day hunter-gatherers have a capacity to consume, transport, and use oxygen[3] that is 50% greater than people of similar age from industrialized cultures. In addition, hunter-gatherers have leg strength 20% greater than industrialized peoples of similar age and weight.[4]

Modern day hunter-gatherers are much smaller than both people living in industrialized societies and the Paleolithic hunter-gatherers who are our ancestors of 25,000 years ago. Although it's difficult to extrapolate the 20-hour workweek backward to our ancestors, it is possible to state that their level of fitness was similar.[5]

Based on an examination of skeletal remains of Paleolithic hunter-gatherers, industrialized humans use about 40% of the energy in physical activity compared to our ancestors. Paleolithic people were over twice as active as industrialized humans. But our ancestors consumed more energy on average than we do—an estimated 45% more.

This only says that hunter-gatherers were more physically active and so compensated by eating more. But that's only the beginning of the story.

The physical activity of our ancestors most resembles what we now call cross training, a routine that mixes exercise that develops strength with exercise that develops cardiopulminary capacity. The first builds muscle and bone and the body's capacity to use energy efficiently. The second builds heart, circulation, and lung fitness—that is, the capacity to consume and efficiently use the oxygen essential for converting fuel to energy. According to physical anthropologist, the physique of the average Paleolithic hunter-gatherer was not like the average modern human. The physique of our average ancestor was like that of an Olympic athlete.

In other words, we have inherited the capacities of high performing athletes from our hunter-gatherer ancestors.[6]

The first article in this section, "Reverse the Aging Process," gives testimony to this inheritance. It describes how strength exercise affects a wide range of gene activity associated with the deterioration in capacity we've come to think of as the inevitable consequence of aging.

Re-enforcement of our inheritance is also found in "Life, Death, and Vegetables" on page 66. You will recall that one of the simple things that extends people's lives is a modest amount of physical activity.

Some scholars argue that the overall decline of modern humans in their stature and physical fitness came with the slow, gradual shift from the hunter-gatherer way of life to the agricultural way of life that occurred as civilizations rose, populations settled, and class societies developed.

With the Industrial Revolution and the successful struggles by the working class for social equity, health and fitness returned.[7] As both life expectancies and physical stature increased throughout most of the modern period, the physical activity of the vast majority of people remained rooted in their work.

However, since World War II a significant shift has taken place in the mix of work so that far fewer people work in physically active jobs where walking, running, lifting, and carrying are required. For example, the fitness of current Marine Corps recruits is markedly less than the recruits of 1946.[8]

This relative decline of physical fitness since World War II is widely acknowledged to be a causal factor in the simultaneous rise in the incidence of chronic illnesses such as heart disease and diabetes. Even the food pyramid now has an exercise component.

Does this mean we all need to become Olympic caliber athletes? Likely not. Nevertheless, we need balance among three factors.
• nutrients consumed
• physical activity using those hunter-gatherer capacities
• resting metabolism

Resting metabolism is the energy you use while at rest, doing things such as keeping the body warm, blood circulating, and the brain working. Most of the energy people use each day is consumed for this purpose, keeping the physiological ship afloat. On average, industrial humans use up 2030 calories each day. Of that 2030 calories, 1450 calories are for resting metabolism—almost 72%.

On the other hand, our Paleolithic ancestors used 2900 calories on average each day of which 1665 calories was for resting metabolism—less than 60%. The reason for the difference is that with their greater relative muscle mass and aerobic fitness, Paleolithic hunter-gatherers (and Olympic athletes) used energy sources more efficiently. In fact, they used nutrients in general more efficiently.

Physical activity level (PAL) is a measure of how efficiently a body is using energy. It is the ratio of total energy used to resting metabolism. For the average industrial human, the PAL is 1.4. For the average Paleolithic hunter-gatherer, the PAL is 1.74.

For PAL, a higher ratio means better fitness and better health.

Adding 60 minutes of physical activity each day that consumes an additional 490 calories[9] would bring the average industrial human's PAL in line with her Paleolithic ancestor. Current recommendations from public health organizations call for 30 minutes of physical activity each day that adds 200 calories used. That results in a slight PAL increase to 1.55.

The second article in this section, "Walking: Think You Know How?" discusses one of our most basic forms of physical activity. It's simple and accessible.

The third article, "Moved to Move," discusses how to make changes that help make greater physical activity part of life. It focuses principally on what each person can do in her personal environment. A considerable literature has evolved around how the built environment[10] and social environment affect physical activity[11] through collective action.

As with food, physical activity is basic to our health. The three principles are the starting place.

Unique Biology

Few of us have the time, inclination, or physical structure to be Olympic athletes. However, we all have the capacity to sustain and improve our muscle strength and cardiovascular fitness. One of the most important things to grasp when improving fitness is that it must be undertaken gradually and within each person's physical constraints.[12] Some people are able to build muscle easily. Others struggle. Some people are able to develop cardiovascular fitness easily. Others cannot.

As with food, if someone is doing exercise that benefits her, she'll feel better. If a form of exercise is painful or makes her feel worse, she should look for something else that feels right. There are a wide range of methods for both strength training and aerobic training.[13]

The Body as an Ecology

Physical activity is another example of how different systems work together. Respiration works with circulation and the heart to distribute oxygen. Eating and digestion work with circulation to store and distribute fuel. Muscle and bone work with fuel and oxygen to create motion.[14]

If any of the areas of a body's ecology are out of balance, the others are threatened with imbalance. For example, it's common for someone to have difficulty with running because her musculoskeletal structure is misaligned. Trying to exercise could cause injury. Often, a good body worker can re-align her structure and enable her to exercise safely—and feel the benefit as she should.

Do the Simplest Things First

Dancing is exercise. Dancing around the house is exercise. Physical activity does not have to be arduous to be beneficial. It can be made easy by integrating it into existing routines—for example, taking a brisk 10-minute walk after breakfast and dinner. Because the body wants to move, simple acts can meet that need. It's just not always easy.[15]

Some of the barriers to physical activity are personal. Some are environmental. As we discuss in "Moved to Move," the key is for each person to discover how to change her personal environment and how she can find or help create built, natural, and social environments that provide the right environmental support for her.[16]

Notes

[1] Donald M. Fisk (2001) "American Labor in the 20th Century."
[2] See Chapter 1 The Original Affluent Society in Marshall Sahlins (2004) *Stone Age Economics* originally published in 1972.
[3] Referred to as aerobic capacity, maximum oxygen consumption, and maximum oxygen uptake. The standard measure is *VO2 max.*
[4] S. Boyd Eaton and Stanley B. Eaton (2003) "An Evolutionary Perspective on Human Physical Activity: Implications for Health" page 155.
[5] Christopher Ruff, et al. (1993) "Postcranial Robusticity in *Homo*. I: Temporal Trends and Mechanical Interpretation."
[6] Christopher Ruff (2000) "Body Mass Prediction from Skeletal Frame Size in Elite Athletes."
[7] See James C. Riley (2001) *Rising Life Expectancy: A Global History.*
[8] Cited in S. Boyd Eaton and Stanley B. Eaton (2003) "An Evolutionary Perspective on Human Physical Activity: Implications for Health."
[9] 490 calories are added to the diet. This isn't a weight-loss scheme. It's a fitness scheme in which physical activity is fueled by matching nutrient load.
[10] For example, Lawrence D. Frank, et al. (2003) *Health and Community Design: The Impact of the Built Environment on Physical Activity* and R. Sturm and D.A. Cohen (2004) "Suburban Sprawl and Physical and Mental Health."
[11] For example, Ming Wen, et al. (2007) "Neighbourhood Deprivation, Social Capital and Regular Exercise during Adulthood: A Multilevel Study in Chicago" and Gary G. Bennett, et al. (2007) "Safe to Walk? Neighborhood Safety and Physical Activity among Public Housing Residents."
[12] See Layna Berman (2002a) "Exercise: An Integrative Perspective."
[13] See Layna Berman (2001) "Exercising Beyond Constraints."
[14] See Layna Berman (2002b) "The Science of Weight Training."
[15] See Layna Berman and Jeffry Fawcett (2007) "Exercise and Disease Prevention."
[16] For example, see James Prochaska, et al. (1995) *Changing for Good: A Revolutionary Six-stage Program for Overcoming Bad Habits and Moving Your Life Positively Forward.*

REVERSE THE AGING PROCESS

The promise sounds thrilling: reverse aging with exercise. Too good to be true? Maybe not.

Although news reports took liberties with the science, research published in *PLoS ONE* describes some remarkable effects from regular weight lifting. Previous research has shown that as we grow older, the protein fibers that make up skeletal muscle deteriorate in quality. What this latest study shows is that there's good reason to believe that this process can be reversed.

It all starts with mitochondria.

Mitochondrial Theory of Aging

As we described in "Healthy Mitochondria" (PHO #9), mitochondria are organelles within each cell. Mitochondria are known best for producing energy. They also control when a cell dies. A tissue type might have few or many mitochondria in each cell—red blood cells have none; muscle cells of the heart are loaded, with about one-third of their weight in mitochondria.

Mitochondria have a set of DNA separate from the cell's DNA. Mitochondria are matrilineal: your mitochondrial DNA comes exclusively from your mother. When a cell divides, its mitochondria divide as well. As you grow older, you go through many generations of cells and mitochondria.

With each generation, mistakes are made in copying cell and mitochondrial DNA. Both the cell's nucleus and the mitochondria in the cell have genes that produce enzymes that proofread DNA as it is copied and correct mistakes. However, with a much more limited number of genes, the mitochondria are much more vulnerable to the proofreading system failing.

In addition to mistakes during cell division, cell nuclear and mitochondrial DNA are subject to oxidative stress. Mitochondria are doubly vulnerable because they produce powerful reactive oxygen species (*ROS*) as a direct result of energy production.

ROS come from our environment and other cellular processes in addition to mitochondrial energy production. However, the mitochondrial production of ROS is constant and high in volume. Fortunately, mitochondria produce powerful anti-oxidants that neutralize ROS, most importantly Coenzyme Q10.

Over time even small amounts of ROS can create mischief by degrading the effectiveness of the enzymes that repair DNA mistakes. As mitochondrial DNA mistakes accumulate over thousands of cell generations, mitochondria decline in their ability to clean up the ROS they create.

With both exposures to ROS from the environment and increasingly inefficient ROS clean up, mitochondria work with declining effectiveness. When the power source for cells don't work well, the cells don't work well. And so we age.

DNA, Young and Old

Aging produces a decline in muscle mass and strength. Many observational studies have found that exercise is beneficial for many of the ails associated with aging. What Simon Melov and his colleagues looked for was the effect of exercise on mitochondria, the engine of aging.

The researchers examined two groups of people: one group in their late teens and twenties and another in their sixties and seventies. They took samples of muscle from each subject and compared gene expression.

Gene expression means the process that leads to some biochemical action such as the creation of an enzyme. An environmental stimulus (such as physical activity, food, stress, pollution) causes a cascade of biochemical reactions that reach a cell's mitochondrial DNA. The DNA for a specific gene unwinds and more biochemistry causes an enzyme or other chemical to be produced: the gene has expressed itself.

The Melov researchers were looking for gene expression that was either more or less active in the older subjects compared to the younger subjects. They found nearly 600 of these (out of a total 24,000). Approximately half showed greater gene activity and half showed less gene activity.

Genes that were less active in older people were associated with mitochondrial function and energy metabolism. Genes that were more active were not strongly associated with any function, although they hovered around DNA repair, cell cycle control, transcription (how DNA is read to produce proteins), and cell death.

In other words, in aged individuals mitochondria are slowing down and activities associated with damage control are increasing—which is what you would expect.

Rejuvenating Mitochondria

All of the subjects in the study were in good health, although the young people were relatively sedentary and the old people were relatively active. This leaves unanswered questions such as what a comparison of young and old DNA would look like were the people studied truly representative of the population as a whole. Nevertheless, the researchers had the older people doing weight lifting for six months. No one was training for the Olympics. There were two sessions per week. Each person did three sets of ten repetitions each on the leg press, chest press, leg extension, leg flexion, shoulder press, lat pull-down, seated row, calf raise, abdominal crunch, back extension, arm flexion, and arm extension.

No mention is made as to whether weight machines or free weights were used. In general, free weights are better because they engage more muscle groups so that muscles are not developed in isolation. In addition, free weights help maintain balance and proprioception—the sense you have of your body's position.

At the end of the six month training period, the gene activity of the old people had improved. Formerly down-regulated genes (associated with mitochondria) were more active. Formerly up-regulated genes (associated with, for example, DNA repair) were less active.

Although their gene activity was not restored to the level of the young people, every older person's gene activity was restored to higher, younger levels. Again, many questions come to mind. Does aerobic exercise of similar intensity have the same effect? What happens as the training period increases to one or more years? What is the profile for people who have been lifting weights from the time they were young?

However, there's no doubt that you can benefit at any age.

The News
Kovner, Guy. 2007. Working Out Reverses Aging, Novato Researchers Find. *Santa Rosa Press Democrat.* May 23, 2007.

The Research
Melov, Simon et al. 2007. Resistance Exercise Reverses Aging in Human Skeletal Muscle. *PLoS ONE.* 2(5): e465. DOI:10.1371/journal.pone.0000465.

Resources
Buck Institute for Aging Research. Access at http://www.buckinstitute.org.
Fawcett, Jeffry. 2006. Healthy Mitochondria. *Progressive Health Observer.* Spring 2006 (9): 2ff.
Your Own Health And Fitness. Resources on Aging. Access at http://www.yourownhealthandfitness.org/topicsAging.php.
Your Own Health And Fitness. Resources on Exercise and Musculoskeletal Health. Access at http://www.yourownhealthandfitness.org/topicsExercise.php.

WALKING: THINK YOU KNOW HOW?

Taking yourself out for a walk not only improves your health, it improves your mood. Even a walk around the block will change your perspective.

The emotional effect of exercise has been studied. Robert Thayer's book *Calm Energy* discusses this effect in detail, but anyone who has taken a "time out" by walking even for ten minutes knows the powerful effect of movement on mood.

So Easy I Forgot To Do It!

Most people don't think they're exercising unless they're uncomfortable. I have good news: ten minutes of walking two to three times a day actually does help your health and conditioning.

Walking for longer stretches at a time works even better because it moves your metabolism into a higher burning rate which makes you use your food calories more efficiently all day. Walking longer and pushing your capacity conditions your heart and lungs, making them stronger and more resistant to disease.

Still, my experience is that if I can get someone to start by walking ten minutes at a time, they run out of excuses for not doing it and they actually find they enjoy walking longer.

Assess Yourself!

Although easy and natural to do, there are things to think about before you take up walking as exercise. It's hard to think of yourself as a beginner when it comes to walking. You've been doing it how long?

First, start at an appropriate level of effort instead of thinking that, since you're an expert at walking, you can do it for long periods of time without getting sore or tired. Any increase of activity requires some training—time for your body to adapt and become more efficient.

When you start a new exercise program of any kind, the first adaptations are neurological. This means that your cells communicate better with each other, including those that control how the food you eat is used. When you're fitter, more of the food you eat will be used for fuel for exercise instead of stored as fat. You will feel and see new muscles after a few weeks of consistent exercise.

The rule of this *training effect* is to increase your duration and intensity slowly to avoid burning yourself out and spoiling the fun. Listening to your proclivities for time and place will improve your experience, too.

Do you prefer to walk while watching TV or does being outside make your heart sing? Investing in a "breathable" rain suit is cheaper than a gym membership or a treadmill, and walking in a downpour is a good way to reconnect with your kid self.

Is walking a solitary experience for you, a time to think things through and get back in touch with yourself? Or is it a great time to spend with a friend?

Answering these questions honestly and following your own inclinations are essential for your success. Forcing yourself to do something you hate isn't discipline, it's self-imposed slavery that's seldom productive. Finding out what you like promotes a healthy relationship with yourself and simply works better.

Feet First

With any form of movement, your body's biomechanics affect how you feel. Understanding your posture and how you move can protect you from injury. It will make the difference between pleasure and pain.

Your feet are where it all begins. How you position and place your feet affects the position of your knees, hips, lower back, and pelvis, and even work its way up your back to your neck.

Some lucky people stand and walk right through the middle of their feet. The rest of us roll in or out. You can check this for yourself.

Stand up with your feet together.

Is there space between your shins?

Do your knees knock together?

Supination, rolling outward on your feet, will create a space between your shins. *Pronation*, rolling in, makes you knock-kneed. Looking at your shoe wear is also a clue: supinators wear down the outside of the soles on their shoes; pronators wear down the inside.

Both of these foot positions, depending on their severity, will put more strain on your knees than standing and walking through the middle of your feet. You can try to train yourself to walk through the middle of your feet, but that can cause some strain if you get too zealous.

The Shoes Have It

Fortunately, having the right shoes can help. Some people even resort to orthotics—shoe inserts commercially available or custom-made by a podiatrist or chiropractor. They might help, but if they're not perfect, they can make things worse.

The key to having the right shoes for a supinator or a pronator is lateral (sideways) stability. Supinators and to some degree pronators wear shoes out faster. It's important to replace shoes that have lost their stability to avoid pain in your knees, hips, lower back, and on up.

For lateral stability, medium weight hikers may be the best solution, with cushioning commensurate with the surface you're walking on. City walkers need more sponge, so running shoes with good stability work well. Rural walkers, on the other hand, may need a solid step to protect their feet on uneven ground.

Walking on uneven ground or soft sand causes foot position changes. In fact, changing terrain during a walk can cause knee or hip pain or even shin splints, a painful condition where the muscles separate from the bone. It heals pretty quickly, but it's murder the day after it happens. Another good reason for good, stable shoes. Extra support around the heel bed and a slightly wider heel base also helps.

The arch of your foot needs to be supported. Those with high archs will need more arch support. Another painful condition that can occur when your foot is insufficiently supported is *plantar fasciitis*, an inflammation of the plantar fascia, the ligament of rope-like tissue that runs along the inside of your sole, connecting your heel to the ball of your foot.

Plantar fasciitis comes on very suddenly. If it hits, you'll feel it the night after a hike. Although very painful, it can resolve by the next day if treated with ice for 8 minutes every hour the first night. You can also pull back on your toes and massage the fascia with a combination of MSM (methylsulfonylmethane) powder, arnica gel, and enough hand cream to dissolve the powder.

People who walk through the middle of their feet will have little or no physical problems walking. Their shoes will last until the cushioning starts to compress. For these people, light hikers or running shoes work great. Running shoes have the advantage of a slightly raised heel, which moves your body weight forward.

Special walking shoes are fine if they feel good and provide the right stability and cushioning and you want to have lots of pairs of special shoes. It's true that boots and shoes last longer when you rotate several pair. There's also a law somewhere that if you find a pair of shoes you love, love, love, the manufacturer will stop making them, so buy two pair!

How Much and How Hard Should I Walk?

As with any exercise question, the answer has to do with what you want your body to do. There's a design rule that applies here: form follows function.

If you're just trying to extend your life, several sessions of walking 10 minutes, 2 or 3 days a week will work. The more you do, the longer it extends your life—unless you do so much that you're not able to recover enough when you rest. More exercise, even walking, means you need more rest since your body responds to good stressors such as exercise when you're asleep.

If a more optimal level of fitness is your goal, shoot for 40 minutes to an hour of walking 5 or 6 days a week, including some hill climbing. And if you want to climb Mount McKinley faster than anyone else your age, you should train by hiking in tall mountains pushing your capacity as you go.

The trick here again is to honestly assess your life and your needs. Optimal fitness will get you around really well, it will improve your strength, energy, and outlook and will add protective muscle.

A word about hill walking or hiking. Going up is great for developing great buttock muscles, but going back down is hard on your knees and hips. The secret is strong muscles around your knees to stabilize them. These muscles will develop as you walk, but have a care going down hill: keep your knees and hips loose; don't lock them out when you straighten your leg stepping down.

Getting in Shape to Walk

If knee pain is a consistent problem, you may want to engage in weight training. Leg extensions can be done on a machine or at home with just the weight of your leg. When working out with gym equipment, make sure the pad on the machine is resting on your ankle, not down on your foot. Leg extensions can put the same kind of strain on your knee as running down a flight of stairs. With the pad on your ankle, you're less likely to hurt your knee.

Your lifting should be slow and even. Don't snap your leg up. And keep your knee soft, not bolt straight at the end of the movement.

If the machine isn't adjustable, you're better off doing this exercise on the floor with just the weight of your leg.

- Do this exercise by sitting on the floor with your back against a wall. The closer your buttocks are to the wall, the harder the lift will be.
- Keep both legs straight.
- Work one leg at a time.
- Start by flexing the foot of the working leg—that is, bring your toes to you or toes-to-nose—turn your toes out very slightly

- Lift your leg a few inches off the floor.
- Then lower it without touching the floor.
- Repeat as many times as you can. This may only be a few times at first.
- Repeat with the other leg.
- Over time, build up so that you can do 2 sets on each leg.

You only need to do this exercise 2 times a week: muscles grow when they're resting! As with any weight lifting, it's important to train both sides of your body equally. Leg lifts train the front of your thighs, while leg curls develop your hamstrings on the back of your thighs.

Use the leg curl machine at the gym for this exercise. As with leg extensions, the weight should be on your ankles and your motion should be slow and even. If you can't use a leg curl machine, you can do a floor exercise.

- Lie on the floor face down with your legs together.
- Curl both your legs, bringing your feet toward your buttocks.
- You don't need to bring your feet all the way to your buttocks. 90 degrees at your knees will do it.
- As you curl your legs, press your pelvis gently into the floor to increase the squeeze you feel in your hamstrings.

Regarding leg weights, don't use them when you walk. Only use leg weights when your body is stabilized, such as when you're sitting or lying down. Walking with leg weights is stressful to your knees. If you want to weight your walking, carry a back pack with books or weights in it.

Benefits Abound

After any exercise, your body's metabolism is speeded up. This lasts for several hours. Which means that you're burning more calories even while you're resting.

A note on walking after meals. Overall, a short walk after meals helps digestion and gut health. However, some people might need to make the walk a very gentle one to avoid an upset stomach.

Diabetics and people with insulin resistance will find that walking after a meal helps keep blood sugars low. For heart patients and people at risk of heart disease, walking after meals decreases clotting incidents and protects you from heart symptoms.

The benefits are even broader. In addition to being good for diabetes and heart disease, 40 minutes of walking 5 to 6 days a week reduces your risk for all diseases of aging such as osteoporosis and lung diseases. It also reduces your risk of developing physical limitations such as difficulty with your balance.

Not only does 40 minutes a day of walking help you live healthier, it helps you live longer. People who walk regularly are less likely to die from diabetes, heart disease, or from any other cause compared to people who don't exercise.

Fuel efficiency, mood elevation, less disease, better health, and a longer life. Doesn't sound too bad when you add it up!

Resources

Berman, Layna. 2003. Exercise How-to. *Your Own Health And Fitness.* Broadcast November 18, 2003.

Thayer, Robert. 2001. *Calm Energy.* New York: Oxford University Press.

MOVED TO MOVE

At least one industry can't wait for Christmas to be over. While most retailers make the bulk of their money in the run up to Christmas, health clubs get their big surge in revenue at the beginning of the new year.

One way or another, many people start the new year with the resolve to exercise. They get a new health club membership or renew their old one. But as the months pass, many falter. By June, 60% of those new exercisers have fallen off the treadmill. By September, 80% to 90% are missing from the gym.

Why can't these people stick with it? Do they have some character flaw? Is it a lack of will power?

Not according to people who study how and why people start and stop exercising. What they know can help you make exercise a part of your life, with or without a health club membership.

How Trainers Motivate Clients

Professional trainers depend on their ability to understand what gets clients to start exercising and what keeps them exercising. Five factors that determine how well someone is able to incorporate exercise into their life.

Feel the Training Effect   You should feel and see the *training effect*. When you start exercising, you need to exercise at the appropriate level to experience the training effect: the tangible and pleasant feeling of your body changing. Too much training and you'll burn out. Too little and you'll get bored.

Inspiration   It's more important than discipline. For example, an advantage to exercising at a gym is that you can watch other people. You can be inspired by how others have developed. You can watch what they do and learn from it. What you do for exercise needs to be something you enjoy doing.

Control   Exercise is one of the few things where the outcome is commensurate with your effort. If you are exercising the right amount, you will see and feel the training effect. It will become part of inspiring yourself.

Biomechanics   You need to exercise from how your body actually works. You can evaluate your biomechanics yourself or have someone else do it.

Support   Your family and social circle have a big impact on your exercising. For example, couples often make silent "deals" to get in or out of shape together.

Pain   "No pain, no gain" is a good motto for masochists, but most people sensibly stop activities that hurt. This isn't being a sissy. It's paying attention to your body.

So the task is to find the kind and level of physical activity that makes you feel good, that you are motivated to do, that you can manage, and that fits into your life.

The "feel good" part is important. Most people start exercising to lose weight. Health improvement is a distant second. But what keeps people going is that exercise makes them feel good both physically and emotionally.

In *Calm Energy*, Robert Thayer develops ways to pay attention to how exercise makes you feel. To the *what* and *how* of exercise, Thayer adds *when*. He advises that you plan exercise on days and at a time of day that work for you: when your energy or mood are at their best and when what you plan doesn't conflict with other commitments.

Getting to "Move"

But how do you get moving in the first place?

The most widely cited approach is called Stages of Change. Developed by psychologist James Prochaska, PhD and his colleagues, Stages of Change has been used to deal with a wide range of issues including exercise. It is based on observing how people who change their habits go about doing it.

The idea is that before you take an action such as joining a health club, you go through stages that prepare you to take that action. Prochaska and his colleagues found five distinct stages that people go through. In each stage, people use stage-specific processes to work through each stage and go on to the next stage. And ultimately get to "move."

Consider our recommendation of 40 minutes of moderate exercise (such as brisk walking) 6 days each week.

If you have been getting this much exercise for more than several months, then you are in the fifth, maintenance stage of change: for example, you walk 45 minutes every day with a friend.

If you just started doing 30 minutes of moderate exercise per day, then you're in the fourth, action stage: for example, during the last month you've taken a 30 minute walk at least 4 days each week.

If you plan to start getting 30 minutes per day in the near future, you're in the third, preparation stage: for example, you're talking with a friend about where and when to walk.

If you're trying to figure out whether to start and how, you're in the second, contemplation stage: for example, you're weighing the opportunites for walking, bicycling, and swimming against the obstacles.

And if you really don't pay much attention to exercise, you're in the first, precontemplation stage: for example, you have a vague notion that more walking would be good but don't have the time.

A major insight is that you need to go through these stages in sequence to successfully make exercise a part of your life. If you jump directly from rationalizing why you don't have time (the first, precontemplation stage) to joining a health club (the fourth, action stage), your chances for success are not good.

People who joined the gym on New Year's Day, then disappeared by June, were not at the right stage.

Stages of Change

To go from the first (precontemplation) to the second (contemplation) stage, one of the most important processes is understanding how you rationalize not changing. Take a close look. You're trying to evaluate the issues honestly, not commit to an exercise routine.

To go from the second (contemplation) to the third (preparation) stage, an important process is finding the emotional spark that helps you to move from evaluating possibilities to deciding how you're going to exercise.

To go from the third (preparation) to the fourth (action) stage, an important process is finding the exercise plan that has the balance of benefits and obstacles that enables you to commit to starting.

Prochaska and his colleagues discovered that in the early stages, perceived obstacles outweigh opportunities by a big margin. As people advance through stages, the balance tips, but in an interesting way: obstacles decline a little, but opportunities increase a lot.

You've already read about what it takes to go from the fourth (action) to the fifth (maintenance) stage of exercise: the right kind of support, an exercise plan you can manage, and most importantly, exercise that make you feel good physically and emotionally.

An important insight is that getting to the fifth (maintenance) stage is not always permanent. People stop exercising for all sorts of reasons. What Prochaska and his colleagues found was that people who stop exercising regularly don't revert back to the first (precontemplation) stage, but some intermediate stage. Often, it seems, you have to go through several "relapses" before change becomes permanent.

That you "relapse" and stop exercising is not a character flaw or lack of will power. It's how you change. It's how we all change.

Consider another realm of physical intimacy: romance. You're not looking for love, but you notice someone and wonder.... You ask them out. Then you're dating regularly. Then you commit to the relationship. And then you move in together. Stages of change. Getting yourself ready for intimacy.

If you don't start living together after the first date, have you failed? Of course not. If you do start living together on the first date, is the relationship likely to last? Anything's possible, but it's a long shot. You need to prepare yourself for intimacy.

So it is with exercise. You learn how to get to "move," you go through stages that prepare you to make regular exercise a part of your life, and nurture a romance with your body.

Resources

Berman, Layna. 1996. The Psychology of Exercise. *Your Own Health And Fitness*. Broadcast July 2, 1996.

Prochaska, James et al. 1994. *Changing for Good*. New York: Quill.

Thayer, Robert. 2001. *Calm Energy*. New York: Oxford University Press.

What role does science play in consumption and lifestyle decisions as they affect health? An example comes from the Silent Spring Institute's Household Exposure Study.[1] This is an ongoing project concerned with breast cancer in women and their exposure to carcinogens in household products. It began as a study of 120 women living on Cape Cod and is now reaching beyond that locale.

As part of the original study of Cape Cod women, sociologists examined how each woman made sense of and took action on three kinds of scientific information:

- her body burden of industrial chemicals (such as PCBs and phthalates),
- exposures to chemicals in her home based on air and dust samples, and
- the association of the air- and dust-born chemicals with common household products.[2]

It is a clear objective of the larger Silent Spring Institute's study to make science accessible to women at risk and help them make better health decisions. One of the unique features of the Silent Spring Institute's study is that it is a community-based, participatory research project. That means the participants were intimately and actively involved with the project, including access to researchers. This might not sound like much, but it's very unusual for a science project to have this participatory structure. It is a good thing.[3]

In addition to the women's participation in the project, researchers took great care to ensure that information was accessible. For example, each woman's results were presented to her in a way that compared her results to the results of the other women in the study and to EPA or other relevant guidelines. In addition, each woman was able to discuss her results at length with researchers.

Virtually all of the women in the study had levels of numerous chemicals in concentrations above EPA or other guidelines. For the most part, the women were surprised by the results—but few were alarmed. Many put the findings in context by talking to people they knew and by doing media research. Some even spoke directly to toxicologists involved with the project.

Contrary to expectations, most of the women made sense of their body burden by attributing it to external sources: polluting industries, dumping, power plants, military installations, and the like.

These women had trouble making sense of the chemicals in their homes' air and dust. They especially had difficulty connecting their body burden to household product exposure.

One of the sociologists' key findings was that, from these women's point of view, the toxic risk of external sources was "common knowledge" whereas the toxic risk from household products was not. Although a simplification, accepting household products as a health risk was not compatible with these women's lifestyles. The sociologists point specifically to norms for housekeeping and the association of particular product types with household tasks.

Another key finding was that most of the women made sense of the health risk from their body burden by comparing their levels to other women, not in relation to the guidelines. In addition, so long as she wasn't at the very top of the range, a woman tended to see her body burden as "normal," as nothing to cause alarm.

Each of these outcomes tells us volumes about the relationship between science and consumption.

First, it seems irrational on the face of it that someone provided with carefully crafted, credible science about health risks would fail to make the "obvious" connection between body burden and exposures to household products. A sense of incredulity seeps into the article at one point when the researchers report, "One participant attributed her exposures to her old house while a can of household insecticide sat, unmentioned, on an end table beside her."[4]

What this finding illustrates is that information is not enough— even the most carefully presented information, let alone what is haphazardly strewn throughout someone's daily life. More accurately, data is not enough. That's because human beings obtain a huge amount of information from what other people think and do, including how other's think.

This fact shows up in the second finding: the women gauged their own risk principally in relation to other women, not in relation to official guidelines and standards—in other words, the human scale weighed more heavily than the scientific scale. Again, this seems irrational. Instead of drawing the "obvious" conclusions from the science, these women chose to draw conclusions from their own and other women's experience.

A clash of cultures is on display here.

On the one hand, the researchers come to the information from the culture of science—what we've referred to as the culture of expertise. That culture has a particular ideology about what counts as a rational decision, represented most clearly in the economic practice of cost-benefit analysis: list the costs and benefits for alternative choices, then pick the one with the highest score.[5] The keystone of this ideology is the privileged position of official, sanctioned science.

On the other hand, the women making decisions in real time are not doing so based on what is obvious to the researchers. Instead, they're making decisions based on a variety of lifestyle and cultural cues as well as what we referred to earlier as local knowledge.

Marketing departments, of course, know this very well.[6] The sociologists conducting the Silent Spring Institute study also know it well. We all know it well. And we're all conditioned to believe that it's irrational, that bad decisions result when we take our eye off the science.

In contrast to this culturally privileged ideology of rationality and science, a growing body of research tells us that humans make decisions based on instinct, hunches, gut feelings, rules of thumb, and similar, essentially emotional, responses to their environment.[7] The most important element of our decision-making environment is other people—not as data sources, but as other minds from whom we take information about what to do. [8]

This repertoire of capacities has been called an adaptive toolbox.[9] It is based on the evolutionary theory that our Paleolithic ancestors had to make decisions quickly based on environmental cues under conditions of limited time and information. Those who had or developed the right capacities survived because they adapted successfully to the threats and opportunities they faced. Come to think of it, modern humans have to do the same thing.

So the women in the Silent Spring Institute study are not making irrational decisions by ignoring obvious and relevant scientific information. They are using their adaptive toolbox, their Paleolithic capacities to act on the science by understanding it in the context of other environmental cues.

Still, the question lingers: wouldn't the women have made better decisions if they had stuck to the science?

The question assumes that sticking to the science is inherently superior. It also assumes the "sticking to the science" is unambiguous. If this book is nothing else, it is a testament to the danger in failing to understand what "sticking to the science" actually means. Both assumptions are the basis for the ideology of expertise. It is just this bias that is being challenged by researchers of the adaptive toolbox.

But shouldn't these women be protected from making decisions based on instincts and emotions that are easily manipulated?

The simplest answer is that, yes, we all deserve to be protected. The critical question, of course, is who is doing the protecting, how are they doing it, and what's the basis for the protector's actions.

The common urge for protection by the culture of expertise assumes that Paleolithic decision-making capacities are inherently faulty. It's a very unscientific assumption. The question for protectors, including each person as a self-protector, should be how to create the right environmental cues for his Paleolithic capacities.

Instead of household products, consider children's food. In the first article in this section, "Starving Children," we discuss issues of manipulation and how food decisions are affected by environmental cues. Food manufacturers manipulate children into demanding Chocolate Frosted Sugar Bombs because they are permitted to create the environmental cues that children read using their Paleolithic adaptive toolbox. Better environmental cues would consist of, for example, edible schoolyard and farm-to-school programs that provide children with a tangible experience of whole foods.[10]

In the second article, "Health and Plastic," we discuss toxic plastics used in children's toys and attempts to reduce exposures. We describe how parents armed with science on toxic risks are met with contrary science by plastics and toy manufacturers and retailers allegedly responding to consumer demand. Most importantly, we challenge the assumption that plastics are a necessary part of modern life. For industry it might be necessary. For consumers, it is more a fact of life, not a lifestyle choice.

On that note, it's worth considering the role of lifestyle and culture as these affect consumption decisions that affect health. The literature on prevention overflows with use of "lifestyle." For example, researchers conducting a long-term study in England frame one of their reports by saying that a "huge body of evidence indicates that lifestyles such as smoking, diet, and physical activity have a major influence on health,"[11] going on to cite 16 studies.

Yet smoking, diet, and physical activity are not lifestyles. The researchers have confused behavior with lifestyle. Consider two people who have identical smoking, eating, and exercise habits. One could have a lifestyle common to the culture of working class Bronx residents while the other could have a lifestyle common to the culture of San Francisco avant-garde artists.

So when researchers talk about the relationship between lifestyle and the risk of illness and injury, they do so from a perspective that is extremely primitive with regard to culture. In other words, it would be extremely valuable to frame research based on how actual lifestyles and cultures affect consumption decisions and ultimately health itself. The most effective way to reduce smoking among working class Bronx residents is likely quite different from the most effective way to reduce smoking among avant-garde San Francisco artists.[12]

One of the few studies to address this issue looked at consumption of certain products that affect the risk of illness (such as smoking, alcohol, and vitamins), comparing consumption to social class. There was a consistent relationship: the "higher" someone's social class, the less likely they are to smoke and drink, and the more likely they are to take vitamins.[13] In another study, the quality of a person's diet (nutrient-dense versus calorie-dense) revealed the same relationship: "high" status people were more likely to have a nutrient-dense diet compared to "low" status people who were more likely to have a nutrient-poor, calorie-dense diet.[14] Is this because "low" status people have poor judgment? Not according to a careful study that found social and physical exposures rather than measures of intelligence to better explain differences in health outcomes.[15]

We introduced the concept of a system of provision in "Food" (on page 71) as integrating the material and cultural forces at work in the production and consumption of food. The concept is applicable to consumption generally and its relationship to health.[16]

The material forces consist of the specific processes for producing, distributing, and consuming products that fulfill human desires: for example, the range of products used to control household pests. The cultural forces consist of the specific social relationships that invest desire with meaning, assign meaning to products that fulfill the desire, and regulate production, distribution, and consumption activities: for example, the significance of toxins in pest control products. These are woven together so that a unique path is created from raw material to the act of consumption itself: for example, the toxic content of pest control products, their choice by consumers, and their use in the home.

There is a range of products available for controlling household pests, each with a unique system of provision. On the one hand, there are the highly commercial, toxin-laden products such as the "can of household insecticide" observed by the researchers. On the other hand, there are the environmentally benign pest control methods described in *Tiny Game Hunting: Environmentally Healthy Ways to Trap and Kill the Pests in Your House and Garden*.[17]

How could the women in the Silent Spring Institute study have made better use of the scientific information presented to them? The simple answer is better environmental cues.

We've already noted how marketing departments are well-versed in the art and science of creating environmental cues. In the past two decades, the discipline of social marketing has developed. Unlike commercial marketing, which is directed at creating desire for products, social marketing is directed at overcoming barriers to doing what is inherently desirable.

The smart practitioners of social marketing apply social marketing techniques as a community-based discipline. In other words, instead of experts manipulating people, the people of the community in question participate in developing ways to overcome barriers to desirable behavior, including what counts as desirable behavior.[18]

An answer to how the women of the Silent Spring Institute study could make better use of the scientific information they received has two parts. The first part consists of identifying the barriers that prevent them from eliminating toxic household products. The second part consists of creating the environmental cues that enable the women to overcome those barriers—for example, what would be needed to make the toxicity of household products common knowledge.

Notes

[1] Silent Spring Institute website http://www.silentspring.org/.

[2] Rebecca Gasior Altman, et al. (2008) "Pollution Comes Home and Gets Personal: Women's Experience of Household Chemical Exposure."

[3] A leading organization in participatory research is the DataCenter website http://www.datacenter.org/.

[4] Rebecca Gasior Altman, et al. (2008) "Pollution Comes Home and Gets Personal: Women's Experience of Household Chemical Exposure" page 425.

[5] Virtually any textbook in conventional microeconomics will have this ideology on full display. In Gerd Gigerenzer (2007) *Gut Feelings: The Intelligence of the Unconscious* pages 4-5, this ideology is illustrated by Benjamin Franklin's advice to his nephew about how to choose a wife and it's utter failure. For a criticism of cost-benefit analysis itself, see Frank Ackerman and Lisa Heinzerling (2004) *Priceless: On Knowing the Price of Everything and the Value of Nothing.*

[6] For example, see S. Ratneshwar, et al. eds (2000) *The Why of Consumption: Contemporary Perspectives on Consumer Motives, Goals, and Desires.*

[7] For example, see George Lakoff and Mark Johnson (1999) *Philosophy in the Flesh: The Embodied Mind and Its Challenge to Western Thought*, Gerd Gigerenzer (2007) *Gut Feelings: The Intelligence of the Unconscious*, Gerd Gigerenzer and Reinhard Selten eds (2001) *Bounded Rationality: The Adaptive Toolbox*, Gerd Gigerenzer (2000) *Adaptive Thinking: Rationality in the Real World*, Malcolm Gladwell (2005) *Blink: The Power of Thinking without Thinking*, and Gary Klein (1998) *Sources of Power: How People Make Decisions.*

[8] For example, see the discussion of how humans read other minds and speak and hear body language in Malcolm Gladwell (2005) *Blink: The Power of Thinking without Thinking* Chapter Six "Seven Seconds in the Bronx: The Delicate Art of Mind Reading," Beatrice de Gelder (2006b) "Towards the Neurobiology of Emotional Body Language," Beatrice de Gelder (2006a) "Toward a Biological Theory of Emotional Body Language," Susan

Hurley (2005) "Social Heuristics That Make Us Smarter," and Dan Sperber and Deirdre Wilson (2002) "Pragmatics, Modularity and Mind-Reading."

9   Gerd Gigerenzer and Reinhard Selten eds (2001) *Bounded Rationality: The Adaptive Toolbox.*

10   See Alice Waters's organization Edible Schoolyard website http://www.edibleschoolyard.org/ and the national organization Farm to School website http://www.farmtoschool.org/.

11   Kay-Tee Khaw, et al. (2008) "Combined Impact of Health Behaviours and Mortality in Men and Women: The EPIC-Norfolk Prospective Population Study."

12   Janet Brigham (1998) *Dying to Quit: Why We Smoke and How We Stop.*

13   Mark Tomlinson (2003) "Lifestyle and Social Class."

14   Nicole Darmon and Adam Drewnowski (2008) "Does Social Class Predict Diet Quality?" In this and most studies, social class is measured by some combination of income, education, and occupation. Wealth and pedigree are rarely used. See John Lynch and George Kaplan (2000) "Socioeconomic Position."

15   John Lynch, et al. (1997) "Why Do Poor People Behave Poorly? Variation in Adult Health Behaviours and Psychosocial Characteristics by Stages of the Socioeconomic Lifecourse."

16   Ben Fine (2002) *The World of Consumption: The Material and the Cultural Revisited.*

17   Hilary Dole Klein and Adrian M. Wenner (2001) *Tiny Game Hunting: Environmentally Healthy Ways to Trap and Kill the Pests in Your House and Garden.* Environmentally benign versions of the other household products are described in Debra Lynn Dadd (2005) *Home Safe Home: Creating a Healthy Home Environment by Reducing Exposure to Toxic Household Products* and *Debra Lynn Dadd Website* website http://www.dld123.com/.

18   See Doug McKenzie-Mohr and William Smith (1999) *Fostering Sustainable Behavior: An Introduction to Community-Based Social Marketing* and Fostering Sustainable Behavior website http://www.cbsm.com/public/world.lasso.

❧

STARVING CHILDREN

Food manufacturers spend $10 billion each year for advertising that targets children. Targets. Our children are targets. Of course, we're targets too, but that's another story.

Much of that money shows up in TV advertising. The Kaiser Family Foundation released a report on just how much children are exposed to food advertising on television. This is an easy punching bag so we'll only linger on a few statistics from the report.

Overall advertising that targets children: for children 2 to 7, 14,000 ads per year totaling 106 hours (that's almost 4½ days); for children 8 to 12, 30,000 ads per year totaling 230 hours (almost 10 days); and for children 13 to 17, 29,000 ads per year for 217 hours (9 days).

That's advertising for everything. For just food advertising that targets children: children 2 to 7, 4,400 ads per year for 30 hours; children 8 to 12, 7,600 ads per year for 50 hours; and children 13 to 17, 6,000 ads per year for 40 hours.

The bulk of foods advertised are candy, processed foods, cereal, and sugar-fortified drinks. There were no ads for fruits or vegetables. None.

Advergaming

A news article in the *San Francisco Chronicle* that covered the release of the Kaiser report opened with the story of a mother who wondered why her 7-year old son, who had been an avid fruit and vegetable guy, started asking for junk food. She spent a half hour with him watching his favorite TV program. Quite a surprise.

She'd have another rude surprise if she followed him to his favorite websites. In July 2006, Kaiser published another report on the new frontier of advertising that targets children: advergaming. As the name suggests, it is a blend of advertising and video games presented on the Internet.

Advergaming and the other methods being developed by those clever people in the marketing departments of our leading corporations employ all of the slick methods of the Internet, methods such as viral marketing—that's when a kid is asked to email a friend about her or his favorite advergaming site.

The virtue of this new frontier, expected to quadruple over the next five years, is that it's cheap compared to TV advertising and it doesn't have even the fangless FCC to oversee it. The industry, of course, has promised to behave itself and so on. Some people have to pretend that they believe it. You certainly shouldn't.

Protecting Children

Last year, the Institute of Medicine issued a report on the topic of advertising that targets children. Their recommendations, adopted by respectable organizations, consist of

* encouraging food manufacturers to use their creative talents to promote healthful diets for children,
* working with industry to develop a better code of conduct, and
* encouraging research to determine just how much marketing actually affects children.

Some obvious questions arise.

Who is going to do the encouraging? Why should corporations cooperate? The encouragers are likely to be the same public and private organizations the industry already works with. Why should we expect a significantly better outcome?

But suppose food manufactures respond. What constitutes a healthful diet for children? The current standard is the USDA guidelines. The food industry carries considerable weight in defining those guidelines. Even beyond that, the standards are a child-sized version of the low fat, low protein, high carbohydrate diet recommended for adults.

Putting children on this diet starves them of essential nutrients for growth, particularly fats. If breast milk is the preferred food for babies, would you not think that other foods should be like it? Breast milk is 55% fat.

As representatives of the Weston A. Price Foundation point out, the USDA's standard diet is very much like the recommended diet for fattening livestock.

As to working on a code of conduct, corporations are chartered to serve the public interest. They don't have a constitutional right to target children. We should apply a public health standard: if there's a possibility of harm, corporations should be prevented from marketing to children.

The same goes for the "more research" action item. The Institute of Medicine recommendations imply that marketing to children might have a small or large influence. What then constitutes too much influence? Why should corporations have any influence over children?

The Institute's recommendations simply dodge responsibility. Consider two alternative ideas.

Kids are very smart. Let's make media studies part of their education and help them become media savvy. Then they will be alert to when they're being manipulated and played for chumps.

On the industry side, let's make them contribute to a fund, $2 for every $1 they spend targeting children. The fund would be used specifically to make kids media savvy and to counter industry advertising with alternative content.

For obvious reasons we should avoid mandating what constitutes a "healthy diet" in that alternative content. Instead of dictating, educate kids to figure it out.

Junk Food, Fat Kids

The impetus for the two Kaiser reports and the Institute of Medicine report is the growing concern that children are too fat: the obesity epidemic among kids caused by junk food. It's a nice, neat causal chain: advertising leads to bad eating habits leads to obesity.

This view is quite wrong. As with adults, the increase in the number of fat kids is a symptom of something more profound. The eating problem behind it is not that kids are eating *too many* calories. The problem is that kids are eating *empty* calories: foods high in calories but lacking in micronutrients.

Recall what's being advertised: candy, processed foods, cereal, and sugar-fortified drinks. Kids are fat because they're malnourished, which doesn't mean too few calories, it means they're not getting the nutrients they need to thrive.

Kids' diets should consist principally of whole, fresh foods. Processed and packaged foods should be at a minimum. It can be done. And children need to be part of the process.

Food advertising that targets children isn't just making kids fat. It's ruining their health because the foods they're being manipulated to eat are empty calories. They're suffering from malnutrition. Our children are starving.

The News

Allday, Erin. 2007. Kids See Hours of Fast Food TV Ads. *San Francisco Chronicle*. March 29, 2007.

Raloff, Janet. 2007. How Advertising is Becoming Child's Play. *Science News Online*. July 29, 2006 (170:5). Access at http://www.sciencenews.org/articles/20060729/food.asp.

The Research

Gantz, Walter et al. 2007. Food for Thought: Television Food Advertising to Children in the United States. *Kaiser Family Foundation Report*. March 2007. Access at http://www.kff.org/entmedia/entmedia032807pkg.cfm.

Moore, Elizabeth. 2006. It's Child's Play: Advergaming and the Online Marketing of Food to Children. *Kaiser Family Foundation Report.* July 2006. Access at http://www.kff.org/entmedia/7536.cfm.

Resources

Your Own Health And Fitness. Resources on Food, Diet, and Nutrition. Access at http://www.yourownhealthandfitness.org/topicsFood.php.

Your Own Health And Fitness. Resources on Children's Health. Access at http://www.yourownhealthandfitness.org/topicsChildren.php.

HEALTH AND PLASTIC

For many people the word plastic suggests something cheap, perhaps tawdry, even unsavory. An article in the San Francisco Chronicle warns readers against going too far, reminding us of how plastics are essential to how we live.

The title of the article ("SF should drop ban on certain toys") suggests that the lunatic fringe governing San Francisco has gone too far and outlawed toys made from plastic.

But the first paragraph of the article makes it plain that the San Francisco Board of Supervisors had not Scrooged out. Instead, they had, as a result of parent activism, outlawed the sale of toys that contain chemicals believed to cause harm, in particular a chemical called bisphenol A or BPA.

No Cause for Concern?

The author of the article, Gilbert Ross, is medical director for a nonprofit named the American Council on Science and Health (ACSH). He argues that San Francisco's concerns are based on bad science and invites readers to his organization's website for a review of the research.

If you take Dr. Ross's invitation and go to his site you'll find one and only one piece of research cited: a literature review paid for by Ross's organization. Otherwise, the "review" consists of unsubstantiated claims about the weakness of BPA science and in particular the science about the health risks from low dose exposures to BPA and other endocrine disruptors.

As you have no doubt guessed, the ACSH is a notorious shill for chemical manufacturers. The American Chemistry Council (the chemical industry's trade organization and patron of the ACSH) was joined by the California Retailers Association, the California Grocers Association, and the Juvenile Products Manufacturers Association to file suit against San Francisco's action. This is the same group that successfully lobbied against statewide legislation.

Big money is at stake.

Bisphenol A

In contrast to the industry-friendly ACSH literature review, the August 2005 issue of *Environmental Health Perspectives* includes a thorough review of BPA research and finds considerable cause for alarm. In examining this research, the authors of the article note that there is a clear divide between independently-funded and industry-funded studies: 90% of independently-funded studies found an effect of low dose BPA exposure while none of the industry-funded studies found an effect.

You should not be surprised. Denial and doubt-mongering from made-up science paid for by business increase in proportion to the financial stake. Unfortunately, you have to wade through this nonsense because the mainstream media and government feel compelled to be, in what is now a heavily abused phrase, "fair and balanced."

Why is this a big deal?

Bisphenol A is literally everywhere. The CDC estimates that 95% of people in the United States have a measurable amount in their body. It is a chemical that hardens plastics. It's used to make toys that babies will inevitably chew on. It's used to make baby bottles that babies drink from. It's also used to line cans and food containers. It's the most common substrate for polycarbonate plastics used for CDs and DVDs, Nalgene bottles, signs, lenses for eyewear, resins used in dental composite fillings, and on and on.

When BPA-containing plastics are exposed to acidic or alkaline environments, the leaching of BPA accelerates. Heat and repeated washing do the same thing. One of the biggest sources of BPA is drinking water where landfills containing plastics (including what's in electronic circuit boards) release BPA into surface and ground water.

BPA exposure is linked to breast cancer and prostate cancer, insulin resistance, miscarriage, and the disruption of children's neurological development. Some scientists compare its potential effects to DES (diethylstilbestrol), a fertility drug given to women that caused incredible damage to the daughters and granddaughter of those treated.

Bisphenol A is a risk. In principle, we accept those risks because of the wonderful things BPA does for us.

Soft, Squishy, and Everywhere

Phthalates are another chemical added to plastics. Instead of making plastics hard, phthalates make PVC (polyvinyl chloride) soft, squishy, and pliable. Phthalates are used in children's toys (think rubber duckies), squeeze bottles, surgical tubing and a wide range of medical devices, floor coverings, and sex toys.

This substance shows up in some places you might not expect, places that you don't immediately think of as soft, squishy, and pliable. Phthalates are used in personal care products such as insect repellants, hair spray, perfumes, nail polish, and lubricants. It's also in car upholstery and accounts in part for the "new car smell." When a car's interior heats up, volatile phthalates outgas from the seats, head-lining, and dash. When the car cools, the phthalates condense and form a greasy film on the interior surfaces, including the windshield.

Most interesting of all, phthalates are used for time-released capsules. A drug or any other substance that is released slowly into your system is delivered in a capsule coated with phthalates that resist digestion.

Like bisphenol A, phthalates are almost everywhere and are a health risk. Exposure in the home affects the development of aller-gies and asthma. Exposure in the womb affects genital and brain de-velopment. Exposure lowers sperm counts and promotes early breast development in girls.

The CDC's 2003 study of chemical exposures found metabolites of phthalates in almost all of the 250 people examined. The Environ-mental Working Group's *BodyBurden* report that same year found traces in all of the nine people they carefully studied.

It's possible to make a rubber ducky (or a sex toy, for that mat-ter) without using phthalates. The reason they're used is that PVC is ridiculously cheap compared to the rubber or latex or other soft, squishy, pliable materials that phthalate-impregnated PVC can re-place.

Do we need the wonderful things BPA and phthalates do for us? No.

There are alternatives, even though the alternatives might mean living differently. But as long as money is involved, there will be lies masquerading as science about the dangers of BPA, about the dan-gers of endocrine disruptors, about the dangers of materials industry finds useful and cheap in making the commodities it's convinced us we need, the commodities it's convinced us we can't live without, the commodities it's convinced us our children can't live without.

It's not enough to ban some toys. We need to choose and create safe alternatives.

The News

Fischer, Douglas. 2007. Scientists Expose Body Toxin Risks: Synthetic Chemicals May Affect Two Generations' Ability To Have Children. *Oak-land Tribune*. February 2, 2007.

Kay, Jane. 2006. Toxic Toys: San Francisco Prepares To Ban Certain Chemi-cals in Products for Kids, but Enforcement Will Be Tough -- and Toymak-ers Question Necessity. *San Francisco Chronicle*. November 19, 2006.

Ross, Gilbert. 2007. SF Should Drop Ban on Certain Toys. *San Francisco Chronicle*. January 7, 2007.

The Research

Andrade, Anderson et al. 2006. A Dose–response Study Following *In Utero* and Lactational Exposure to Di-(2-ethylhexyl)-phthalate (DEHP). *Toxicology.* October 29, 2006 (227:3): 185-92.

Bornehag, Carl-Gustav et al. 2005. The Association Between Asthma and Allergic Symptoms in Children and Phthalates in House Dust. *Environmental Health Perspectives.* October 2004 (112:14): 1393-7. DOI:10.1289/ehp.7187.

Centers for Disease Control and Prevention. 2003. *Second National Report on Human Exposure to Environmental Chemicals.* Atlanta, GA: National Center for Environmental. NCEH Pub. No. 02-0716.

Hauser, Russ et all. 2004. Medications as a Source of Human Exposure to Phthalates. *Environmental Health Perspectives.* May 2004 (112:6): 751-3.

vom Saal, Frederick and Claude Hughes. 2005. An Extensive New Literature Concerning Low-Dose Effects of Bisphenol A Shows the Need for a New Risk Assessment. *Environmental Health Perspectives.* August 2005 (113:8) 926-33. DOI:10.1289/ehp.7713.

Resources

Baillie-Hamilton, Paula. 2005. *Toxic Overload.* New York: Avery.

Colborn, Theo, et al. 1996. Our Stolen Future: Are We Threatening Our Fertility, Intelligence, and Survival? A Scientific Detective Story. New York, Dutton.

Environmental Working Group. 2005. *Skin Deep.* Access at http://www.ewg.org/reports/skindeep/.

Houlihan, Jane et al. 2003. *BodyBurden: The Pollution in People.* Environmental Working Group. Access at http://www.ewg.org/reports/bodyburden1/.

Health Care Without Harm, PVC and DEHP. Access at http://www.noharm.org/us/pvcDehp/issue/.

Our Stolen Future, About Phthalates. Access at http://www.ourstolenfuture.org/NEWSCIENCE/oncompounds/phthalates/phthalates.htm#.

Our Stolen Future, About Bisphenol A. Access at http://www.ourstolenfuture.org/NEWSCIENCE/oncompounds/bisphenola/bpauses.htm.

147

Why are products scented with fragrances cooked up in a lab? The list includes hand soap, dishwashing soap, all-purpose cleaners, laundry detergent, fabric softener, dryer sheets, room fresheners, scented candles, shampoo, hair conditioner, cologne, after-shave, synthetic perfume, deodorant, and make-up.

The simple answer is that it promotes sales. What has happened over the past several decades is that the addition of artificial fragrance to products has become the norm. It is the default. It is what our noses expect, like it or not. The absence of fragrance is more likely to be noticed than its presence—unless, of course, you're one of the many people who react badly to artificial fragrance. This is not a small number—one estimate puts it at 30% of the population.[1]

Little research has been done on the health effects of these pervasive substances. What research there is should concern us.

The most systematic study to date[2] by Dr. Anne Steinemann at the University of Washington found a significant number of toxic substances not listed on household product labels. These ingredients were also not on the manufacturer's material safety data sheet (MSDS), a document used by the Occupational Safety and Health Administration (OSHA) to protect workers who handle materials used in manufacturing.

In other words, even a very careful shopper or worker could not determine his toxic exposure from these products.

If these ingredients aren't listed anywhere, how did the researcher identified them? Two standard processes for analyzing chemicals were used: gas chromatography and mass spectrometry. These methods work specifically on volatile organic compounds—VOCs. So the results of the analysis were limited to what these products put into the air but not chemicals transferred by direct contact.

Six products were analyzed: three air fresheners and three laundry products. The air freshener products tested were a solid disk commonly used in lavatories, a wall-mounted mister used in schools and medical institutions, and an evaporator that plugs into an electrical socket used in both homes and institutions. The laundry products tested were a dryer sheet, a liquid fabric softener, and a liquid detergent.

Fifty-eight separate VOCs were found, including ethanol, acetaldehyde, acetone, benzaldehyde, chloromethane, ethyl acetate, and many, many more that are regulated as toxic or hazardous by one or another Federal regulatory agency. The research article discusses the regulatory environment for these products with regard to consumer protection. Because the formulas to artificial fragrances are heavily protected as trade secrets, manufacturers are free to put whatever artificial fragrance they want in their products and tell no one about it.

The Fragrance Materials Association of the United States is the fragrance industry's trade organization, to fragrance what the AMA is to medicine. A representative of the Association responded to this research by saying, "We are certain that, when used in compliance with standards, these fragrance ingredients are safe and can be used ... with confidence."[3]

What standards? There are, for all practical purposes, none.

We're being told to pay no attention to the science. Our clothes smell fresh and bright. Our homes and workplaces and our children's schools smell like a spring day. Isn't that great? And best of all, we get to enjoy artificial fragrance everywhere you go!

Researchers at UC Berkeley's Indoor Environment Laboratory prepared a report for the California Air Resources Board on the indoor air chemistry of common cleaning products.[4] Many of the VOCs released from these products are toxic just by themselves. But once in the air these chemicals do what chemicals like to do: they react with each other. So two non-toxic chemicals can react to produce a third that is toxic. Or two toxic chemicals can react to produce a third that is more toxic than the sum of the original two alone.

When we interviewed her, Dr. Steinemann acknowledged that she was unable to evaluate these secondary atmospheric reactions, but that they are almost certainly going on. She also noted that we know virtually nothing about the long-term effects from exposures to these ubiquitous chemicals.[5]

The people who react to artificial fragrance might be lucky. They avoid fragranced products like the plague. For those who don't suffer an acute reaction and so don't avoid artificial fragrance, what happens to their health after 20 to 40 years of exposure? What happens to children who spend there entire lives exposed?

As in too many instances, industry is conducting an uncontrolled medical experiment. And in this case it's for absolutely no good purpose, other than to improve sales. We don't need it. It's acutely toxic to many people. And it's likely to have chronic health effects for the rest of us.

This is not an instance of ill-informed consumers making imprudent choices. It's not possible for consumers to be informed at all. The case of artificial fragrance is only an extreme example in a system of industrial production based on unequal knowledge that favors business. There are two principle reasons.

First, consumers must stay informed on a vast array of products in their spare time while businesses need only pay attention to information that affects their product, recorded as a cost of doing business covered in the selling price paid by consumers. In other words, consumers pay to be kept in the dark and then, in order to overcome that ignorance, must spent time to educate themselves. Second, businesses have considerable control over what information reaches consumers, as Dr. Steinemann's research illustrates.

The economist Joseph Stiglitz, now famous for his critique of corporate globalization, received a Nobel prize for his work in showing that this information bias in favor of business is systematic and prevents markets from working effectively in the absence of external intervention.[6] Nevertheless, influential voices argue for the basic dynamic of business culture as the best way to achieve health-conscious products and production by bolstering well-informed consumers.[7]

In addition to the dynamics we discussed in "Consumption" (on page 131) that are at work when consumers make decisions, the production side of systems of provision have their own dynamic. The cynical version of that dynamic is that businesses pursue profits to the exclusion of all else. That's only half the story, half the problem, and indicates where much more than half the solution is to be found.

In addition to making as much as they can as fast and they can, businesses have to do two other things: first, they have to design a product that people will actually buy and, second, they must do what needs to be done in order to stay in business. Neither is a trivial task.

Consider product design. Many detergent manufacturers are responding to demand for "green" products by offering unscented cleaners. However, as Dr. Steinemann describes, "unscented" does not mean "without fragrance." So-called unscented products have chemicals added to mask the scent of the detergent. In other words, the manufacturers were solving a production problem, not solving a problem as conceived by consumers.

This problem is not peculiar to the health effects of fragranced products, industrial chemicals, or chemical wastes from production processes generally.[8] Fundamental to any business production process, however well intentioned, is an insurmountable conflict. On one side, people have needs to meet—including the need to avoid health risks. On the other side, businesses must make money, stay in business, and design products that sell. As we are all too frequently reminded, "products that sell" does not mean "meets peoples' needs," particularly as it concerns health effects.

For example, "green" and "sustainable" have become common selling points for products.[9] The dynamic is an old one: producers see an advantage in selling products to consumers who associate, for example, "green" and "sustainable" with desirable lifestyle and cultural practices. This dynamic has given rise to the practice of greenwashing, in which producers misrepresent their products and practices as environmentally responsible.[10]

Some well-intentioned businesses might attend to reconciling this conflict. However, the world of business in general does not. Instead, a wide range of actors intervenes to reconcile what people need to what businesses are able to sell. The two most important are government agencies and citizen activists—and it is virtually always citizens who prompt government take action.

For example, baby bottle manufacturers have pledged to cease use of bisphenol A after a long campaign by parents and environmental groups, extensive media coverage, and focused attention by lawmakers about the health risks.[11] And although Dr. Steinemann describes how the use of fragrance is virtually unregulated, it's likely that we are in the early stages of a process that will lead to better regulation.

The limitations of the regulatory process are illustrated by the US Food and Drug Administration. Pharmaceuticals are designed to have specific, allegedly beneficial effects. The FDA requires pharmaceuticals to be both effective (beneficial use) and safe (designed to minimize any negative effects). It's a regulatory requirement that pharmaceutical companies have to meet in order to stay in business. Yet even under this allegedly tight regulation, the toxic effects of pharmaceutical products are widespread.

The following are some examples. One study found that adverse drug reactions during hospitalization killed approximately 181,000 people each year.[12] A study in a highly computerized (and presumably tightly managed) hospital found that over half of the patients were admitted because of an adverse drug reaction.[13] A study of hospital emergency rooms found that over 700,000 visits (about 2.5% of the total) were due to adverse drug reactions.[14] Finally, the Florida Medical Examiners Commission announced in its 2007 annual report that prescription drugs killed four times as many people as street drugs.[15]

This litany is intended to illustrate the limits of regulation as a mediator between human need and business practices in the wide variety of medical systems of provision. The two articles in this section illustrate others.

The first article, "Chemical Exposures and Breast Cancer," examines how current practices divert breast cancer research, media attention, and, to a great degree, citizen activism away from risks posed by industrial chemicals in products and production. As the article discusses, this is an ongoing failure of cancer research in the

United States. It raises the issue of why cancer institutions are not in the forefront of the fight to reduce chemical exposures but instead focus almost exclusively on treatments.

In the second article, "Pollution, Body Fat, and Blood Sugar," we discuss how pesticides commonly used in industrial agriculture contribute to the rise in body weight (diagnosed as overweight and obesity) and blood sugar derangement (diagnosed as diabetes, insulin resistance, and metabolic syndrome). Once again, research, media, and activist attention are focused on treatments instead of the prevention of environmental causes.

The lesson is complementary to that found in "Consumption:" information, lifestyle, and culture shape the production side of systems of provision. So doing the simplest thing first on the production side consists of attending to those activities outside the marketplace that promote responsible production practices.

This takes some imagination. We offer two ideas here.

The regulatory environment in Europe is diverging from that of the US. In 2007, the European Parliament passed legislation that created REACH—a tortured acronym for **R**egistration, Evaluation, Authorisation and Restriction of **Ch**emical Substances. In essence, REACH makes the precautionary principle the criteria for the use of chemicals in products: before a chemical can be used, it must be proven safe.[16] Ironically, this new practice has caused the US to become a dumping ground for toxin-laden products that can't be sold in Europe and other countries that conform to REACH.[17] Unfortunately, as Dr. Steinemann reported in our interview with her, REACH does not cover fragrance.[18]

The basis of REACH is the precautionary principle.[19] Although stated in a variety of ways, the basic idea is that when taking action, the objective should be met using technologies known to be safe. Through the advocacy of citizens, many local governments are adopting the precautionary principle for how they plan, build, and purchase.[20]

With regard to product and process design itself, a growing number of engineers and designers are actively promoting the idea of non-toxic, non-polluting product and process design. Some believe that producers have an incentive to adopt such cradle-to-cradle, sustainable products and processes in order to lower costs by reducing waste, create more appealing products, and avoid health risks that threaten business stability.[21] Whether or not that is the case, the cradle-to-cradle concept is less about protecting businesses than it is about creating production processes that are inherently low risk. Along a complementary line, a group of biologists working under the conceptual umbrella of biomimicry promote sustainable product and process design based on biological processes.[22] So it seems that not only does the body act as an ecology but so can the processes that meet our needs.

Notes

1 Stanley Caress and Anne Steinemann (2009) "Prevalence of Frangrance Sensitivity in the American Population."
2 Anne Steinemann (2008b) "Fragranced Consumer Products and Undisclosed Ingredients."
3 Lynette Evans (2008) "Forget the Fragrance."
4 William W Nazaroff, et al. (2006) *Indoor Air Chemistry: Cleaning Agents, Ozone and Toxic Air Contaminants.*
5 Anne Steinemann (2008a) "Foul Fragrance."
6 Joseph E. Stiglitz (1987) "The Causes and Consequences of the Dependence of Quality on Price."
7 For example, Paul Hawkin, et al. (1999) *Natural Capitalism: Creating the Next Industrial Revolution.*
8 For example, Philip Shabecoff and Alice Shabecoff (2008) *Poisoned Profits: The Toxic Assault on Our Children,* Mark Schapiro (2007) *Exposed: The Toxic Chemistry of Everyday Products and What's at Stake for American Power,* Gerald Markowitz and David Rosner (2002) *Deceit and Denial: The Deadly Politics of Industrial Pollution,* and Dan Fagin, et al. (1996) *Toxic Deception: How the Chemical Industry Manipulates Science, Bends the Law, and Endangers Your Health.*
9 However, "green" and "sustainable" do not necessarily mean that a product is without health risks. See Layna Berman and Jeffry Fawcett (2007) "Does Green Mean Non-Toxic?"
10 For example, Greenpeace, Greenwashing http://stopgreenwash.org/.
11 Lyndsey Layton (2009) "No BPA for Baby Bottles in U.S.."
12 Donald Barlett and James Steele (2004) *Critical Condition: How Health Care in America Became Big Business and Bad Medicine,* pp 55-6.
13 Jonathan R. Nebeker, et al. (2005) "High Rates of Adverse Drug Events in a Highly Computerized Hospital."
14 Daniel S. Budnitz, et al. (2006) "National Surveillance of Emergency Department Visits for Outpatient Adverse Drug Events."
15 Damien Cave (2008) "Legal Drugs Kill Far More Than Illegal, Florida Says" and Medical Examiners Commission (2007) *Drugs Identified in Deceased Persons by Florida Medical Examiners: 2007 Interim Report.*
16 Mark Schapiro (2007) *Exposed: The Toxic Chemistry of Everyday Products and What's at Stake for American Power.*
17 Mark Schapiro (2008) "Why the US Is Importing Toxic Products."
18 Anne Steinemann (2008a) "Foul Fragrance."
19 See Mary O'Brien (2000) *Making Better Environmental Decisions: An Alternative to Risk Assessment.*
20 Science and Environmental Health Network http://www.sehn.org/.
21 See Michael Braungart, et al. (2007) "Cradle-to-Cradle Design: Creating Healthy Emissions E a Strategy for Eco-Effective Product and System Design" and William McDonough and Michael Braungart (2002) *Cradle to Cradle: Remaking the Way We Make Things.*
22 See Janine M. Benyus (1997) *Biomimcry: Innovation Inspired by Nature,* Biomimcry Guild http://www.biomimicryguild.com/, and Biomimcry Institute http://www.biomimicryinstitute.org/.

CHEMICAL EXPOSURES AND BREAST CANCER

There are over 80,000 chemicals not found in nature that are in commercial use in the United States. Of these, the Environmental Protection Agency has developed estimates of the toxicity for only a tiny fraction. The Occupational Safety and Health Administration requires medical surveillance for exposure to only 11 of the 80,000 chemicals.

In 2007, the *Los Angeles Times* carried news with the headline "Common chemicals are linked to breast cancer." Three studies published in the online edition of the journal *Cancer*, a publication of the National Cancer Institute, were the subject of the *Times* article. The studies were not original research but instead were reviews of the science available on the association between breast cancer and chemicals and nutrition.

Only 152 instances of research on the association of chemicals to breast cancer were found. In contrast, over 1,500 instances of research on the relationship between diet and breast cancer were identified.

Fewer Studies, Greater Risks

In the 152 studies of the relationship between chemicals and breast cancer, 216 separate chemicals were examined. The reviewers of this research found a strong and consistent association. However, when the reviewers examined research on diet and breast cancer, no comparably strong and consistent relationship was found.

The reviewers of these studies were quick to point out that the strong and consistent association of chemicals with breast cancer didn't prove conclusively that, for example, a common solvent such as methylene chloride causes breast cancer. What exactly does that caution really mean?

It means that conclusive proof is required before action is necessary. What they're waiting for is a series of repeated clinical studies showing the biological mechanisms that lead from methylene chloride to breast cancer. Without that smoking gun, the cancer establishment doesn't want to do anything extreme such as restricting the use of the chemical or enforcing special precautions in handling the material. And they would never call for the outright banning of a chemical.

This, of course, is utter nonsense. If there's a suggestion of harm, then a reasonable person would take steps to minimize the risk.

What these 152 studies really show is that a great deal of time and money has been thrown at the relationship between women's diets and breast cancer whereas the effect of those 80,000 chemicals has received crumbs. However, with these studies you might think that the cancer establishment is finally waking up to the dangers of our chemical-laden world. You'd be wrong.

Wake Up Call

The National Cancer Institute didn't fund these studies. They were funded by a private foundation called Susan G. Komen for the Cure, an organization dedicated to breast cancer activism. The reviews were not conducted through the National Cancer Institute but by researchers at the Silent Spring Institute. In addition to the studies, a database of the chemicals is available on their website (see Resources).

It is alarming that methylene chloride and the other 215 chemicals that have been studied might cause breast cancer. It is even more alarming that the remaining 79,784 chemicals haven't been studied at all. Are all of them harmful? Are all of them safe?

A more important question is why we have to prove, conclusively or otherwise, that any of these chemicals cause cancer or any other kind of biological mischief. Why don't manufacturers of methylene chloride and the rest have to prove that they don't cause harm?

REACH

These are exactly the questions being asked in the European Union by regulatory agencies. This year they launched the Registration, Evaluation, Authorisation, and Restriction of Chemical Substances (REACH) system that now requires all new chemicals to have science to showing they're safe to use. Over the next 10 years, all existing chemicals currently in use must have science showing that they're safe. If they fail the test, they cannot be used.

REACH is one of the many ways in which the precautionary principle is being implemented in Europe—that is, when a substance or technology is about to be introduced into our environment, the burden of proof is to show that it is safe. In large part this is a consequence of Europe's public health tradition, far stronger than that of the United States.

As journalist Mark Schapiro discusses in his book *Exposed*, what's happening in Europe affects what happens in and to the United States. The dark prospect is that the chemical Wild West of the United States will become a dumping ground for chemicals and products containing those chemicals that manufacturers can't sell in

Europe. The bright prospect is that the United States will be forced to step up to the higher European standards.

Before you stand and cheer for the precautionary principle, note that we as individuals are in the same boat with chemical manufacturers. Air pollution from burning fossil fuels includes polycyclic aromatic hydrocarbons, which are associated with breast cancer.

Then there are the more complicated problems of dealing with chemicals that are byproducts such as dioxins. That would require eliminating use of any material that when burnt produces them. Finally, there are legacy chemicals such as PCBs (polychlorinated biphenyls) that haven't been produced in years, yet they're still floating around and bioaccumulating in body fat and breast milk. PCBs are also associated with breast cancer.

It sounds overwhelming and guilt-ridden. But the situation is neither. It simply calls for doing what you are able to do using your own best judgment and the resources at your disposal.

But don't expect the National Cancer Institute and the American Cancer Society to lead the way. "Prevention" is not in their vocabulary.

The News

Cone, Maria. 2007. Common Chemicals Are Linked to Breast Cancer. *Los Angeles Times*. May 14, 2007.

Raloff, Janet. 2007. How Advertising is Becoming Child's Play. *Science News Online*. July 29, 2006 (170:5). Access at http://www.sciencenews.org/articles/20060729/food.asp.

The Research

Brody, Julia et al. 2007. Environmental Pollutants and Breast Cancer. *Cancer*. June 15, 2007 (109: 12 Suppl): 2667–711.

Clapp, Richard et al. 2007. *Environmental and Occupational Causes of Cancer: New Evidence, 2005–2007*. Lowell, Massachusetts: Lowell Center for Sustainable Production, University of Massachusetts.

Rudel, Ruthann et al. 2007. Chemicals Causing Mammary Gland Tumors in Animals Signal New Directions for Epidemiology, Chemicals Testing, and Risk Assessment for Breast Cancer Prevention. *Cancer*. June 15, 2007 (109: 12 Suppl): 2635–66.

Resources

Collaborative on Health and the Environment, Breast Cancer Working Group. Access at http://www.healthandenvironment.org/working_groups/br_cancer.

Schapiro, Mark. 2007. *Exposed: The Toxic Chemistry of Everyday Products and What's at Stake for American Power*. White River Jct, Vermont: Chelsea Green Publishing.

Silent Spring Institute. Access at http://www.silentspring.org/.

Susan G. Komen for the Cure. Access at http://cms.komen.org/komen/index.htm.

Your Own Health And Fitness. Resources on Cancer. Access at http://www.yourownhealthandfitness.org/topicsCancer.php.

Your Own Health And Fitness. Resources on Environmental Health. Access at http://www.yourownhealthandfitness.org/topicsEnvironment.php.

POLLUTION, BODY FAT, AND BLOOD SUGAR

It is somewhat old news that we are in the midst of an obesity and diabetes epidemic. Less well publicized is the dramatic increase in insulin resistance, a precursor to both.

The percentage of people diagnosed with diabetes has been growing steadily for at least half a century. The percentage of people classified as obese has been growing steadily for four decades.

Conventional medicine has been quick to apply pharmaceuticals and surgery to these health problems. As for prevention, public health officials have wrung their hands over imprudent diets and lack of exercise. The causes have been cast as the result of the personal sins of gluttony and sloth.

A search is in progress for the genetic causes of the obesity and diabetes epidemics as well, principally it seems to screen for those at risk and to develop designer drugs for them. However, as we have said many times, genes do their work in response to an individual's environment.

Unfortunately, research on the relationship between environmental pollution, body fat, and blood sugar derangement has been paltry compared to the well-financed research into gluttony and sloth. This is quite surprising since the rapid rise in obesity and diabetes are clearly the result of environmental changes.

Persistent Organic Pollutants

Following the Vietnam War, the Veterans Administration (VA) found a disproportionate number of soldiers diagnosed with diabetes along with a wide range of other ailments. These were men and women who had been exposed to Agent Orange, an herbicide used to defoliate the Vietnamese countryside.

After almost two decades of struggle, afflicted veterans were able to force the VA to acknowledge exposure to Agent Orange as a presumptive cause of diabetes. As a consequence, vets could be treated through the VA.

The principle active ingredient in Agent Orange is dioxin. For some time it was used domestically in herbicides. However, its toxic effects caused it to be outlawed from use in the United States.

"Dioxin" describes a class of chemicals rather than a single chemical. So it is more accurate to refer to the plural dioxins. Although no longer available in the United States, dioxins pollute our environment as byproducts of manufacturing and burning of plastics. Dioxins are only one class among many persistent organic pollutants (POPs).

POPs are organic because they are carbon compounds, not because they are in any way "natural." They are persistent because it takes a long time for natural processes to turn them into chemicals that are not toxic. They are also persistent because they accumulate in body fat.

Body Burden

The Centers for Disease Control and Prevention (CDC) now maintains a program for monitoring the level of POPs in our bodies. The database tracks 148 chemicals found in the blood of people participating in the National Health and Nutrition Examination (NHANES). NHANES is a detailed examination of the health and illness status of a large sample of people. The sample is representative of the entire US population.

The latest CDC study in this series was published in 2005. It used blood and urine samples taken from NHANES participants to look for levels of 148 chemicals, including POPs. This number is small in comparison to the estimated 80,000 unique chemicals that are released into the environment by human activity. Although the CDC study did not find all 148 chemicals in every blood sample, it did find all 148 chemicals in one group of people or another. In other words, these toxins are widespread in our blood.

Using the same NHANES data source, Duk-Hee Lee and her colleagues examined the relationship between the level of a very limited number of POPs and the incidence of insulin resistance and diabetes. They found a strong dose-response relationship for some but not all of the POPs and the chance that an NHANES participant was either diabetes or insulin resistant.

What that means is that as the concentration of POPs increased, the number of people with diabetes or insulin resistance increased. Virtually every chemical studied was associated with diabetes. Fewer were associated with insulin resistance. Because insulin resistance is the most common condition leading to diabetes, this result suggests that the unique biology of some individuals makes them particularly vulnerable to POPs as a disruptor of energy metabolism.

The Environmental Working Group's BodyBurden study found that even people who are very health conscious test positive for these chemicals. The Lee research group found that concentrations were greater for people with low income.

Detoxification

Obesity has been made the whipping boy for diabetes and insulin resistance. The Lee study seems to confirm that view and became a highlight of the news reports on this study. What the Lee group found was that POPs concentrations tended to increase with waist circumference.

However, unique biology seems to be at play here as well. The relationship of POPs to body weight is only striking at the extreme highs of POP concentrations or waist sizes. The question that goes begging is whether POPs have an effect on obesity itself, a hypothesis that conventional researchers have shunned.

We can see this weakness in the CDC and Lee research. Both are based on the level of POPs to which tissues are exposed as detected in people's blood but not what they're carrying in their fat tissue. In other words, these studies measure what a person's body is actually capable of clearing from her or his body. The toxin could come from an immediate exposure (for example, breathing a toxic vapor) or from clearing of the toxin from fat cells.

Left unanswered is the relationship of toxins sequestered in fat tissues to obesity, insulin resistance, and diabetes. We know from animal studies that POPs bioaccumulate so it's reasonable to assume they bioaccumulate in humans too. It's also unlikely that every person sheds these accumulated toxins with equal efficiency.

The lesson to learn from these studies is that we should avoid exposures. They also suggest that detoxification makes sense. Many people have been mistakenly convinced that fasting and purging programs labeled "detox" are the way to remove toxins. Such methods can be dangerous by exposing the person fasting to large doses of toxins released from fat cells. And they're unnecessary.

As we discuss in the Your Own Health And Fitness show "Detoxification," there are many safe and natural ways to promote detoxification. These methods support the body's innate capacity to remove toxins. As this latest research suggests, aggressive detoxification risks increasing your exposure to toxins.

The News
Coghlan, Andy. 2006. Diabetes Spotlight Falls onto Fish. New Scientist. September 30, 2006.

Pearson, Aria. 2007. Obesity's Helper in Triggering Diabetes. New Scientist. April 14, 2007.

The Research
Centers for Disease Control and Prevention. 2005. Third National Report on Human Exposure to Environmental Chemicals. Atlanta, Georgia: National Center for Environmental Health. NCEH Pub. No. 05-0570. July 2005.

Houlihan, Jane et al. 2003. BodyBurden: The Pollution in People. Washington, DC: Environmental Working Group. January 2003. Access at http://www.ewg.org.

Lee, Duk-Hee et al. 2007. Association Between Serum Concentrations of Persistent Organic Pollutants and Insulin Resistance Among Nondiabetic Adults. Diabetes Care. March 2007(30:3): 622-8. DOI:10.2337/dc06-2190.

Lee, Duk-Hee et al. 2006. A Strong Dose-Response Relation Between Serum Concentrations of Persistent Organic Pollutants and Diabetes. Diabetes Care. July 2006(29:7): 1638-44. DOI:10.2337/dc06-0543.

Resources

Berman, Layna. 2006. Detoxification. Your Own Health And Fitness. Broadcast September 19, 2006.

Colborn, Theo, et al. 1996. Our Stolen Future: Are We Threatening Our Fertility, Intelligence, and Survival? A Scientific Detective Story. New York, Dutton.

Fawcett, Jeffry. 2007. Blood Sugar Derangement. Progressive Health Observer. Winter 2007 (11): 7.

Our Stolen Future. Access at http://www.ourstolenfuture.org.

Your Own Health And Fitness. Resources on Detoxification and Addiction. Access at http://www.yourownhealthandfitness.org/topicsDetox.php.

The idea that health comes from how each person's unique biology responds to its environment is making headway in the scientific literature. The causation works in the other direction as well—our unique biology calls upon us to change our environment. It's an ongoing dance.

As an example, a study reported in the *Public Library of Science Genetics* argues that the environment can affect genes, those bits of DNA that allegedly define our biological uniqueness. The research is not about alterations in the DNA sequence that result from exposures to toxins. Instead, the research shows how gene expression itself is changed in response to geography and culture.[1]

The researchers studied a Moroccan people called the Amarigh. DNA sequencing identifies them as genetically very homogeneous. The Amarigh live in three distinct environments, each with a distinct culture: urban slum, mountain settlement, and desert nomad.

When the researchers looked at each population's white blood cells, they found a significant difference between which genes were at work, despite the significant similarity in the Amrigh's individual genes. What this means is that her immune system worked differently depending on where an Amarigh lived. It also means that simply having a specific version of a gene does not by itself put someone at a greater or lesser risk of disease and injury. What matters is how gene versions respond to their environment.

For example, the gene that produces immune factors involved with asthma were significantly more active in urban Amarigh compared to mountain dwellers and nomads. In other words, an Amarigh who moved from the city to the mountains would downregulate genes associated with asthma—that is, asthma genes would be less active. This is an example of what we discussed in "Epigenetics and Proteomics" on page 34.

It's no surprise that changing the environment to which a person is exposed will change her health. However, what this and related research suggests is that her unique biology, the very way in which her body responds to an environmental provocation is changed.

This raises a number of salient questions. What environments promote health? How can they be found? How can they be created?

This and the following three sections look at these issues. In effect, we will be discussing the environmental cues that are the basis of health decisions. In this section, we examine how someone's personal environment affects his health and his risk of illness and injury. In subsequent sections, we look at how built environments, natural environments, and social environments affect health and the risk of illness and injury.

By *personal environment* we mean that realm over which a person has a high degree of control. In other words, the environmental cues he creates for himself. Some examples...

- what's in his refrigerator
- how he controls pests that show up in his kitchen
- how he decorates his living space
- how he arranges his work space
- how he decorates himself
- where his living space is located
- electrical and electronic devices he uses
- whether he allows smoking in his living space
- scented products he uses

Each of these is a particular kind of exposure that can affect his health and risk of illness and injury. Careful consideration of each suggests that they are not entirely up to him. For example, what's in his refrigerator depends on what he can afford and his access to alternative food sources. So we're not promoting the tired idea that someone's health is entirely up to him. We know enough about the social determinants of health to avoid that pit. We'll discuss that side of the issue in the next three sections.

Two news items highlight the issue of how each person can adapt his personal environment for better health and lower risk of illness and injury. They also highlight the barriers to do so.

The first item reported on yet another weight loss study.[2] The newsworthy piece of this research was that people who were better at keeping a food diary tended to lose more weight.[3] There are many things wrong with the design of the study, not least of which is the obsession with weight gain as a disease rather than a symptom of metabolic imbalances.

We believe that metabolic disruptions that appear as weight gain, the so-called obesity epidemic, and diagnoses such as metabolic syndrome, insulin resistance, and type 2 diabetes are caused by physiological stress that is caused principally by environmental exposures and psychosocial stress from social inequity.[4]

On its face, both the news and the research leads us to believe that someone who keeps track of what he eats will change his eating pattern more easily that someone who does not. It is a simple idea about how to change someone's personal environment. It sounds very appealing, which should cause immediate suspicion.

In social research there's a well-known phenomenon called the Hawthorne Effect, discovered over one hundred years ago. When researchers observed how people did their jobs, they noticed that their work performance improved. And when the observation stopped, work performance dropped back to its previous level. The Hawthorne Effect is now generalized to include any temporary change in a person's environment that elicits an equally temporary change in behavior.[5]

When the weight loss study ends, what happens to the food diaries?

For the study, everyone was supposed to keep a diary. Some were more diligent that others. Those who were more diligent diarists lost more weight. Was it the diary or the diligence or something else that preceded both?

This is an obvious demonstration of the alternative ways in which people create their personal environment. Some people in the study took to keeping a diary; some did not. For the people who didn't, what other method might have worked as well for them? To the extent that the diary served as a cue for some participants to pay attention to the diet, what other kind of cue would work more effectively for non-diarists? Some examples...

• a cookbook for the diet permanently placed on the kitchen counter
• music that inspires the dieter in preparing a meal
• artwork that's a visual or tactile reminder of nutrient goals

When trying to make things better, the challenge is to shape the personal environment in a way that works for a specific person and that moves her through the stages of change.[6]

In another study, the issue of *avoiding* change that affects health and risk is examined. Researchers studied what might predict whether a child at age 12 who doesn't smoke would become a smoker by age 16.[7]

Several factors are already known to affect the risk of a child becoming a smoker:

• whether a parent smokes,
• a parent's approval of smoking,
• the child's awareness of cigarette advertising, and
• the child's curiosity and willingness to take risks.

In addition to these, the researchers found that two things added to the risk of a child becoming a smoker:

• how easily the child thought he could get cigarettes and
• whether the child had friends who smoked.

Although the study discussed various public health policies for reducing these factors and their impact, it seems critical to ask what methods a child could find to control his own personal environment in order to avoid cigarette addiction. This is thick soup. Children in this particular age group typically have a strong desire for control over their personal environment.

The answer is not the age-old strategy of proscribing a child's association with peers who are a "bad influence." The answer is enabling a child to have a sense of agency by refusing to take up smoking. An early anti-smoking commercial took this approach by depicting the tobacco industry as a Marlboro Man wrangling and branding teens.[8]

There's an important piece of information buried in this research on what gets children hooked on smoking: the vast majority of children did not try smoking and fewer still became smokers after trying. Of the 1,027 young people in the study, 177 tried smoking and only 109 became regular smokers over the 4 year duration of the study: about 1 in 6 tried and about 1 in 10 got hooked.

Why didn't 5 out of 6 try smoking? Why didn't 9 out of 10 become addicted smokers? What did these young people do for themselves that helped them resist becoming a smoker? What would research look like that identified the factors that strengthen that capacity?

These two studies tell us that people can adapt their personal environment in ways that improve or undermine health and increase or decrease the risk of illness and injury. Those adaptations, those self-directed changes in environmental cues are nothing other than lifestyle and cultural choices, which are choices about the person he wants to be.

The first article in this section, "Nicotine Addiction," discusses the physiological effects of nicotine. We also discuss proven methods for kicking the habit. To quit smoking is one of the most important changes that anyone can make for improving health and reducing risk.

In the second article, "A Good Night's Sleep," we discuss a pervasive problem in our culture: rest and recovery. We describe the physiology of sleep, its effect on health and risk, and how to develop a healthy sleep pattern.

"The Multitasking Myth," the third article in this section, describes how the culturally popular idea of multitasking actually has physiological limits. It is also a complement to the preceding article on sleep: the consequence of a culture that promotes staying busy for its own sake. In particular, we look at the contribution of electronic devices such as cell phones to the multitasking myth and the urgency felt for staying busy.

Finally, "A Pill to Stop Your Period" discusses how hormone imbalance is being sold as a convenience. By portraying menstruation as a problem, pharmaceutical companies are encouraging women to take synthetic hormones that have significant long-term health risks. In this instance, the culture of the eternally busy appears as the culture of convenience—menstruation as an interference in the lifestyle fulfillments.

Notes

[1] Youssef Idaghdour, et al. (2008) "A Genome-wide Gene Expression Signature of Environmental Geography in Leukocytes of Moroccan Amazighs."

[2] Jack F. Hollis, et al. (2008) "Weight loss during the intensive intervention phase of the weight-loss maintenance trial."

[3] For example, Erin Allday (2008) "To Drop Pounds, Write Down Everything You Eat."

[4] That issue is discussed in detail in "Obesity: A Social Disease" on page 229. On the relationship between stress and obesity, see Per Bjorntorp (2001) "Do Stress Reactions Cause Abdominal Obesity and Comorbidities?" and Per Bjorntorp ed (1992) *Obesity*. For a general critique of the science behind the obesity epidemic, see Paul Campos (2004) *The Obesity Myth: Why America's Obsession with Weight is Hazardous to Your Health* and Michael Gard and Jan Wright (2005) *The Obesity Epidemic: Science, Morality, and Ideology*.

[5] The Hawthorne Effect, its origins, and its place in the shaping of the industrial workforce is describe in Harry Braverman (1974) *Labor and Monopoly Capital: The Degradation of Work in the Twentieth Century*.

[6] We discussed the stages of change concept in "Moved to Move" on page 127.

[7] Chyke A. Doubeni, et al. (2008) "Perceived Accessibility as a Predictor of Youth Smoking."

[8] Stanton A. Glantz and Edith D. Balbach (2000) *Tobacco War: Inside the California Battles* page 340-1.

NICOTINE ADDICTION

The good news is that fewer young people even try smoking. The bad news is that of those who do give it a try, an increasing percentage become addicted. Tobacco companies know this. They've known it for a very long time.

The results of the survey on kids, reported in *Science News*, confirms what we suspect: some people are more likely than others to get hooked. We don't have to go to theories of addictive personalities or other forms of blaming the victim. What we also suspect is confirmed by research: addiction is physiological. An article in *Science* identified the specific biochemistry of how nicotine addiction works.

Nicotine Biochemistry

Nicotine affects your nervous system by disrupting neurotransmitters, the molecules responsible for signaling among nerve cells and between nerve cells and the rest of your body. Neurotransmitters can also signal the release or suppression of other neurotransmitters.

One of the principle effects of nicotine is to stimulate the release of dopamine. Norepinephrine and dopamine are the primary catecholamines produced in your brain. Catecholamines get and keep you alert. They are released when you are under stress. While norepinephrine stimulates sustained alertness, dopamine stimulates spurts of euphoria and your ability to focus.

Neurotransmitters such as the catecholamines do their work by attaching to receptors on nerve cells. Each receptor is designed to recognize a specific kind of neurotransmitter: catecholamine receptors are designed for catecholamines and not for the neurotransmitter serotonin, for example.

Receptors are proteins that stretch from the outside of a cell membrane to the inside. When a dopamine molecule attaches to a catecholamine receptor on the outside of a nerve cell, it starts a chemical reaction on the inside of the cell. The cell responds by contributing to your sense of pleasure and alertness.

The *Science* article identified a specific receptor in mice to which nicotine molecules attach and which leads to addiction. The receptor is one of four, all of which are called nicotinic acetylcholine receptors because they respond to nicotine. A single nicotinic acetylcholine receptor that accounted for the addictive behavior of the mice they experimented on. Exposure of this receptor to nicotine produced all of the symptoms of chronic nicotine use: behavioral tolerance, sensitization, dependence, and withdrawal.

The researchers found a dramatic increase in dopamine (the short-term, excitatory neurotransmitter) in the nicotine sensitive mice. The news reports of the research inaccurately portrayed this as the primary mode of addiction. In the next section we describe how much more than dopamine is affected.

Although the *Science* researchers conclude only that their methods open up new possibilities for studying nicotine addiction, the news reports went further. What they implied was a silver bullet: the development of pharmaceuticals that could block the body's actions.

Nutrients to Kick the Habit

Dr. Charles Gant, an innovator in the use of nutrients to treat addiction, paints a much broader canvas. He describes how "nicotine's effects quickly spread to each of the four major neurotransmitters." In addition to dopamine, nicotine affects GABA (mental relaxation), serotonin (emotional relaxation), and endorphins and enkephalins (pain relief).

Gant's approach is to look at the entire milieu of neurotransmitter effects (the many faces of addiction). He doesn't look for a pharmaceutical silver bullet, but instead looks to your body's own mechanisms and the nutrients that will help your body heal.

Gant's regimen consists of two stages. In stage one you restore your neurotransmitter balance disrupted by nicotine.
- B vitamins (cofactors for neurotransmitter production)
- Minerals (calcium, magnesium, potassium, zinc, manganese, copper, chromium, selenium, and molybdenum)
- Phosphatidyl choline (raw material for acetylcholine)
- L-tyrosine (raw material for catecholamines)
- 5HTP (raw material for serotonin)
- L-glutamine (a relaxant that also soothes your gut)

None of these requires a prescription. None are pharmaceuticals. However, Gant cautions that using some of these nutrients depends on your physical condition—for example, people with a thyroid disease such as Grave's or Hashimoto's should not take tyrosine.

Another caution is that phosphatidyl choline sold as a supplement is made from soy sludge. DMAE (dimethyl-amino-ethanol) is also a precursor to acetylcholine. And egg yokes are loaded with phosphatidyl choline.

In stage two you detoxify. Nicotine, after all, is a poison. A very powerful poison. Detoxification could include chelation to remove toxins. In all cases, you provide nutrient support for your liver and gut, and lots of antioxidants.

Nicotine and Emotional Disruption

Addiction has an emotional as well as a physiological component. An interview survey of 43,000 people published in the *Archives of General Psychiatry* reports that over half of smokers (55%) suffer from mental disorders from mild to severe. In other words, if you are psychologically troubled, you are not only more likely to smoke, you will likely smoke more than other smokers.

This simply says something else we suspect: nicotine addiction is self-medication that eases the smoker's troubles.

The authors of the *Archives* article concluded that the mental disorders have to be treated as well as the nicotine addiction. Newspapers dutifully echoed them: more treatment. Meaning, treatment with pharmaceuticals.

The first question to ask, however, is the extent to which re-establishing balance from nicotine addiction affects the associated mental disorder. After all, many of the neurotransmitters affected by nicotine affect the user's mental and emotional life. And as the work of Dr. Abram Hoffer and Dr. Eva Edelman suggests, nutrient imbalance is at the heart of mental and emotional disorders.

Kicking nicotine addiction is about restoring balance, not about bombarding your body with drugs.

Resources

Bower, Bruce. 2001. Youthful Nicotine Addiction May Be Growing. *Science News*. September 22, 2001, 160(12): 183.

Edelman, Eva. 2000. Natural Healing for Mental Disorders. *Your Own Health And Fitness*. Broadcast November 7, 2000.

Edelman, Eva. 1998. *Natural Healing for Schizophrenia and Other Common Mental Disorders*, 2nd edition. Eugene, Oregon: Borage Books.

Hoffer, Abram (1999). *Dr. Hoffer's ABC of Natural Nutrition for Children with Learning Disabilities, Behavioral Disorders, and Mental State Disorders* Kingston, Ontario: Quarry Health Books.

Gant, Charles and Greg Lewis. 2002. *End Your Addiction Now*. New York: Warner Books.

Gant, Charles. 2004. End Addictions with Nutrient Therapy. *Your Own Health And Fitness*. Broadcast February 10, 2004.

Grant, Bridget. 2004. Nicotine Dependence and Psychiatric Disorders in the United States. *Archives of General Psychiatry*. November 2004, 61(11): 1097-1103.

Henderson, Diedtra. 2004. Nicotine Research Points to Key Molecule. *The Washington Post*. November 4, 2004.

Tapper, Andrew, et al. 2004. Nicotine Activiation of α4* Receptors. *Science*. November 5, 2004; 306: 1029-32.

A GOOD NIGHT'S SLEEP

Healthy, Lively Larks. Sleep Savvy Seniors. Dragging Duos. Overworked, Overweight, and Over-Caffeinated. Sleepless and Missin' the Kissin'. These are the too-cute names assigned to American sleep habits by WB&A Market Research.

The market researchers conducted a poll of Americans on their sleep habits for the National Sleep Foundation. The results are reported in the Foundation's *2005 Sleep in America*. The cute names reflect the patterns that the market researchers observed in the poll results.

The report is part of a growing recognition of sleep as a major health issue. As one would expect, overt sleep disorders such as sleep apnea receive the bulk of attention. But less acute sleep problems are far more pervasive and weave themselves into a wide range of chronic illnesses.

Sleep In America

According to the National Sleep Foundation's report, about ½ (48%) of the people polled have a "healthy" sleep-life, while the other ½ (52%) have sleep troubles of one sort or another. Looking at the actual numbers in the survey tell a somewhat different story.

In clinical research on sleep, humans left to their own devices will sleep about 9 hours per day. Yet few people in the National Sleep Foundation survey get anything close to that much sleep. The average was 6.8 hours per night, with little variation among the 5 cutely named categories: from a high average of 7.3 (seniors) to a low of 5.7 (overworked).

Despite this 2 to 3 hour gap in sleep, almost ½ (43%) of the people surveyed felt that they get *more* sleep than they need. Which group felt they get the most "unnecessary" sleep? The "healthiest" sleepers, 2/3 (67%) of whom thought they got more sleep than they needed.

The people who get the least sleep are also the people who are more likely to have a medical condition such as high blood pressure, arthritis, depression, diabetes, or heart disease. These people are also more likely to smoke, drink alcohol and caffeinated beverages, and work longer hours at part-time jobs with irregular work hours.

One subgroup consists of people who are more likely to be men, a person of color, and overweight. Another subgroup are predominantly women who work in service sector jobs, have their sleep dis-

rupted by their partner's sleep habits (especially snoring), and who feel most acutely the effect of their sleep problems during the day. Two important points:
- "healthy" sleepers have medical conditions, smoke and drink, and all the rest, just less frequently than the "unhealthy" sleepers; and
- medical conditions, smoking and drinking, and so on can be the cause of poor sleep health or they can be the consequence of poor sleep—in other words, they can be bound up in a vicious cycle.

Sleep Debt

Sleep is not as easy as it looks. Sleep researchers such as William Dement, PhD, have found that our sleep metabolism consists of two opposing forces: one creates pressure for us to sleep, the other keeps us alert.

Mammals such as mice, when left undisturbed to sleep when they want, will drift in and out of sleep repeatedly during the day. The sleep periods tend to be short and shallow.

This sleep-wake cycle is the result of *sleep debt*. From the time you or any other mammal wakes up, your body starts to build the need to sleep. Like the need to eat and the corresponding sensation of hunger, when the sleep debt reaches a threshold, a mammal will become "hungry" for sleep. In the absence of overt stimulation, a mouse curls up and dozes. Researchers measure sleep debt by how long it takes a mouse or human or other mammal to fall asleep.

Humans and other primates, unlike mice, stay awake during the daylight hours and sleep during the night. Our sleep is uninterrupted and includes the deep REM (rapid eye movement) sleep that puts us into a state of physical paralysis and the land of dreams.

Humans are able to achieve this by overcoming the sleep debt that builds during the day with *biological clock-dependent alerting*. Your biological clock consists of two clusters of nerves located in your brain directly above each optic nerve. Each cluster consists of about 10,000 nerve cells—about the size of a pinhead.

Because of its location next to your optic nerve, your biological clock is affected by light. But it can also operate independently of light. That means light can work to reset your biological clock, but once set it will arouse you in a regular pattern over a 24 hour day.

Typically, clock-dependent alerting occurs twice during the day: once at the beginning of the day to wake you up, then again in the late afternoon and early evening to keep you going. Each alerting peak counteracts the urge to sleep that builds continuously over the day. In between the two alerting peaks, the urge to sleep emerges in the early afternoon: siesta time.

For some people, the wake-up call comes early and the late afternoon "second wind" also comes early. For some people, alerting comes later. Morning people and night people.

Clock-dependent alerting is your body's way of keeping you awake during the entire day. But with civilization, we have other, external forms of stimulation that can overwhelm our urge to sleep: artificial light, night shift jobs, stimulating entertainment before bed, caffeine, stress, and the belief that sleep is wasted time. As we discuss in "The WiFi Blues" (page 188), wireless technologies provide an added burden to sleep disruption.

The caveat to *2005 Sleep in America* is that the average age of the people surveyed was 47. Teenagers are an entirely different matter. The biological clock for teens runs late: late to bed and late rising with longer periods of sleep required. An important piece of work that the National Sleep Foundation pursues is to adjust school hours to the sleep needs of children and teenagers in particular.

Get a Good Night's Sleep

It is unfortunate, yet understandable that discussions of sleep in the conventional media focus on overt sleep disorders such as sleep apnea (when you stop breathing while asleep), severe snoring, insomnia, and narcolepsy (when you pass out into a REM state).

But the more pervasive problem is that we don't get enough sleep and rest. This situation isn't helped by a culture that devalues sleep as being for sissies: "If you snooze, you lose" is the motto. So we suck it up and overcome our sleep debt with stimulants and stimulation and pushing ourselves past tired.

Even if we don't consciously succumb to the "sleep is for sissies" mindset, we are too often unable to give in to the urge to sleep. We don't feel sleepy, just tired. We don't fall asleep at the wheel, but we make mistakes. Some mistakes are disastrous: the crash of the Exxon Valdez and the explosion of the space shuttle Challenger are only two of the most dramatic mistakes owing to sleep debt.

Special health conditions interfere with your ability to sleep. Hormone imbalance in both men and women can be particularly disruptive for sleep. Too much or too little estrogen or thyroid and, as we already mentioned, too much cortisol interfere with sleep. Since testosterone balances the effects of estrogen, low testosterone can have the effect of raising estrogen and its consequent sleep disruption. On the other hand, progesterone is calming and helps with sleep. High cortisol counteracts progesterone's calming effects.

People with chronic pain such as fibromyalgia and conditions of chronic inflammation (heart disease, diabetes, and arthritis) tend to have elevated stress hormones (*cortisol*) and so are likely to have difficulty sleeping. The irony is that chronic stress, which produces chronically high levels of cortisol, promotes these same conditions.

Pharmaceuticals can also affect sleep. For example, asthmatics who take steroidal inhalants are getting a dose of cortisol. In addition, sleep medications and antidepressants, which are frequently prescribed as sleep aids, become addictive because they disrupt your bodies own sleep chemistry without treating the basic cause of sleep troubles.

The information that follows is for you to get better sleep, even if you don't have a diagnosed sleep disorder. The resources listed below will give you more in-depth information.

- Have a sleep routine that includes going to bed and waking at approximately the same time.
- Set your time to bed and time to rise to correspond to available daylight—go to bed between 10pm and 11pm.
- Succumb to the urge to sleep during the day: take naps. You can "catch up" on your sleep you've lost because you've been pushing yourself or for some other reason have built up a sleep debt.
- Make your sleep environment quiet, comfortable, and dark.
- Establish "going to bed" rituals.
- Avoid activities that stimulate you right before bed (such as work-related problem-solving).
- Avoid caffeine after mid-day.
- Avoid pushing yourself past tired. Getting yourself over-tired raises cortisol which in turn counteracts hormones that help you relax and get to sleep.
- When you wake up, try to get out into bright sunlight.

Resources

Berman, Layna. 2003. Insomnia. *Your Own Health And Fitness*. Broadcast September 23, 2003.

Coren, Stanley. 1997. *Sleep Thieves*. New York: Free Press.

Dement, William. 1999. *The Promise of Sleep*. New York: Delacorte Press.

Dement, William. 2001. Sleep. *Your Own Health And Fitness*. Broadcast December 4, 2001.

National Sleep Foundation. 2005. *2005 Sleep in America*. Access at http://www.sleepfoundation.org.

National Sleep Foundation. 2000. *Adolescent Sleep Needs and Patterns*. Access at http://www.sleepfoundation.org.

THE MULTITASKING MYTH

Efficiency is a virtue in our culture. People take pride in their ability to pack as much as possible into every minute. Even greater pride is taken by people who can multitask, packing more into each minute.

Unfortunately, the sense of efficiency you might have in multitasking is likely more a matter of faith than fact. It seems that the very biology of our nervous system limits how much information we can act on within a fixed amount of time.

Attention has focused on the common practice of talking on a cellphone while driving. In 2005, traffic accidents caused by cellphone use resulted in approximately 2,600 deaths and 330,000 injuries. Many law enforcement and traffic safety agencies are calling for outlawing the practice. Some state legislatures have responded.

Beyond the use of cellphones while driving, less lethal multitasking activities hang on the belief that you can do several things simultaneously with no loss in efficiency, thereby saving precious time. The science suggests otherwise.

The Bottleneck

Rene Marois and his colleagues have demonstrated what's called the central bottleneck. Their investigations use simple tests to identify neurological limitations to responding to multiple stimuli.

First, they conducted two simple stimulus-response tests.

In one test people were asked to respond to a colored dot that appears randomly on a screen by pressing a specific letter with a specific finger: red dot, index finger presses the letter J; blue dot, pinky presses the letter P. In very little time, these people able to respond in about one half second.

In another test this same group of people were asked to respond to a sound with a vocalization: bird song, say "ba"; electronic sound, say "ko." Again, response time quickly settled at one half second.

Then Marois combined the two stimuli in various sequences. When the dot and sound occurred at the same time, people responded to one stimulus then the other in sequence. The total time was simply the sum of the two separate responses. The same was true when the second stimulus was delayed. In other words, each person's brain created a response queue.

Marois identifies three causes for the delay, each of which indicates that we neurologically focus on one thing at a time.

First, we have to identify the stimulus in what's called the attentional blink. That's a few tenths of a second.

Second, once we've identified a stimulus we put it in short-term memory. Short-term memory can take up to about four items, fewer if the items are complex. So once identified, we need to sort out what's there.

Third, we have to choose a response. While focused on a response to one stimulus, our brain ignores what to do about other stimuli.

Some researchers believe that these neurological limitations can be overcome. These researchers have shown that, with enough practice, two tasks can be performed without a bottleneck. However, these tasks are extremely simple and it took people 2,000 repetitions to achieve duel-tasking efficiency.

In the real world of complex stimuli, even these skeptical researchers think it's impossible to talk on a cellphone and drive without increased risk.

Rub Your Tummy, Pat Your Head

It turns out that some stimulus-response combinations can be affected by training and some cannot. For example, visual stimulus-motor response (in the eye, out the hand) and hearing stimulus-verbal response (in the ear, out the mouth) combinations improve with practice. On the other hand, visual stimulus-verbal response and hearing stimulus-motor response combinations do not improve with practice.

Our experience tends to confirm this experimental result. The speculation is that humans have adapted to learn in some combinations and not in others: learn to move by watching, learn to talk by listening. So we would be neurologically adapted to combine these responses.

Not surprisingly, age affects the capacity to respond to stimuli and multitask. The capacity seems to peak in the twenty-somethings, declines mildly through the fifty-somethings, then declines markedly in the sixty-and-older-somethings. Practice, however, does improve performance in sixty-and-older-somethings.

The simplicity of the stimulus-response tasks, the physiological matching of the response to the stimulus, and the age of the actor are not the only things that affect multitasking. The ability to focus on tasks further affects performance.

As a kind of corollary to the central bottleneck, researchers investigating how easily someone is distracted found that the stimulus load can make people equally susceptible to distractions. Some people are more easily distracted than others, acknowledge as much, and test out that way when what is called their perceptual load is low. But when their load is increased, they are no more distractible than people who are not easily distracted.

The explanation is in the ability of people to focus. When a task requires a high degree of focused attention (as is the case with a high perceptual load) everyone is equally distracted. In essence, we come up against our neurological limits when we are saturated with stimuli.

Drunk Driving

David Strayer and his colleagues found that drivers on cellphones are as likely to have an accident as a driver who is at the legal limit for alcohol. The reasons for the susceptibility differ: cellphone users are slower to react and less decisive due to slower reaction time, while drinkers are more prone to tailgating, tracking, and over-reacting.

We're all well aware that people who reassure us that a few drinks haven't affected their ability to drive are kidding themselves. The science is there to back up this bit of common sense. Researchers looking at multitasking find the same phenomenon: people often pride themselves on their effectiveness at multitasking, believing they've performed tasks simultaneously in less time than it would have taken them to perform them one after another. In fact they do not.

Likewise with cellphone users. They feel fully competent to talk and drive while in fact they are impaired—and a risk to themselves and others. More generally, we live in a culture that saturates us with stimulation. Many people actively seek it out, feeling that they are effective and efficient as they multitask through their day. That's not what the science tells us. It suggests that we should attend more to the quality of our time rather than how much we can pack into it.

The News

Motluk, Alison. 2007. How Many Things Can You Do at Once? *New Scientist.* April 7, 2007: 28-31.

The Research

Forster, Sophie and Nilli Lavie. 2007. High Perceptual Load Makes Everybody Equal: Eliminating Individual Differences in Distractibility With Load. *Psychological Science.* 18:5: 377-81.

Langer, Peter et al. 2005. Hands-free Mobile Phone Conversation Impairs the Peripheral Visual System to an Extent Comparable to an Alcohol Level of 4-5g 100ml. *Human Psychopharmacology.* 20: 65-6.

Marois, Rene and Jason Ivanoff. 2005. Capacity Limits of Information Processing in the Brain. *Trends in Cognitive Sciences*. June 2005 (9:6): 296-305. DOI:10.1016/j.tics.2005.04.010.

Sigman, Mariano and Stanislas Dehaene. 2006. Dynamics of the Central Bottleneck: Dual-Task and Task Uncertainty. *PLoS Biology*. July 2006 (4:7): e220. DOI:10.1371/journal.pbio.0040220.

Strayer, David et al. 2006. A Comparison of the Cell Phone Driver and the Drunk Driver. *Human Factors*. Summer 2006 (48:2): 381-91.

Resources

Your Own Health And Fitness. Resources on Radiation: Wireless, EMR, RFR, and Ionizing Radiation. Access at http://www.yourownhealthandfitness.org/topicsRadiation.php.

A PILL TO STOP YOUR PERIOD

Karl Marx once said, "Social progress can be measured by the social position of the female sex."

The FDA has approved Lybrel made by Wyeth Pharmaceuticals. Lybrel suppresses menstruation. Lybrel uses the same ingredients as Wyeth's standard birth control pill, but it's formulated so that a woman can take these pills every day of the year and not only stop ovulation to prevent pregnancy but stop menstrual bleeding altogether.

Planned Parenthood thinks this is a great idea. According to their Vice President for Medical Affairs, Vanessa Cullins, MD, "FDA approval of Lybrel is great news for women who want or need to safely suppress their menstrual cycle, and now they have the convenience of a full year's birth control prescription to do it."

According to the news reports of Lybrel's approval, Wyeth found that one third of the women they surveyed want their periods to go away. But the news reports also include voices of caution from women's advocates and researchers concerned with the long-term health effects of doing away with a woman's periods.

Should we celebrate as social progress the ability of a woman to chemically stop her period?

Get Rid of It

Researchers working on suppressing periods emphasize that they're concerned with treating women who have difficult menstruation: heavy bleeding, cramps, mood disorders, and more. Wyeth expresses concern for these issues as well, but its marketing strategy is much broader. In addition to difficult menstruation, Wyeth clearly intends to promote Lybrel as a straight-on birth control method and as a drug of convenience.

In a presentation to Wall Street analysts, Wyeth's director of women's health recited a litany of problems women commonly have with their periods then asked, "So who wouldn't want to get rid of this?"

A considerable body of feminist research has shown that our culture makes menstruation into something negative: unclean, painful, shameful. That's reinforced by health research into menstruation that frames it as a negative event.

The vast majority of research focuses on premenstrual changes and PMS, not on menstruation itself. What little research exists is framed in terms of menstruation "management." In other words, the assumption that menstruation is a "problem" is built into the research itself.

This research bias seems invisible because it feeds on cultural biases that fail to portray menstruation as an essentially healthy event. For example, advertising for "feminine hygiene products" reinforces the negative framework associated with menstruation.

The bias starts early. Girls are not adequately educated about menarche. Girls receive an education that is predominantly abstract. They're taught physiology, but not practical issues such as what menstrual bleeding actually feels like. Instead of actual experience, the practical aspect of sex education typically focuses on products that "manage" the problem of menstruation.

It's no surprise that many girls have a more negative attitude after menarche than before.

Wyeth knows what it's doing. Their marketing to the idea that they have a solution to a problem: menstruation. They reinforce the bias and at the same time sell to it.

Body Image

Feminist researchers have found that women who feel positively about menstruation are more likely to have accurate knowledge about menstruation, to have positive health habits, and to have a positive body image. It therefore seems sensible to ask whether the problem is menstruation or instead how women feel about their bodies.

This only serves as a backdrop to Wyeth's marketing. The makers of Lybrel promote it under the guise of freedom and control. Freedom and control are good things. Women have struggled for them interminably.

A generation ago cigarette manufacturers developed and marketed products to the same sense of freedom and control. They marketed one brand of cigarette under the slogan "You've come a long way, baby."

The outcome of that campaign for women's freedom and control is smoking rates equivalent to men's and the accompanying increases in lung cancer and heart attacks. With the advent of Lybrel we can expect an equally horrific effect on women's health.

In his book *What Your Doctor May Not Tell You About Premenopause*, the late John Lee described the health risks associated long-term use of birth control pills. These include increased risk of
- stroke
- heart attack
- cervical, breast, endometrial, ovarian, liver, and thyroid cancer

- birth defects in children born to users
- uterus and ovary removal
- anxiety, depression, and sleep disorders.

Indicator of Health

What promotion of this "solution" threatens to drown out is the concept that menstruation is normal and an indicator of health. Problem menstruation is a symptom, not a deficiency of pharmaceuticals. For the most part, the root cause is hormone imbalance, particularly a deficiency in progesterone.

The progesterone a woman's body produces has a wide range of beneficial effects in addition to its role in menstrual cycles. Metabolites of progesterone calm the brain, promote cardiovascular health, and reduce the risk of breast cancer.

On the other hand, the progestins that are the synthetic version of progesterone used in Lybrel and birth control pills have none of these beneficial downstream effects. In fact, progestins *increase* the risk of breast cancer.

One of the most common things women on birth control pills report is that they just don't feel right. That's because their natural biochemistry has been disrupted by the introduction of synthetic estrogen and progestins.

Bioidentical progesterone can be purchased over the counter and, used properly, can supplement what a woman's body is already producing. But progesterone deficiency comes from somewhere. The most common cause is insulin resistance caused by stress, a high starch diet, and exposure to endocrine disrupting chemicals. Birth control pills actually make insulin resistance worse.

Social progress doesn't come from chemicals that give women a false sense of freedom and control over menstruation, even difficult menstruation. It comes from restoring and maintaining hormone balance and real reproductive health.

The News

Bridges, Andrew. 2007. Birth-Control Pill Halts Women's Periods. *San Francisco Chronicle.* May 22, 2007.

Lerner, Maura and Josephine Marcotty. 2007. No-period Pill: Is It Meddling, or Convenience. *Minneapolis-St. Paul Star Tribune.* May 28, 2007.

Stein, Rob. 2007. Pill that Suppresses Periods OK'd. *Washington Post.* May 23, 2007.

The Research

Beral, Valerie et al. 1999. Mortality Associated with Oral Contraceptive Use. *British Medical Journal.* Volume 318 (January 9, 1999): 96-100.

Hitchcock, Christine et al. 2004. Evidence About Extending the Duration of Oral Contraceptive Use to Suppress Menstruation. *Women's Health Issues.* November-December 2004 (14:6): 201-11. DOI:10.1016/j.whi.2004.08.005.

McPherson, Marianne and Lauren Korfine. 2004. Menstruation Across Time: Menarche, Menstrual Attitudes, Experiences, and Behaviors. *Women's Health Issues.* November-December 2004 (14:6): 193-200. DOI:10.1016/j.whi.2004.08.006.

Resources

Lee, John. 1999. *What Your Doctor May Not Tell You About Premenopause.* New York: Warner.

Your Own Health And Fitness. Resources on Hormones, Women's Health, and Men's Health. Access at http://www.yourownhealthandfitness.org/topicsHormones.php.

Zava, David. 2007. Menstrual Suppression Cautions. *Your Own Health And Fitness.* Broadcast May 29, 2007.

In 2008, the Los Angeles City Council passed an ordinance banning fast food restaurants from South LA[1]—the area of the city that has the lowest average income and the highest percentage of people of color. With 45% of the restaurants serving fast food, the area is the highest in the city. The Northeast around Pasadena comes in second with 33%. The hip and wealthy Westside has the lowest at 19%.

The fast food ban is based on two ideas—one right, the other not. South LA has the highest rate of obesity in the city. The conventional thinking is that obesity is a disease. In that way of thinking, the high rate of obesity in South LA is a public health crisis caused by unhealthy eating habits and lack of physical activity. So take away fast food and you help reduce obesity.

This idea is wrong because obesity is a symptom, not a disease.[2] And while unhealthy food aggravates that symptom, fast food should be banned because it's unhealthy, because it lacks nutrient density, because it causes malnutrition. Obesity, on the other hand, is the consequence of stress—psychosocial stress caused by social inequity and physiological stress caused by toxic exposures, fast food only one of many.[3]

The good idea behind the ban is that it is entirely appropriate for the City Council or any local government to modify the built environment specifically to attain a positive health effect. The Council member responsible for the moratorium, Jan Perry, represents a portion of South LA. She worked for six years to pass the moratorium because "there are not a lot of food choices in South LA."[4] In addition to the moratorium on fast food restaurants, a separate piece of legislation provided for actively encouraging grocery stores and restaurants with table service to move into the neighborhood.

To no one's surprise, the National Restaurant Association objected to the moratorium, as did conservatives concerned about government "meddling into the very minutiae of what people are putting in their mouths."[5]

Eating fast food contributes to obesity and other medical problems because it is an adaptation to stress.[6] In other words, it is a form of self-care that is a response to circumstances that induce a physiological stress response—although, as in too many cases, the self-care turns out to be a maladaption because the food contains anti-nutrients that block or otherwise interfere with the proper metabolism of nutrients the body needs. Nevertheless, changing circumstances by changing the concentration of fast food restaurants is a good thing.

A more comprehensive view of obesity as an adaptation the body makes in response to stress places it with a wide variety of other stress-related illnesses such as heart disease and diabetes.[7] As a physiological stressor, malnutrition from fast food doesn't cause obesity—but it does turn up the volume on the body's already stressed state. So from this perspective as well, changing the built environment to reduce exposure to malnourishing foods and to increase exposures to nutrient dense foods is a good thing.

Unfortunately, halting the spread of fast food restaurants and promoting grocery stores and restaurants with table service in South LA is a weak contribution to reducing malnutrition. The problem that needs to be solved is how to change the entire food infrastructure in the area.

Nutrition and food security will not be well served by simply maintaining the status quo on the number of fast food restaurants. Nor will it be fully served by the limited alternatives that are being encouraged. Why not promote and even subsidize farmers markets and urban gardens?[8]

But a more fundamental problem needs to be addressed: what makes sense of the fact that people in South LA use fast food as a food source in disproportionate numbers? The answer is not that they don't know what's good for them. Instead look to their rationality in the face of a specific political economy of which the food infrastructure is only a part.

Posing the problem in this way gives us the opportunity to change what we mean by a healthy built environment. Currently, the people of South LA are forced to protect themselves from the risk of illness posed by fast food. Instead, they should have the tools that will enable them to actively shape their food infrastructure in order to create health benefits.

Avoid the risk of illness versus create health benefits.

Of course, our food infrastructure is only one aspect of our built environment that exposes us to health risks.

A traditional example is illustrated by the Environmental Protection Agency's Risk-Screening Environmental Indicators (RSEI)[9] database that links air pollution to risks of illness in specific neighborhoods throughout the US. As the Chicago Tribune revealed,[10] this information is a well-kept secret. In response, the Tribune published its own web page[11] to enable better access to this information so people can better understand the risks posed by the built environment that surrounds them.

A less traditional example is noise pollution. Researchers concerned with the issue have compared secondhand noise to secondhand smoke as a risk for illness and injury.[12] In addition to hearing loss, noise pollution is associated with sleep disruption, chronic stress, cardiovascular disruption, and impaired cognitive development in children. San Francisco's Department of Public Health has developed a model of noise pollution caused by traffic.[13] The model will be used by the city for building codes as well as for land use (particularly transportation) policy and planning. Such actions aim to modify the forces that shape our built environment in order to reduce risks. The problem, however, seems to be the shaping itself.

There's no doubt that we have to take action as communities to protect ourselves from a wide variety of risks. But that fact is not a result of the natural order of things. Who gets to build what and where is a consequence of who has money, political power, and cultural power.[14]

It's also a consequence of how each community regulates its political economy. It's a consequence of a culture that celebrates the virtues of the so-called free market in which the default regulation is: you can change the built environment unless it turns out to be harmful.

Instead, the correct default regulation should be: you can change the built environment, but only if you can prove it's safe. Better yet, the default should be: you can change the built environment, but only if it makes the community a healthier place to live. Otherwise, go away.

The articles in this section cover various aspects of the built environment and its health effects.

In "Smog: Deadlier than Ever," we discuss the health effects of air pollution and how researchers continue to reveal ways in which our health is impaired. We make the point that the fundamental problem is our transportation system.

"The WiFi Blues" discusses what is becoming one of the most serious and most underexamined public health issues worldwide. Although wireless technologies appear to be personal consumer products, in fact the telecommunications infrastructure in the built environment that supports the consumer products creates public health risks.

Finally, "Sick Buildings" discusses how the construction practices used for our homes and workplaces can creates risks of illness and injury. As with transportation and communication, shelter is a major aspect of our built environment that cries out for a positive principle: you can build it, but only if it makes the community a healthier place to live.

Notes

[1] Kim Severson (2008) "Los Angeles Stages a Fast Food Intervention."

[2] For a critique of the conventional thinking on obesity, see Paul Campos (2004) *The Obesity Myth: Why America's Obsession with Weight is Hazardous to Your Health*, Michael Gard and Jan Wright (2005) *The Obesity Epidemic: Science, Morality, and Ideology* .

[3] Per Bjorntorp (2001) "Do Stress Reactions Cause Abdominal Obesity and Comorbidities?" See also the articles "Obesity, a Social Disease" on page 229 and "Fat and Death" on page 274.

[4] Quoted in Kim Severson (2008) "Los Angeles Stages a Fast Food Intervention."

[5] Quoted in Ibid..

[6] Mary F. Dallman, et al. (2003) "Chronic Stress and Obesity: A New View of 'Comfort Food'."

[7] See Layna Berman and Jeffry Fawcett (2007) "Stress Related Illness."

[8] For example, see Community Food Security Coalition. Access at http://www.foodsecurity.org.

[9] Risk-Screening Environmental Indicators (RSEI). Access at http://www.epa.gov/oppt/rsei.

[10] Michael Hawthorne and Darnell Little (2008) "Chicago's Toxic Air."

[11] How Clean is Your Air? Access at http://www.chicagotribune.com/news/local/rsei-database,0,3220483.htmlstory.

[12] Lisa Goines and Louis Hagler (2007) "Noise Pollution: A Modern Plague," Stephen A Stansfeld and Mark P Matheson (2003) "Noise Pollution: Non-auditory Effects on Health," and Louis Hagler (2008) "Noise Pollution and Health."

[13] Rachel Gordon (2008) "SF Traffic Noise Risks Health of 1 in 6."

[14] For example, see the classic Jane Jacobs (1993) *The Death and Life of Great American Cities*.

SMOG, DEADLIER THAN EVER

The California Air Resources Board (CARB) has passed rules that would severely limit carbon dioxide emissions from cars and trucks.

Fred Webber of the Alliance of Automobile Manufacturers complained that the new rules were utopian folly: Californians will pay a king's ransom for no environmental benefit and the technology can't be developed in the time. Peter Welch, president of the California Motor Car Dealers Association, worried about the limits to consumer choice and that the added expense would be 3 times what CARB projected.

Other states, particularly New York and the New England states, are likely to follow California's lead. In air pollution control, California holds a unique position: because California regulated air pollution before passage of the 1968 Clean Air Act, California can set standards higher than EPA's national standards. Other states can use either the EPA standards or California's tougher standards.

Mr. Webber and Mr. Welch were singing an old song. Automobile manufacturers and dealers, as well as industrial polluters, argue that regulations are too expensive, won't do any good, and are not technically feasible.

What has driven air pollution control is another old song: smog kills.

Smog and Your Heart

In April 2004, the American Heart Association (AHA) officially included air pollution as a risk factor for cardiovascular disease. The AHA likened the effect of air pollutants to the effects of smoking.

The specific air pollutants cited by the AHA were carbon monoxide, oxides of nitrogen, ozone, particulate matter, and sulfur dioxide. The first four come mostly from cars and trucks and are the result of combustion. Sulfur dioxide comes mostly from industrial polluters burning coal.

A study of the 90 largest US cities showed that for each increase of 10 micrograms of particulate matter per cubic meter of air
- total deaths increased by 0.21%
- and cardiovascular deaths increased by 0.31%.

These are small percentages. In the cities studied, the daily concentration of particulate matter ranged from 26 to 534 micrograms per cubic meter. In the San Francisco Bay Area, about 7,400 people die each year from heart attacks and strokes. Reducing particulates by 10 micrograms per cubic meter would save 23 lives each year.

The worst elements of air pollution are heavy oxidizers. Small particles, principally from diesel engines, are especially dangerous. Called "reactive oxygen species," they cause direct oxidative injury to both lungs and heart. Although the body responds with anti-oxidants, for some it's not enough.

Smog, Asthma, and Lung Development

In the last 25 years, the percentage of people diagnosed with asthma has doubled, from about 3.5% to 7.2%. The number of kids with asthma is about 20% greater than the number of adults.

In August 2004, Environmental Defense (EDF) released *Dangerous Days of Summer*, a report on the risk kids face from air pollution. They ranked 50 metropolitan areas by an index for the number of asthmatic children at risk.

Los Angeles was first, then Riverside-San Bernardino, New York City, Philadelphia, Houston, Washington, DC, Chicago, Baltimore, Atlanta, Detroit. Fresno, Sacramento, and Bakersfield.

It's likely that the danger is underestimated. For their risk index, EDF used the national average for the percent of children with asthma. But in Fresno, asthma in children occurs twice as often as the national average, no doubt because of agricultural contaminants such as pesticides. And in Harlem, asthma in children is triple the national average, the effects of economic and racial inequality.

There's a strange dance around what causes asthma. The EDF report is agnostic. However, one study has shown that smog causes healthy rats to become asthmatic. Given what we know about the inflammatory effect of smog and particulates on lung and heart tissue, it's not a great leap to say that air pollution causes asthma, by itself and in concert with exposure to smoking, molds, dust mites, and allergens.

Physiologically, asthma is an inflammatory process that permanently changes your body's reaction to lung irritants. Susceptibility comes from genetics and the developmental effects of air pollution and other environmental factors.

In an 8-year study of children in 12 Southern California communities, kids in smoggier communities suffered permanently reduced lung capacity. Diminished lung capacity puts these children at greater risk of asthma and other chronic illnesses.

The effect of air pollution on our kids' developing lungs is creating a huge health bill that will come due in the future.

Exposure and Protection

You can protect yourself in two ways: reduce your exposure and support your body.

Reduce your exposure to air pollution.

- Move to a cleaner community. This is a very big deal and requires you to research the cleanliness of your new community.
- Live as far away from major traffic as possible, especially truck routes and congested stop-and-go traffic.
- Use an air purifier in your living and work space. Not air filters or dehumidifiers. Purifiers react with the contaminants in the air to make them inert and precipitate them out.
- Keep your living and work space free of dust, molds, and allergens.

Support your body against the effects of air pollution.

- Include plenty of anti-oxidants in your diet. Take supplements and eat nutrient-rich foods.
- Recover from stress with rest, particularly when your immune system is challenged.
- Support your immune system with a modality that works well for you (such as homeopathy and herbs).
- Identify and eliminate allergenic foods from your diet.

Resources

Balbus, John and Yewlin Chee. 2004. Dangerous Days of Summer. *Environmental Defence*. Accessed at www.edf.org.

Brook, Robert D., et al. 2004. Air Pollution and Cardiovascular Disease. *Circulation*. 109: 2655-2671). Accessed at www.circulationaha.org.

Gauderman, W. James, et al. 2004. The Effect of Air Pollution on Lung Development from 10 to 18 Years of Age. *New England Journal of Medicine*. 351(11), September 9, 2004, 1057-67.

THE WIFI BLUES[1]

Philadelphia, the city of brotherly love is going to have it; many in San Francisco want it: Wireless broadband Internet access (*WiFi*).[2] It seems too good to be true. At relatively low cost, anyone can get on the Internet anywhere in a city. All the city needs to do is install a network of WiFi antennas.

An often-repeated argument in favor of citywide WiFi is that it will help close the digital divide: the poorer you are, the more limited your access to the Internet and its wealth of information resources. Cities such as Philadelphia and San Francisco are actively trying to close the digital divide. One option is WiFi.

Yet in weighing the options, virtually nothing is heard about the potential health risks. Saturating an entire city with WiFi adds to the existing burden of radio frequency radiation (*RFR*). That burden, called *electrosmog*[3] by some, consists of long-term exposure to low-levels of nonionizing electromagnetic radiation in the radio frequency and microwave range from familiar sources such as radio and TV broadcast signals, radar, and the ubiquitous cell phone.

Health Risks

Henry Lai, PhD has been researching the biological and health effects of RFR for 35 years. His research focuses on the effects of RFR in the range used by cell phones and other wireless technologies. His laboratory at the University of Washington in Seattle is the single remaining lab in the US that conducts such research. Ten years ago it was one of four.

There is no funding in the United States for research of the biological and health effects of RFR and EMF. No foundation, government agency, or corporation will lay down money to help clarify the science behind concerns about WiFi, cell phones, and other wireless devices. Dr. Lai keeps his lab going by doing cancer research, some of it concerning the use of electromagnetic radiation to treat cancer.

In Europe there are many well-funded projects in RFR research. Citizens are more organized. Public figures have championed the issue. And the European Union has a much greater public health orientation than the United States. These days we have to rely on the Europeans for the science of wireless technology health risks.[4]

It was not always so. For example, in the early 1990s the Cellular Telecommunications and Internet Association (CTIA) came up with $25 million for research into the potential health effects of cell phones.

The CTIA is the cell phone industry's trade organization. Their intention was to lay concerns about cell phones to rest. The Wireless Technology Research (WTR) program administered the funds and research program. When the $25 million was spent, the WTR final report submitted in 2000 recommended further study. The CTIA cut a deal with the FDA to spend another $1 million to review further research.[5]

The money is still there. The FDA has been waiting since 1999 when the deal with CTIA was cut to spend the money.

> FDA plans to convene a meeting in the near future to evaluate all completed, ongoing and planned research looking at health effects associated with the use of wireless communication devices and identify knowledge gaps that may warrant additional research.[6]

Initially, the WTR found no cause for concern. But in 1995 Dr. Lai and his colleague NP Singh, PhD found that exposing the brain cells of rats to RFR at a level similar to cell phones produced breaks in strands of DNA. Their discovery was a turning point in the research and in the CTIA's enthusiasm for the project. Dr. Lai and Dr. Singh had uncovered a mechanism that explained how RFR exposure might cause health effects.[7]

Since 1990 Dr. Lai has maintained a database of research on the effects of RFR on humans, lab animals, and cell cultures. He has amassed over 300 studies published in peer reviewed scientific journals. To avoid bias, he excludes his own research from the database.

Of these studies, 56% show a biological or health effect[8] from exposure to RFR. These effects include
- cancer,[9]
- genetic effects such as damage to DNA,[10]
- cellular and molecular effects such as a reduction in enzymes critical to the central nervous system,[11]
- changes in electrophysiology such as reduced activity between nerve cells,[12] and
- physiological and behavioral changes such as impairment of peripheral vision.[13]

Biased Research?

An interesting thing happens when the studies from Dr. Lai's database are placed in two stacks: one of studies funded by the wireless industry (30% of the studies), the other stack of independently funded studies (70%). Of the studies that show a biological or health effect from wireless RFR, 14% are industry funded while 86% are independently funded. Of studies showing no effect, 49% are industry funded while 51% are independently funded.

To make the point another way, of industry funded studies, only 27% found an RFR effect. Independently funded studies found an RFR effect 68% of the time. This discrepancy is consistent among the effects listed. Of studies that found an effect on cancer, 11% were industry funded, 47% were independently funded. Cellular and molecular effects: 19% industry, 69% independent. Electrophysiology effects: 33% industry, 77% independent. Physiological and behavioral effects: 57% industry, 83% independent.

If Dr. Lai's research were included in the tally, the percent of studies showing an effect from RFR would be even greater. But when Dr. Lai is asked about these statistics, he often says that 50% of the studies show an effect. And then he points out that 50% is a significant number, significant enough to justify a precautionary approach that minimizes exposures.

The differences between the industry funded stack of studies and the independently funded stack suggest bias. Bias enters research through the way a study is designed, the methods used in the study, how data is collected, and how results are interpreted. It might be that some independently funded researchers are biased because they are consumed by a burning passion to eliminate RFR exposures or, even more sinister, destroy the wireless industry. They might have consciously or unconsciously designed their studies, chosen methods, collected data, and interpreted the results to show health effects from RFR. However, the rewards for doing so are not great. Many researchers who advise precaution regarding RFR have been ostracized or their research funding has been slashed. Careers have been stalled and in some cases terminated—hardly circumstances that would encourage jumping on that particular bandwagon. [14]

The rewards for producing industry-friendly results are obvious: funding, professional recognition, a clear career path, and employment opportunities in industry. This is not to say that these researchers are dishonest. It is to say that rewards are more likely as a consequence of producing the "right" answers. In other words, researchers typically aren't corrupted into conducting biased research. More often they're already biased and the rewards flow to them as a consequence. [15]

Within each group, whether industry or independently funded, results don't always agree—some studies show an effect while others do not regardless of who did the funding. That difference suggests another kind of problem: scientists don't know enough yet to conduct decisive experiments that can produce something like a professional consensus regarding the biological and health effects of wireless RFR. Many of the scientists who work in this field and who believe that there's ample reason for concern will say that the science is not yet conclusive. [16] This drives some activists crazy. Yet it is a true statement about the state of the science.

We should not be surprised that this lack of conclusive science has led the wireless industry to claim that cell phones and other wireless technologies are safe. The FDA is with them, stating that

> [t]he available scientific evidence does not show that any health problems are associated with using wireless phones. There is no proof, however, that wireless phones are absolutely safe.[17]

This carefully constructed statement is intended to reassure us. Yet Dr. Lai's database puts the lie to the first sentence: it's simply false. The framework set up for us is that a technology should be adopted unless there's conclusive evidence that it does harm. Not all regulatory agencies think this way.

The UK's equivalent to the FDA, the Health Protection Agency (HPA), has declared a voluntary moratorium of marketing cell phones to children as a precautionary measure.[18] The moratorium has so far been observed by the UK cell phone industry. The HPA opens its discussion of the health risks from cell phones by saying that

> There is a large body of scientific evidence relating to exposure to radio waves and there are thousands of published scientific papers covering studies of exposed tissue samples (e.g. cells), animals and people. It is not difficult to find contradictory results in the literature, and an important role of the HPA Radiological Protection Division (RPD) is to develop judgments [sic] on the totality of the evidence in controversial areas of the science.[19]

Unlike the FDA, the HPA points to contradictory science regarding cell phone radiation. The reassurance is that they're paying attention, not that cell phones very likely don't cause harm. The HPA goes on to cite the National Radiological Protection Board (NRPB), which reviews the science and recommends standards. The NRPB and with it the HPA explicitly adopt a precautionary standard. With regard to children, the NRPB's 2004 report recommends that

> in the absence of new scientific evidence, the recommendation in the Stewart Report on limiting the use of mobile phones by children remains appropriate as a precautionary measure.[20]

In 2004 the International Association of Fire Fighters (*IAFF*) decided that they will not permit cell phone antennas on fire houses. The decision was made by resolution at the IAFF's annual delegate assembly. The resolution directed the International to review the potential health risks from cell antennas. If the science demonstrated a risk, then the union would oppose the use of fire stations as sites for cell antennas until further science demonstrated that cell antennas are safe.[21]

The resolution was passed in August 2004. In April 2005 the union's Health and Safety Department completed the review of the science. They found more than ample evidence to conclude that the union should oppose cell antennas on fire stations. The position paper included 49 references and a bibliography of 40 citations.[22] Based on that evidence, the resolution cites a wide range of effects experienced by fire fighters:

- slowed reaction times,
- lack of focus,
- lack of impulse control,
- severe headaches,
- anesthesia-like sleep,
- sleep deprivation,
- depression,
- tremors, and
- vertigo.[23]

Three things are worth noting about the substance of the resolution and the union's official position. First, the fire fighters were focused on their ability to do their job. Second, fire fighters were involuntarily exposed to a health risk. And third, the fire fighters oppose cell antennas on fire stations until they are proven safe.

The decision that the fire fighters faced—a decision we all face—is how to evaluate the safety of wireless technologies and decide what level of involuntary risk we are willing to take.[24]

- Use it unless there's good evidence that it's harmful.
- Or don't use it until there's good evidence that it's safe.

So consider this: 47% of independently funded studies found cancer effects, 69% found effects on cell function, 77% found effects on electrical signaling in the body, and 83% found physiological and behavioral effects. Suppose you have several hundred marine biologists study your swimming pool. 47% (or 69% or 77% or 83%) of the biologists say you've got a shark in your pool. Would you dive in? Would you let your kids dive in?[25]

RFR Exposures

Citywide WiFi is only the latest RFR wireless technology to place us involuntarily at risk. Cell phone networks are the best known, which include personal digital assistants (*PDAs*) such as the Blackberry™. Wireless networks at home and at the office are newer than cell phones and are another RFR exposure. Even if you don't have one, your neighbor might and that will expose you. Also relatively new are the Bluetooth technologies used for applications such as hands-free telephone headsets which operate using RFR. The familiar cordless phone is another RFR exposure that might put you at as much risk as a cell phone.[26]

What these technologies share is reciprocal receiving and transmitting of RFR signals between an end-user device and antennas that link the device to a network. There are three characteristics of these RFR signals that are believed to contribute to the biological and health effects of wireless technologies: signal strength, frequency, and modulation.[27]

Signal strength is measured in watts, a standard unit of energy. Although less in signal strength compared to cell phone antennas, citywide WiFi nevertheless uses a signal strength sufficient to blanket a wide area. Wireless networks for the home and office have less signal strength (although they can be increased with boosters). Bluetooth devices have even less strength. And while older cordless phones had low signal strength, current models emit radiation equivalent to cell phones.

All of these technologies use roughly the same frequency band: 0.3 to 3 GHz. *GHz* stands for *gigahertz*. A *hertz* is a standard measure of electromagnetic radiation created by sending an alternating electrical current through an antenna that is one cycle per second. A gigahertz is one billion cycles per second. The higher the GHz, the faster the current alternates.

An alternative way of measuring RFR is in wavelength. Wavelengths have an exact and inverse relationship to frequency: higher frequencies correspond to shorter wavelengths. Visible light is electromagnetic radiation with higher frequencies and shorter wavelengths than RFR, with red light having a lower frequency and longer wavelength than blue light.

Modulation refers to whether the signal comes at a constant frequency (as in AM radio and analog cell phone systems) or in pulses (as in FM radio and digital cell phones). All digital wireless technologies are pulsed. Risk increases with signal strength. But risk also increases at low signal strength where a breakdown in the blood-brain barrier has be demonstrated.

The frequencies used by wireless technologies are to some extent "ideal" for affecting our bodies because the wavelengths are at a human scale. Digital (pulsed) signals are of greater risk than analog signals.[28]

Short-term, high-intensity exposures to wireless RFR have received the most research attention, in particular the acute affects of cell phones. Far fewer studies have looked at long-term effects of cell phone use let alone the use of other wireless devices. Even less studied are the effects of the low-intensity, persistent exposure to RFR from cell phone and WiFi antennas.

Electrohypersensitivity

Much of the discussion about RFR health effects is framed as a concern with people who are electrohypersensitive. Unlike immune-mediated hypersensitivity that responds to allergens, electrohypersensitivity is a reaction to nonionizing electromagnetic radiation from video display monitors, cell phones, cordless phones, wireless routers, or other RFR source. Characteristic symptoms of electrohypersensitivity can include:[29]

- localized heat and tingling,
- dry upper respiratory tract and eye irritation,
- brain fog, headache, and nausea,
- swollen mucus membranes,
- muscle and joint pain,
- heart palpitations, and
- progressively severe sensitivity to light.

Critics argue that electrohypersensitivity is not a physical ailment but a psychological one. Research led by Olle Johansson, MD at the Karolinska Institute in Stockholm identified changes in mast cells in electrohypersensitives.[30] So Dr. Johansson exposed rats to RFR exposures similar to his human subjects, assuming that the rat psyche is not predisposed to produce the symptoms of electrohypersensitivity. The study produced results similar to what he found in human subjects: enlarged mast cells aggregated close to the surface of the skin.

Dr. Johansson went further and tested both electrohypersensitives and nonsensitives human subjects in similar exposures. Though the nonsensitives had no hypersensitivity symptoms, the mast cells in their skin showed the same behavior as electrohypersensitives, although the effect was less severe.[31] Based on this research, Dr. Johansson and his colleague Shabnam Gangi proposed one mechanism for the health effects of RFR as an immunological response, hypothesizing as to how this mechanism affects internal organs such as the cardiovascular and neurological systems.[32]

In *The Invisible Disease*,[33] Finnish journalist Gunni Nordström associates electrohypersensitivity with multiple chemical sensitivity and chronic fatigue syndrome. People in Sweden made electrohypersensitivity a public health issue when cathode ray tube-based video display monitors were introduced into offices. The rise of Silicon Valley—both in the original Silicon Valley and the many Silicon Valleys that have developed around the world—gave rise similar health effects among computer manufacturing workers. Researchers observed a relationship between materials used in products and their synergistic reaction with electromagnetic radiation.[34] But both funding for research and data collection on occupational health quickly dried up when these issues came to light.

Electrohypersensitives are not an unlucky few. They are likely harbingers in a complex landscape of environmental risks. Just like any other environmental stressor, RFR affects some people more than others. And as with other environmental stressors, the greater the overall burden, the greater the risk of becoming one of the "unlucky few."

Citywide WiFi adds to the existing burden of RFR.[35] Just as burning more fossil fuels adds to the level of smog, adding more RFR adds to the level of electrosmog. You don't have to expose your home or your city to the increased burden created by WiFi. There's a viable alternative: a wired Internet access and network. The hype might make it seem less convenient and more expensive. But what's a good night's sleep worth? Or reducing your risk of cancer?[36]

Postscript

Since the publication of this article a group of researchers calling themselves the Bioinitiative Working Group[37] has published a report on the health effects of electromagnetic radiation. Their *Bioinitiative Report*[38] assembles the research on the health effects of RFR. The *Report* argues that current exposure standards are at least one thousand times greater than is justified by the science the author's review. The *Bioinitiative Report*, published in August 2007, was widely publicized in Europe and had an immediate effect: the European Environment Agency, the European Union's equivalent of the US Environmental Protection Agency, called for an immediate re-examination of RFR exposure standards.[39] Subsequently, the European Parliament took up the issue and is headed for legislation to lower exposure standards. No mention of the *Report* was made in the US media and no major public official has taken it up as a call to action.

Notes

1. Originally published in the *Townsend Letter* July 2007.
2. See Wireless Philadelphia (http://www.wirelessphiladelphia.org) and San Francisco TechConnect (http://www.sfgov.org/techconnect/)
3. The term is more familiar in Europe than in the US because of the greater political attention paid to the issue by citizen groups and politicians who support them. Beginning in Sweden in the 1980s, citizens suffering from *electrohypersensitivity* have been vocal advocates for research into the health risks from non-ionizing electromagnetic radiation and for the reduction of electrosmog. See the Swedish Association for the Electrosensitive (http://www.feb.se/index_int.htm).
4. Louis Slesin (2006) "EMF Health News."
5. George Carlo and Martin Schram (2001) *Cell Phone: Invisible Hazards in the Wireless Age: An Insider's Alarming Discoveries about Cancer and Genetic Damage.*
6. FDA, Cell Phone Facts: Consumer Information on Wireless Phones (http://www.fda.gov/cdrh/wireless/braincancer040606.html).
7. The original Lai and Singh research was published in 1995 (Henry Lai and Narendra Pal Singh (1995) "Acute Low-intensity Microwave Exposure Increases DNA Single-strand Breaks in Rat Brain Cells"). The next year they published a paper showing even more alarming effects on DNA: double

DNA strand breaks (Henry Lai and Narendra Pal Singh (1996) "Single-and Double-strand DNA Breaks in Rat Brain Cells after Acute Exposure to Low-level Radiofrequency Electromagnetic Radiation"). Subsequent research has confirmed these findings and found that the breaks can persist in cell cultures through multiple mitotic cycles—Gursatej Gandhi (2005) "Genetic Damage in Mobile Phone Users: Some Preliminary Findings."

8 The phrase "biological or health effect" is common in this literature. Some research is focused specifically on illness while other research simply looks at effects on the organism which might have a downstream health effect.

9 For example Lennart Hardell, et al. (2006) "Pooled Analysis of Two Case-control Studies on Use of Cellular and Cordless Telephones and the Risk of Malignant Brain Tumours Diagnosed in 1997-2003."

10 For example Elisabeth Diem, et al. (2005) "Non-thermal DNA Breakage by Mobile-phone Radiation (1800mhz) in Human Fibroblasts and in Transformed GFSH-r17 Rat Granulosa Cells *In Vitro*" and Gursatej Gandhi (2005) "Genetic Damage in Mobile Phone Users: Some Preliminary Findings."

11 For example Mario Barteri, et al. (2005) "Structural and Kinetic Effects of Mobile Phone Microwaves on Acetylcholinesterase Activity."

12 For example Shujun Xu, et al. (2006) "Chronic Exposure to GSM 1800-mhz Microwaves Reduces Excitatory Synaptic Activity in Cultured Hippocampal Neurons."

13 For example Peter Langer, et al. (2005) "Hands-free Mobile Phone Conversation Impairs the Peripheral Visual System to an Extent Comparable to an Alcohol Level of 4-5 g 100 ml" and David L. Strayer, et al. (2006) "A Comparison of the Cell Phone Driver and the Drunk Driver."

14 A telling example is described in the November 2005 edition of *Microwave News* (http://www.microwavenews.com). Louis Slesin (2005) "When Enough Is Never Enough: A Reproducible EMF Effect at 12 Mg." Beginning in 1992, seven separate research projects have demonstrated an effect on breast cancer cell metabolism from extremely low electromagnetic radiation, intensities much lower than current standards and well below intensities that are supposed to have any effect. The effect disrupts cell signaling. Each report was ignored. The original researcher was, as Louis Slesin describes it, "drummed out of the EMF profession." The others have had funding cut and endured other harassments. An even more chilling example is described in Gunni Nordstron (2004) *The Invisible Disease: The Dangers of Environmental Illnesses Caused by Electromagnetic Fields and Chemical Emissions*. She describes how the once promising career of Olle Johansson, MD, a leading dermatological researcher at the Karolinska Institute in Stockholm, Sweden, has been damaged. With over 400 peer reviewed publications and major discoveries in dermatology, Dr. Johansson has been refused promotion to full professorship, denied research funding, and denied research facilities for his continued interest in RFR health effects and for his advocacy for electrohypersensitives.

15 The notorious example of how pharmaceutical companies shape medical research and medical practice is described by two insiders: Marcia Angell, MD, a former editor at the *New England Journal of Medicine* and John Abramson, MD, a professor at the Harvard School of Medicine—Marcia Angell (2004) *The Truth about the Drug Companies: How They Deceive Us*

and What To Do About It. and John Abramson (2004) *Overdosed America: The Broken Promise of American Medicine.*

[16] Dr. Lai's 2005 review article is a good example. It describes the many issues in the field that remain unresolved. Henry Lai (2005) "Biological Effects of Radiofrequency Electromagnetic Fields."

[17] Fda, Cell Phone Facts: Do Wireless Phones Pose a Health Hazard? (http://www.fda.gov/cellphones/qa.html#22).

[18] In April 1999 the UK's Ministry of Health formed the Independent Expert Group on Mobile Phones to evaluate the safety of cell phones. Chaired by Sir William Stewart, the commission of independent scientists (which became known as the Stewart Group) reported in May 2000 that enough scientific evidence existed to be concerned about health risks from "subtle effects on biological functions, especially those of the brain." The Stewart Group noted in particular that children would be more susceptible to harm. See the Stewart Group's report Independent Expert Group on Mobile Phones (2000) *Mobile Phones and Health.*

[19] Health Protection Agency. Mobile Telephony and Health: Health Protection Advice (http://www.hpa.org.uk/radiation/understand/information_sheets/mobile_telephony/health_advice.htm).

[20] National Radiological Protection Board (2004) *Mobile Phones and Health 2004*, page 11.

[21] International Association of Fire Fighters (2005) *Position on the Health Effects from Radio Frequency/microwave (RF/MW) Radiation in Fire Department Facilities from Base Stations for Antennas and Towers for the Conduction of Cell Phone Transmissions.*

[22] Ibid. page 13-38. Dr. Lai's database was used as a resource.

[23] Ibid. page 13.

[24] For an excellent discussion of how to evaluate environmental risk, see Mary O'Brien (2000) *Making Better Environmental Decisions: An Alternative to Risk Assessment.*

[25] Some might rightfully howl at this analogy. An "exposure" to a shark is nothing like an exposure to RFR. No analogy is perfect. So consider another. Hundreds of microbiologists test your pool water for cholera and 47% find it. Or hundreds of chemists test your pool water for a powerful toxin with both short-term and long-term effects, something such as mercury, and 47% find it at various concentrations. Sharks are just so much more dramatic. And the analogy makes the same point: how much agreement among scientists do you need to be assured that something is safe?

[26] At the time of the research cited below, the signal strength from cordless phones is far less than cell phones, people tend to use them for longer periods of time: exposure per unit time is less for the cordless phone, but the total exposure is equivalent to that of a cell phone. A European study found equivalent cancer risks for cell phone users and cordless phone users. Lennart Hardell, et al. (2006) "Pooled analysis of two case-control studies on use of cellular and cordless telephones and the risk of malignant brain tumours diagnosed in 1997-2003."

[27] Henry Lai (2005) "Biological Effects of Radiofrequency Electromagnetic Fields."

[28] Ibid..

[29] See Olle Johansson (2004) "Screen Dermatitis and Electrosensitivity: Pre-

liminary Observations in the human skin," Gunni Nordstron (2004) *The Invisible Disease: The Dangers of Environmental Illnesses Caused by Electromagnetic Fields and Chemical Emissions*, and the Swedish Association for the Electrosensitive (http://www.feb.se/index_int.htm).

[30] A mast cell is a type of immune cell that stores histamine crystals which are released during an allergic response. The skin of the electrohypersensitives Dr. Johansson examined had an abnormally high concentration of mast cells close to the skin's surface that also had high loads of histamine. In other words, these subjects' immune-mediated response is in a reactive state.

[31] Olle Johansson (2004) "Screen Dermatitis and Electrosensitivity: Preliminary Observations in the Human Skin" and Olle Johansson, et al. (1999) "A Case of Extreme and General Cutaneous Light Sensitivity in Combination with So-called 'Screen Dermatitis' and 'Electrosensitivity' - A Successful Rehabilitation after Vitamin A Treatment - A Case Report"

[32] Shabnam Gangi and Olle Johansson (2000) "A Theoretical Model Based Upon Mast Cells and Histamine to Explain the Recently Proclaimed Sensitivity to Electric And/or Magnetic Fields in Humans."

[33] Gunni Nordstron (2004) *The Invisible Disease: The Dangers of Environmental Illnesses Caused by Electromagnetic Fields and Chemical Emissions.*

[34] Joseph LaDou (2006) "Occupational Health in the Semiconductor Industry."

[35] The total burden of already existing electrosmog goes beyond send-receive wireless technologies such as WiFi and cell phones and includes pedestrian technologies such as radio and television broadcast signals. Research by Dr. Johansson and his colleague Örjan Hallberg at the Karolinska Institute looked at the incidence of cancer and other 20th Century illnesses in Europe and the US and found a striking association between the increase in certain cancers during the 20th Century and exposure to RFR as measured by radio and TV broadcasts. Örjan Hallberg and Olle Johansson (2002a) "Cancer Trends during the 20th Century," Örjan Hallberg and Olle Johansson (2002b) "Melanoma Incidence and Frequency Modulation (FM) Broadcasting," and Örjan Hallberg and Olle Johansson (2005) "FM Broadcasting Exposure Time and Malignant Melanoma Incidence."

[36] See Sage, Cindy (2009) "Regulating Wireless Radiation," B. Blake Levitt (2008) "Safe Cell Tower Siting," Cindy Sage and David O. Carpenter (2007) "Bioinitiative: Standards for Electrosmog,"B. Blake Levitt and Cindy Sage (2006) "Where You're Exposed and What To Do: EMF and RFR," Louis Slesin (2006) "EMF Health News," Magda Havas (2006) "Dirty Electricity and EMF Health Dangers," Olle Johansson (2006) "The Science of RFR Health Risks," B. Blake Levitt and Janet Newton (2006) "Wireless Public Health Crisis," Olle Johansson and Doug Loranger (2005) "Electrosmog," and Cindy Sage (2005) "Smart Exposures: Understanding Risks from EMF and RFR."

[37] Bioinitiative Working Group (http://www.bioinitiative.org).

[38] Bioinitiative Working Group et al (2007) *Bioinitiative Report: A Rationale for a Biologically-based Public Exposure Standard for Electromagnetic Fields (ELF and RF).* The principal authors of the *Report* were interviewed on *Your Own Health And Fitness* (Cindy Sage and David O. Carpenter (2007) "Bioinitiative: Standards for Electrosmog").

[39] Geoffrey Lean (2007) "EU Watchdog Calls for Urgent Action on Wi-Fi Radiation."

SICK BUILDINGS

Most of us work in a building. If you're an employee, you work in your employer's building. Even if you're independent, you often have to work in your client's building.

Most office buildings, especially those constructed in the last half century, cause sick building syndrome. Although sometimes categorized as "unexplained illness," along with illnesses such as multiple chemical sensitivity and fibromyalgia, significant elements of the syndrome can in fact be explained. One problem is that conventional science is unable to grasp the multi-system effects that characterize these illnesses.

The relationship between exposures and how they affect specific people needs to be untangled. Understanding how a building and what's in it can cause acute symptoms such as headache is difficult enough. It's even harder to connect a building and what's in it to the emergence of a chronic illness.

With these limitations, clinicians and researchers struggle to come up with diagnostic criteria. Those who are sympathetic try to make sense of symptoms that can include a range of allergic and immune reactions, toxic reactions, and neurological effects, both acute and chronic. Those who are not sympathetic work to show that it's imagined by the sufferer.

Focus on Acute Suffering

As a diagnosis, sick building syndrome focuses on acute symptoms. What distinguishes it from chronic illnesses, such as multiple chemical sensitivity, is that symptoms stop when the sufferer leaves the sick building.

Somehow this seems to suggest to researchers that sick building syndrome is not a chronic illness. However, research shows that symptoms have a well-defined dose-response relationship and that the people who are most likely to react also have physiological markers that point to conditions such as compromised immunity. It's like saying you're allergic only when you're sneezing.

On top of that, there seems to be little research into the long term implications for health. If someone works in a sick building for 20 years without having symptoms, are they at greater risk of compromised health or early death?

An example...

One study found that increased smog outside increases the incidence of sick building syndrome reactions. What's called ozone is a principal bad player (it's not just the molecule ozone, but other molecules that are heavy oxidizers). The explanation of what's going on is quite frightening.

Volatile organic compounds (VOCs) are everywhere in buildings. They come from paint, carpet, furniture, computer equipment, you name it. Some of these materials have been shown to contribute directly to acute sick building syndrome reactions. What the oxidizers in smog do is oxidize materials that would otherwise be stable and non-toxic and turn them into toxins. Ventilation systems then circulate the old and the new toxins throughout the building.

The ventilation system contributes in another way. Most filters on ventilation systems are made from polyester. Ozone reacts with polyester and produces VOCs that are then blown into the building. Researchers estimate that the ill effect of ozone indoors is ten times its effect outdoors because of these reactions.

Chronic Suffering

Back to long-term effects. It's well established that long-term exposure to smog increases the risk of diabetes, heart attacks, and stroke not to mention asthma, emphysema, and other lung diseases. Long-term exposure to VOCs increases the risk of liver, kidney, and nerve damage. Short-term exposures to VOCs are strongly implicated in creating multiple chemical sensitivity, fibromyalgia, and other multi-system chronic illnesses.

Linking long-term exposures to chronic illness is difficult. A case reported in *Scientific American* describes just how difficult.

Two long-time workers at an engine manufacturer died of brain cancer in their mid-50s. Their families pressed for an investigation, suspecting the oils, greases, and solvents to which these men were exposed.

This has led to a multi-million dollar epidemiological study that has to solve such problems as identifying who worked in which manufacturing plant and when they worked there, what substances each person was exposed to, and the state of each person's health. An additional part of the puzzle is that many chronic illnesses have a latency period (it doesn't show up immediately after) and have a dose response relationship (longer exposure causes greater risk).

So the researchers working on this project have to piece together all the parts. This points to what is a basic problem in workplace health and safety: there's no easy way to bring together data on exposures with data on who's sick and what they're sick with. What that means is that it's very difficult for researchers to reliably establish relationships between workplace conditions and worker long-term health—or for that matter worker short-term health.

Joseph LaDou, a researcher in occupational health, has argued that the workers' compensation system actively prevents us from understanding these relationships. Instead, he advocates a single payer medical care system that is able to track people's ill health and injuries with their exposures across place and time. Such a change would also enable people to get the medical care they need without the dynamics of the workers' compensation system putting pressure on them to choose between health and income.

In other words, we don't know nearly as much as we could about how buildings and the materials in them affect the people who work in them—or the people who live in them. However, we know enough so far to say that, since you probably spend about half your waking life working in a building that is very likely sick, there's little doubt you're at risk. So the next time you start looking for a better job, you'd be wise to check out the health of the building you'll be working in. Come to think of it, you should check out that better house or apartment you're about to move into.

The News

Biello, David. 2008. Smog Can Make People Sick, Even Indoors: When the air is thick with pollution, "sick building" complaints become more common. *Scientific American*. January 29, 2008.

Bass, Carole. 2008. Solving a Massive Worker Health Puzzle. *Scientific American*. March 2008:86-93.

The Research

Apte, Michael et al. 2008. Outdoor ozone and building-related symptoms in the BASE study. *Indoor Air*. April 2008 (18):156-70.

Buchanan, Ian et al. 2008. Air filter materials, outdoor ozone and building-related symptoms in the BASE study. *Indoor Air*. April 2008 (18):144-55.

Chao, H. Jasmine et al. 2003. The Work Environment and Workers' Health in Four Large Office Buildings. *Environmental Health Perspectives*. July 2003 (111:9): 1242-8.

Hodgson, Michael. 2002. Indoor Environmental Exposures and Symptoms. *Environmental Health Perspectives*. August 2002 (110:Supplement 4): 663-7.

Ladou, Joseph. 2006. Occupational and Environmental Medicine in the United States: A Proposal to Abolish Workers' Compensation and Reestablish the Public Health Model. *International Journal of Occupational and Environmental Health*. April/June 2006(12:2):154-68.

Resources

Architects / Designers / Planners for Social Responsibility Northern California Chapter, Green and Healthy Building. Access at http://www.adpsr-norcal.org/menu/ResourceGuide/booksgreenbldg.html.

Healthy Building Network. Access at http://www.healthybuilding.net.

Natural Building Network. Access at http://www.naturalbuildingnetwork.org.

Pall, Martin. 2007. *Explaining Unexplained Illness.* Binghamton, NY:Harrington Park Press.

Your Own Health And Fitness. Resources on Environmental Health. Access at http://www.yourownhealthandfitness.org/topicsEnvironment.php.

Does the heavy perfume of spring lift your spirits? Do the short, cold days of winter slow your pace and turn your attention inward? Do you have an animal companion? Do you have houseplants? Do you tend a garden, large or small?

Our connection with the natural world and its effect on our health is even more intimate than the emotional effect of "nature." For example, it turns out that parasites—specifically round worms—can be good for you.[1] A body of research has developed on how roundworms elicit an immune response that protects against diseases of inflammation. In addition to conferring protection against allergies, these parasites promote immune protection against inflammatory bowel disease, asthma, multiple sclerosis, and diabetes.[2]

Two decades ago, researchers noticed that in populations where the incidence of roundworm infestations decreased, the incidence of inflammatory bowel disease increased. By following that trail, the researchers have achieved some clinical successes in curing inflammatory bowel disease and other diseases of inflammation by exposing patients to these parasites.

According to the media, one of the original researchers—Dr. Joel Weinstock of Tufts University—"foresees new worm-based drugs." And although Dr. Weinstock also says, "We're part of our environment; we're not separate from it" the media missed the point entirely, instead paraphrasing him as saying, "You are a community of interacting organisms."[3]

You aren't a community. You're a *member* of a community of interacting organisms.[4] And please keep the drug companies away.

Twenty-five years ago, Edward O. Wilson published *Biophilia*.[5] His hypothesis is that humans have an innate attraction to other organisms, whether plant or animal. A limited amount of research sprang up around this idea, from which emerged the concept of *biophobia*: humans' innate aversion to some organisms. So in its full-blown version, the hypothesis is that humans are naturally drawn to some organisms, naturally repulsed by others, and indifferent to still others because these adaptations conferred an evolutionary advantage to our ancestors. Those who had the capacity to learn quickly to approach or avoid certain plants, animals, or habitats had a better chance to survive and pass on that capacity.

Out of this scientific literature another literature emerged that connects biophilia to health outcomes. No doubt the currency of both increased because of the rising concern for environmental issues.

One of the earliest pieces of research was conducted in a hospital's post-operation ward.[6] Some beds looked out at a grove of trees. Other beds looked out on a brick wall. Patients who looked out on trees took less medication, stayed in the hospital on average one day less, and were rated by the nursing staff as in better spirits than patients who looked out on the brick wall.

Subsequently, a limited amount of research has examined the ways in which health and illness are affected by exposure to natural environments.[7] The following are some of the exposures that have had beneficial effects:

- viewing animals and plants,
- contact with animals and plants, and
- access to and contact with specific landscapes, in the city, country, and wildlands.

For the most part, the research consists of associating environmental exposures with a reduced risk of illness and an improved rate of recovery from illness and injury. The explanations tend to be in the realm of psychology: the beneficial, stress reducing effects of having direct or indirect contact with natural environments. As we discussed in "The Body as Ecology" and "The Hormonal Consequences of Starch and Stress," the body's stress response is manifested in physiological responses that increase risks of illness.

It makes good sense that stress reduction would have a beneficial health effect. There is speculation that such effects come from evolutionary adaptations that conferred Darwinian fitness on those who preferred certain environments.

For example, humans evolved from primates that originated on the African savannah, an environment characterized by grasslands having collections of trees and the occasional body of standing or running water spread throughout a rolling grassland. It sounds like a golf course or urban park—which is just the point.

When people are offered a variety of landscapes to choose from in experimental settings, most respond positively to savannah-like environments. This has been the result of studies in North America, Europe, Asia, and Africa. People in these studies report increased feelings of well-being when viewing these landscapes.[8] Such scenes reduced fear and anger and increased mental alertness, attention, and mental performance.[9]

However, these speculations on evolution and the observation of the beneficial effects of natural environments don't take us much further than the admonitions of 19th Century Transcendentalists such as Henry David Thoreau and early conservationists such as John Muir. Not only is no one looking for the biophilia gene, no one is looking at the physiology of how natural environments affect health—except polluted environments. As one advocate has noted, environmental health is almost exclusively about how we are poisoning ourselves by poisoning our environment.[10]

In addition to asking how we are poisoning ourselves and how to stop it, we should be asking how natural environments and their features confer health benefits directly. For example, the roundworm researchers should be asking how to benefit from the knowledge of how roundworms train the immune system to ward off inflammatory diseases. Few researchers are asking that question directly. Instead, they focus on how to replicate the effect using pharmaceuticals.

It's likely that a big reason no one's asking about the direct health effects of natural environments is that a community of organisms isn't easily replicated by a pharmaceutical or medical device.

Another reason is a weakness that too much of the biophilia research shares with the round worm research. They see natural environments as objects to which we are exposed. There's talk in the biophilia literature about the effect of landscapes and habitats and animal or plant "encounters." That perspective leads to a search for better health through better stage management of the theatre in which we perform—essentially, better environmental mood music. The perspective that's needed would ask how we can best make our way in the community of organisms of which we are members.[11]

The articles in this section are written in the "how we're poisoning ourselves" vein. The first, "Allergic Nation," discusses the rise in allergies and asthma as due to increased exposures to industrial toxins.

The second article, "Drugs in the Water," describes hidden damage done by pharmaceuticals: drugs that end up in waste water systems and eventually in drinking water.

Finally, "The Light Brown Apple Moth" describes a glaring example of bad politics and bad science that threatens health: the aerial spraying to eradicate a moth alleged to be a threat to agriculture with a material known to have toxic effects.

Notes

[1] Covered in the media by Moises Velasquez-Manoff (2008) "The Worm Turns" and Elizabeth Svoboda (2008) "The Worms Crawl In."

[2] David Elliott, et al. (2007) "Helminths as Governors of Immune-mediated Inflammation."

[3] Quotes from Moises Velasquez-Manoff (2008) "The Worm Turns."

[4] A point made with even greater force in "Intestinal Ecology" on page 50.

5 Edward O. Wilson (1986) *Biophilia* and the collection of papers in Stephen R. Kellart and Edward O. Wilson eds (1993) *The Biophilia Hypothesis.*

6 Roger S. Ulrich (1984) "View Through a Window May Influence Recovery from Surgery."

7 For example, see Howard Frumkin (2003) "Healthy Places: Exploring the Evidence," Colin D. Butler and Sharon Friel (2006) "Time to Regenerate: Ecosystems and Health Promotion," and Konstantinos Tzoulas, et al. (2007) "Promoting Ecosystem and Human Health in Urban Areas Using Green Infrastructure: A Literature Review."

8 Roger S. Ulrich (1993) "Biophilia, Biophobia, and Natural Landscapes."

9 Carolyn M. Tennessen and Bernadine Cimprich (1995) "Views to Nature: Effects on Attention" and Terry Hartig, et al. (1991) "Restorative Effects of Natural Environment Experiences."

10 Howard Frumkin (2001) "Beyond Toxicity: Human Health and the Natural Environment."

11 For example, see Frederick Steiner (2002) *Human Ecology: Following Nature's Lead* and Janine M. Benyus (1997) *Biomimcry: Innovation Inspired by Nature.*

ALLERGIC NATION

Asthma has become a critical health problem. In all major industrialized countries, the number of people with asthma increases each year. In the US, the prevalence of asthma has doubled in the last two decades.

Much attention has been given to the effect of environmental stressors on asthma (especially fine particulate air pollution; see "Smog, Deadlier Than Ever" on page 183). However, less attention is paid to the prevalence of allergies generally, with asthma as the most extreme form.

Allergy "attacks" are triggered by contact with an *allergen*. In the classic case of seasonal hay fever, the allergen is a protein from a pollen particle. Although asthma is classified as a form of allergy, attacks can be triggered not only by common allergens but by anything that irritates the lungs—especially fine particulates from fossil fuel exhaust.

Allergies and asthma, referred to as *type 1 hypersensitivity*, are immune responses to otherwise "innocuous" substances. Your body responds as if it were under attack. Allergy symptoms are your body's attempt to get rid of the invader.

Being allergic tends to run in families—if your parents have allergies, you're more likely to have allergies. However, you might not be allergic to the same things. What you inherit is an immune system that tends to overreact. And if you're allergic to one thing, you're more likely to be allergic to others.

This idea led Dr. Samuel Arbes and his colleagues to investigate whether the increase in asthma is from more allergens or greater sensitivity. Are more people having allergic reactions just because there's more stuff provoking them? Or are we becoming more sensitive to our environment?

Sensitivity Rising

The Arbes study was limited and only provides partial answers, but it strongly suggests that we are in fact becoming more allergic to our environment. The study's findings are consistent with similar studies in Japan, the United Kingdom, and Denmark.

Arbes looked at data from the two latest National Health and Nutritional Examination Surveys—referred to as *NHANES II* and *NHANES III*—conducted from 1976 to 1980 (NHANES II) and from 1988 to 1994 (NHANES III).

NHANES II and NHANES III each conducted allergy skin tests for common allergies. Only six were the same in both surveys: ragweed, rye grass, Bermuda grass, oak, cat dander, and the fungus *Alternaria alternata* that's common on plants and crops.

What Arbes found was that the percentage of people who reacted to at least one of these allergens doubled between NHANES II and NHANES III. And the percentage of people who reacted to each of the individual allergens increased from a low of 2.1 times for ragweed to a high of 5.5 times for cat dander.

Change in percentage of people who react to six common allergens

Allergen	Percent who reacted in		Change
	1976-80	**1988-94**	
Ragweed	12.5%	26.2%	+2.1
Rye	11.9%	26.9%	+2.3
Oak	5.8%	13.2%	+2.3
Fungus	4.5%	12.9%	+2.9
Bermuda	5.2%	18.1%	+3.5
Cat	3.1%	17.0%	+5.5

There is no indication that our exposure to any of these allergens has increased. The increase can only be explained by an increase in sensitivity. The implication for asthma is that although our exposure to environmental triggers such as air pollution has increased, our susceptibility has also increased.

Why have we become more sensitive?

Immunity and Allergy

Type 1 hypersensitivity (allergy) is an immune response. The job of the immune system is to recognize unwanted substances and organisms and prevent them from doing harm.

Antibodies are a familiar part of the immune system. They are a kind of memory of unwanted organisms. Specialized white blood cells called *B cells* (because they're produced in bone marrow) produce antibodies that recognize an invader such as a virus. The antibody latches onto the virus and attracts *macrophages* (another kind of white blood cell) that destroy the virus. Antibody production is orchestrated by another kind of white blood cell: a type 1 helper T cell (produced in the thymus) also referred to as a *Th1 cell*.

This classic immune response is typically accompanied by inflammation. The purpose of inflammation is to mobilize the immune system's resources. When the *endothelial cells* that form the outer surface of a tissue sense a foreign substance, they send out chemical signals called *cytokines*. In sending the signal, three things happen that make up the inflammatory response:

- blood flow increases to the tissue;
- white blood cells are attracted to the site; and
- the small blood vessels (capillaries) that supply the tissue become more permeable, permitting white blood cells to get to the tissue.

Antibodies are created from biochemicals called *immunoglobulins*. The three most common immunoglobulins are designated IgG, IgA, and IgM. IgG is present throughout the body and composes 75% of all immunoglobulins. IgA is in mucous membranes. IgM is in blood.

The principal antibody in type 1 hypersensitivity is IgE, a minor fraction of total immunoglobulin. Not surprisingly, it is located primarily in the tissues that come into contact with the outside—mucous membranes and skin.

When your sinuses, lungs, gut, or skin contacts an allergen, IgE acts toward the allergic protein as an antibody would toward a virus: it latches onto it and triggers an immune response by *mast cells*, yet another specialized white blood cell.

Mast cells are fat with histamine granules—"mast" means "well fed" in German. When triggered by IgE, mast cells degranulate, releasing histamine. This causes inflammation. Like IgE, mast cells are concentrated where your body meets the outside—mucous membranes and skin.

Just as an antibody "remembers" a virus, an allergen-specific form of IgE "remembers" that allergen. The more exposure to an allergen in the environment, the more inflammation and allergy symptoms occur. Unlike antibody-mediated reactions, IgE-mediated reactions do not involve B cells. But the process is orchestrated by a type 2 helper T cell (*Th2 cell*).

IgE's principal role in the normal function of the immune system is in defending against parasites. In regions where parasites such as hookworm are common, blood levels of IgE are 100 times greater than in regions low in parasites. In a sense, an allergy attack happens when your immune system mistakes an allergen for a parasite.

Why the Increase in Sensitivity?
Two theories have been offered to explain the increase in allergic

sensitivity: the hygiene hypothesis and the environmental stressor theory.

Proponents of the hygiene hypothesis originally argued that Western cultures have sanitized their environments so much that their immune systems don't develop properly. That is, early exposure to pathogens and allergens helps build immunity and low rates of allergy.

While credible research supports the theory, many critics point out significant instances where it does not hold up. For example, the higher rate of asthma among minority populations (unless one assumes they're more hygienic simply by virtue of their race) and the higher rate of asthma in "dirty" urban populations compared to the "clean" suburbs.

And while rural rates of allergy are lower than urban rates, exactly the opposite is true for infectious disease. In other words, the hygiene hypothesis would suggest that difference in antibody and allergy immune response would be the same, but they're not.

As described by Garry Hamilton in *NewScientist*, this has led some research to rethink the hygiene hypothesis. The current version says that it is exposure to certain innocuous microorganisms that trains the allergy immune response. Rural children have those exposures, while urban children do not. Attention has turned to a new kind of T cell called a suppressor T cell (*Ts cell*).

Before the recent discovery of the Ts cell, immunologists believed that Th1 and Th2 cells had to be forced into action. However, it appears that in fact they have to be held back by Ts cells (hence suppressor T cell). If suppressor T cells are underdeveloped, the other T cells can get out of control. And contact with innocuous microorganisms seems to have something to do with suppressor T cell development.

Environmental Stressors

The theory that environmental stressors actively and permanently disrupt our immune response is as much a complement as it is an alternative to the hygiene theory. Air pollution has received considerable attention as an environmental stressor. The evidence suggests that various forms of air pollution not only trigger asthma attacks, but alter the immune system in a way that promotes the IgE-mediated allergic response. Other research implicates exposure to common herbicides and pesticides.

An example is recent research from Sweden by Carl-Gustave Bornehag, PhD and his colleagues. Bornehag found a significant relationship between *phthalates* and asthma and allergies. Phthalates are a class of chemicals used to make plastic soft and pliable (specifically, polyvinyl chloride or PVC). It is used in a wide variety of products such as electrical cable, fake leather, IV bags, nail polish, latex adhesives, and vinyl and carpet tile.

Other Swedish researchers, Olle Johansson, PhD and his colleagues have investigated the health effects of electromagnetic frequency radiation (*EMF*). Over the last 50 years, electrical appliances and electronic devices, radio and television signals, and most recently cell phones and wireless communications technologies have made our environment thick with EMF. Among his findings is an association between EMF and asthma.

Johansson argues that the biological mechanism for the effect is that EMF causes an increase in the number of mast cells, a higher concentration of histamine in those mast cells, and a greater reactivity of those cells. So the same exposure to an allergen today compared to 50 years ago results in a stronger allergic response.

Protection and Prevention

We can reduce the risk of developing allergies and, for those with asthma and allergies, reduce the incidence of attacks. The strategy has two aspects: support of the immune system and protection against exposures.

The first place to start is with diet. Undiagnosed food allergies are common. The symptoms are often ascribed to a disease state such as chronic fatigue. The simplest way to test for food allergies is to go on an allergy elimination diet for two or three weeks in which you eliminate commonly allergic foods, especially grains, soy, dairy, and corn. When you reintroduce a food to which you're allergic, you'll have palpable symptoms.

Once you've identified allergic foods and taken them out of your diet, you're immune system is likely to quiet down and will be less likely to react to other allergens.

Asthma and other allergies are often aggravated by oxidative stressors such as air pollution. Oxidative stress is also created by carbohydrates: compared to protein and fat, starchy foods need more oxygen to metabolize. The oxidative process creates free radicals which challenge your body's ability to mobilize the antioxidants needed to neutralize the free radicals. A diet (including supplements) rich in antioxidants contributes to lowering the inflammatory effect of allergies. The most important antioxidants are vitamin C and E, coenzyme Q10, and lipoic acid.

Omega 3 fatty acids are also important in your diet for reducing inflammation, as is using fats and oils for cooking that are rich in saturated fat. Polyunsaturated fats are easily damaged when heated, unlike saturated fat. Those damaged fats contribute to the inflammatory process.

The second place to look is your home environment and the potential exposures to allergens there. Dust is not neutral. It consists of potential allergens. Regularly clean surfaces that collect dust. Replace carpet (which collects dust) with washable rugs. Because mold is a major allergen, keep rooms warm and dry.

Air purifiers can help by precipitating allergens out of the air. However, choose one that doesn't produce ozone—it's an air pollution that creates oxidative stress.

Finally, there are the things you can do to support your body and reduce the effects of allergens. Herbal preparations of stinging nettle taken regularly during pollen season reduces or eliminates symptoms for many. Homeopathic remedies for general and specific allergens are available over the counter. And traditional techniques such as a neti pot that keeps sinuses moist also helps support your body's first line of defense.

Resources

Allergy Resources International. Access at www.allallergy.net.

Arbes, Samuel et al. 2005. Prevalence of Positive Skin Test Responses to 10 Common Allergens in the US Population. *Journal of Allergy and Clinical Immunology*. 2005; 116: 377-83. DOI:10.1016/j.jaci.2005.05.017.

Berman, Layna. 2005. Allergy Alternatives. *Your Own Health And Fitness*. Broadcast April 19, 2005.

Berman, Layna. 2005. Indoor Air Pollution. *Your Own Health And Fitness*. Broadcast March 1, 2005.

Berman, Layna. 2004. The Hunter-Gatherer Diet. *Your Own Health And Fitness*. Broadcast March 2, 2004.

Bornehag, Carl-Gustav et al. 2005. The Association Between Asthma and Allergic Symptoms in Children and Phthalates in House Dust. *Environmental Health Perspectives*. October 2005; 112: 1393-7. DOI:10.1289/ehp.7187.

Hamilton, Garry. 2005. Filthy Friends and the Rise of Allergies. *NewScientist*. 2495; April 16, 2005.

Solomon, Gina. 2003. Asthma and the Environment. *The Collaborative on Health and the Environment*. April 10, 2003. Access at http://www.protectingourhealth.org/newscience/asthma/2003-04peerreviewasthma.htm

DRUGS IN THE WATER

The cops burst in. The drug dealers dash to the nearest toilet. If the cops are fast, they nab the criminals and their stash. If they're slow, the dealers flush the evidence away.

If you indulge in the guilty pleasure of police dramas, you've seen this scene many times. When those drugs get flushed away, where to they go? Into the waste treatment system.

The treated water from municipal systems is ultimately released into some body of water, typically a river. Sometimes treated wastewater is used for irrigation or simply sprayed onto the ground where it percolates into groundwater.

Wastewater is treated for biological agents. It's not treated to remove heroin. No agency tests for street drugs in wastewater as it's released into waterways. Nor is drinking water that is taken from those waterways or the groundwater fed by those waterways.

Street drugs are the least of it. The normal use of toilets is a continuous source of drugs in the water. It's measurable. And research is only just starting on what its effects might be.

It's Only Tap Water

The San Francisco *Chronicle*'s business section carried a series on the business of bottled water. It's a very big business indeed: $11 billion in sales and 8.3 billion gallons consumed in the United States alone during 2005. According to the article, that's "more than any other commercial beverage except soda. More than milk. More than coffee. More than beer."

The journalist who wrote the series of articles, David Lazarus, seems taken aback that the product itself is "only" tap water that's been treated. $7.50 per gallon for treated tap water? Because it allegedly tastes better? Even though a taste test revealed that few people could actually tell the difference between the top brands and plain tap water? Oh foolish consumer!

The food (sic) giants Coca Cola and PepsiCo lead the market in bottled water: Dasani (Coke) and Aquafina (Pepsi). $7.50 per gallon does seem a stiff price for tap water. However, it is not as the article says that "the water undergoes a variety of filtration treatments to remove chlorine and most dissolved solids." The water is purified using carbon and reverse osmosis filtration.

Tap water might need it. Tap water has bioactive chemicals that are added to it—some unintentionally (for example, fuel additives such as MTBE) and some intentionally (for example, fluoride). Filtration with carbon combined with reverse osmosis is the best way to remove these substances, as is distillation.

A Pharmaceutical Cocktail

These water purification systems also help remove some of the pharmaceuticals (and street drugs) that end up in your tap water. Researchers have already found biological effects from pharmaceuticals in streams where municipal wastewater systems dump effluent from their treatment processes. So far the study areas have focused on areas downstream of nursing homes where the elderly residents are often taking more that 10 distinct drugs.

Let's review. Your liver doesn't read labels. As far as it's concerned, the drug you just took, a chemical fabricated in a lab and not found in nature, is a poison. So your liver tries to send the chemical out. "Out" usually means into a toilet, which empties its contents into a system that takes it to a waste treatment plant somewhere. Let us not forget the spilled or intentionally discarded pharmaceuticals that are dumped down the drain or toilet without the assistance of the police breaking down the door.

No one has yet studied the actual effect of drug tainted waters on human health. There might be none. By the time a pharmaceutical has swirled down the drain, through the waste treatment process, swirled again down a stream or percolated into the soil, found its way to the intake of a municipal water system, and finally out your faucet and into your glass, it might be transformed into something utterly harmless.

Or not.

Especially in light of time release drugs. A capsule or tablet containing the drug is coated with a type of chemical called a phthalate that slows down the absorption process. Does that mean time released drugs take longer to degrade in the environment?

One of the few researchers in this area, Christian Daughton, has recommended a cradle-to-cradle approach to this problem. Some examples of solutions include drugs designed to degrade quickly or that require lower doses, use of traditional medicines that have chemistry that *is* found in nature and so would degrade more readily, use of individualized therapy that again reduces usage, packaging that minimizes waste of doses, and processes for the return of doses that are not used.

In the meantime, drinking purified tap water seems like a good alternative to being an involuntary participant in a medical experiment.

Purifying What You Drink

According to Colin Ingram, author of *The Drinking Water Book*, distillation combined with a carbon block filter does the most complete job of removing contaminants from drinking water. A drawback to distilled water is that it will tend to leach chemicals from storage containers. This is because distillation demineralizes water so thoroughly that it becomes *aggressive* and actively seeks to remineralize itself.

Reverse osmosis is almost as thorough as distillation in removing chemicals. The process works by forcing water through a membrane that has extremely small pores, so small that only water-sized molecules can get through. But that still allows molecules such as chlorine and some elemental metals and minerals to get through. That's why reverse osmosis systems typically include other filters: a carbon block filter for chemicals such as chlorine and a redox (reduction/oxidation) filter for metals such as lead and mercury.

Bottled water, water from vending machines, and bulk water are typically treated with reverse osmosis systems. However, you should "read the label."

Bottled water that you purchase should be certified by the International Bottled Water Association (IBWA) and should be labeled as either "drinking water" or "purified water." Although the IBWA is the industry's trade association, the certification is performed by the independent NSF International (formerly the National Sanitation Foundation). These assurances aside, the Natural Resources Defense Counsel warns that the Food and Drug Administration's regulatory oversight of bottled water manufacturers is lax to non-existent.

Similarly with water from vending machines. Well-maintained systems that use reverse osmosis or distillation can produce high quality water. However, the systems need to be well maintained. Like most bottled water, vending maching water is treated tap water.

Financially, consumers would probably be smart to install a reverse osmosis filtration or distillation system at home for drinking water and for water used for cooking, with a reusable water bottle to tote around home-grown purified water.

Although these systems cost a few hundred dollars, an average year's worth of bottled water would go quite a way toward paying for it. On average, Americans drink 28 gallons of commercial bottled water each year. At $7.50 per gallon, that's $210 in potential savings in one year. The economics are a little more complex than that, but you get the idea.

The News

Lazarus, David. 2007. How Water Bottlers Tap into All Sorts of Sources. *San Francisco Chronicle*. January 19, 2007: C1ff.

Royte, Elizabeth. 2006. Drugging the Waters. *OnEarth*. Fall 2006: 26-31.

The Research

Daughton, Christian. 2004. Non-regulated Water Contaminants: Emerging Research. *Environmental Impact Assessment Review*. 24 (2004): 711-32.

Daughton, Christian. 2003. Cradle-to-Cradle Stewardship for Drugs for Minimizing Their Environmental Disposition While Promoting Human Health. *Environmental Health Perspectives*. May 2003 (111:5): 757-74.

Hemminger, Pat. 2005. Damming the Flow of Drugs into Drinking Water. *Environmental Health Perspectives*. October 2005 (113:10): A679-81.

Resources

Blue Planet Project. Access at http://www.blueplanetproject.net.

Environmental Working Group. 2005. National Tap Water Quality Database. Access at http://www.ewg.org/sites/tapwater/.

Ingram, Colin. 2006. Safe Drinking Water. *Your Own Health And Fitness*. Broadcast October 3, 2006 on KPFA 94.1 FM Berkeley, CA.

Ingram, Colin. 2006. *The Drinking Water Book*. Berkeley, CA: Celestial Arts.

THE LIGHT BROWN APPLE MOTH

When the jets flew into the Twin Towers on September 11, 2001, the volume on fear in this country was cranked way up, much of it with the intention of manipulating us and unfortunately with considerable success. One of the cooler heads was Mr. Rogers. What he told children (and adults who were smart enough to listen) was "Pay attention to the helpers."

In a society dominated by the culture of expertise, that's really good advice. For well over a century, what governments do in the name of public health and environmental protection has been shaped and administered by experts informed by science. Being anointed as an expert can be a highly political process, particularly when the government's actions affect commerce. Likewise, what counts as science is highly political when powerful business interests are at stake.

Local knowledge has been the counterweight to this historical trend of top down science. Local knowledge is a practice long identified with the emergence of the environmental movement: citizens affected by pollution or subject to other environmental threats have used their own experience to affect both political and scientific change.

Large sections of Santa Cruz County and Monterey County in California have been sprayed from airplanes with a chemical intended to control the light brown apple moth. This little guy was of such concern to large agricultural interests and the experts at the California Department of Food and Agriculture and the United States Department of Agriculture that they persuaded Governor Schwartzenegger to declare an emergency—not that it took much. What that meant was that the Food and Ag department didn't have to go through the cumbersome process of performing an environmental review before Santa Cruz Monterey got bombarded.

Concerned citizens raised a fuss. Although the aerial spraying was postponed, these citizens ultimately lost. A core issue for these citizens is the health effect of the repeated overhead spraying that the Food and Ag department is conducting.

Inert Ingredients

The active chemical used is a pheromone that keeps the light brown apple moth from reproducing. It's a substance commonly used to control the moth. However, the normal mode of use is to tie little plastic cords saturated with the pheromone to trees not spray it all over the place. When sprayed from planes, the pheromone is delivered with so-called inert substances that cause the pheromone to be released over time. The product used in Santa Cruz and Monterey is called CheckMate.

Citizens were very concerned about these supposedly inert ingredients. They were also concerned about the time-release delivery system, which consists of plastic beads impregnated with the pheromone. The beads are of particular concern because, despite assurances to the contrary by the manufacturer and the Food and Ag Department, they are so small that they qualify as fine particulate air pollution. This is a type of air pollution that is of increasing public health concern.

The Food and Ag Department first would not release information about CheckMate's ingredients citing trade secrets. CheckMate's manufacturer Suterra threatened to sue anyone who published the information.

Finally the Food and Ag Department relented. First they said one of the ingredients was toxic. Then they corrected themselves and said the substance wasn't toxic. The department and the governor continued to maintain that there was an emergency, after all, and besides there wasn't anything in CheckMate to worry about.

The Bugman

One of the best technical responses to all of this came from a syndicated column called Ask the Bugman. In response to someone from Santa Cruz, The Bugman said aerial spraying was a bad idea for many reasons. Referring to one of the allegedly inert ingredients he said "According to the Pesticide Action Network North America ... it is considered "moderately toxic" to insects, "highly toxic" to fish, and "very highly toxic" to zooplankton."

That got the Food and Ag department's underwear in a twist. Their PR guy Steve Lyle wrote The Bugman and his editor demanding corrections. Among other things, Mr. Lyle pointed out that the principle inert ingredient is urea, a common and harmless substance. In a subsequent column, the Bugman cites the OSHA Material Safety Data Sheet for urea. Turns out that it's not so harmless after all, especially from exposures such as aerial spraying.

The Bugman went on to describe how he "asked him [Mr. Lyle] about the people who are getting sick after the initial spraying of this noxious material. He said he tells people to go to the doctor if they get sick. That's it? Go to a doctor?"

To back up to the beginning, this is a spraying program forced on Santa Cruz and Monterey because there's a supposed agricultural emergency. Yet the scientific basis for that declaration is flimsy at best.

What Emergency?

Testifying before a California State Senate subcommittee investigating this issue, UC Davis entomologist David Carey argued that this alleged pest had obviously been around for decades without causing any noticeable damage. In addition, based on his long research experience into eradicating agricultural pests, the Food and Ag Department's approach couldn't possibly achieve their state goal of eradication.

At the same hearing Daniel Harder, executive director of the UC Santa Cruz Arboretum, testified about an enlightening visit he made to New Zealand. Originally alarmed because of the Arboretum's value, he sought the advice of people who've been dealing with the light brown apple moth for a century. The only time New Zealand had a problem with the moth was when their natural predators were killed off by industrial strength agricultural pesticides. Today natural predators control the moth in New Zealand.

As a final example, Hawaii has had the light brown apple moth for 100 years. No disasters. And the moth helps control other pests.

And if you think this is just about something bad happening in Santa Cruz, think again. The Food and Ag Department's bombardment campaign is coming to all the counties surrounding the San Francisco Bay. And states as far away as Maine are paying attention to what's going on in California.

The Bugman is Richard Fagerlund, PhD. He's a board certified entomologist at the University of New Mexico. He's an expert. He's one of Mr. Rogers's helpers. The experts at the Food and Ag Department and the USDA are not.

Participatory Science

As part of their community organizing efforts against the aerial spraying program, citizens of Santa Cruz and Monterey had to become their own experts. In addition to enlisting the help of anointed experts like The Bugman, citizens conducted their own research into the moth, the spray, and the risks from aerial spraying.

For example, a citizen of Monterey not prone to activism had to take his son to the hospital immediately after the first spraying. That motivated him to start and maintain an adverse events registry that recorded over 600 events. That's significant because it undercounts the acute health effects by a factor of 10—that is, in reality the health of up to 6,000 people was affected by the first round of spraying in Monterey County.

As another example, a Santa Cruz business executive formed an action team around the issue, divvying up task around legal issues, media relations, government and regulatory affairs, as well as science. They were instrumental in actions taken in court that halted future spraying until environmental, economic, and health impacts are evaluated.

One of the great absurdities of this bureaucratic rush to dump gallons toxic substances on urban as well as agricultural areas is that it's justified as economically necessary to save California's agricultural economy. Yet a careful analysis of all of the economic benefits and loss suggests the economic losses in other sectors, particularly in organic farming, would be ten times the estimated damage to crops from the light brown apple moth. And those crop damage estimates are likely gross overestimates.

Although this continuing battle illustrates how industry frequently trumps health through the culture of expertise, it also demonstrates how participatory science holds a strong hand.

The News

Fagerlund, Richard. 2008. Moth Spraying Likely To Harm More than Help. *San Francisco Chronicle*. February 23, 2008.

Davis, Aaron C. 2008. Moth-spraying PR Deal Suspended Amid Questions. *San Francisco Chronicle*. March 13, 2008.

Kay, Jane. 2008. Experts Question Plan To Spray To Fight Moths. *San Francisco Chronicle*. March 6, 2008.

McKinley, Jesse. 2008. California Holds Off on Crop-Spraying Plan. *New York Times*. April 25, 2008.

The Research

California Alliance to Stop the Spray. 2008. Light Brown Apple Moth (LBAM) Economic Impacts and Solutions. *CASS Economics Research Summary*, May 5, 2008. Access at http://www.cassonline.org.

Cummins, Joe and Sam Burcher. 2008. Sex Hormones and City Life. *Institute of Science in Society*. May 16, 2008. Access at http://www.i-sis.org.uk/sexHormonesInCityLife.php.

Danthanarayana, Wijesiri. 1983. Population Ecology of the Light Brown Apple Moth, Epiphyas postvittana (Lepidoptera: Tortricidae). *The Journal of Animal Ecology*, February 1983 (52:1):1-33.

Werner, Inge et al. 2007. *Toxicity of Checkmate® LBAM-F and Epiphyas postvittana Pheromone to Ceriodaphnia dubia and Fathead Minnow (Pimephales promelas) Larvae*. November 28, 2007. University of California Davis, School of Veterinary Medicine.

Resources

Berman, Layna and Jeffry Fawcett, PhD. 2008. Aerial Spraying and Detoxification. *Your Own Health And Fitness*. Broadcast February 26, 2008.

California Alliance to Stop the Spray. Access at http://www.cassonline.org.

Commoner, Barry. 1971. *The Closing Circle: Nature, Man, and Technology*. New York: Random House.

Ecological Options Network. 2008. *Stop Them Before They Spray Again*. Access at http://www.eon3.net/.

Fischer, Frank. 2000. *Citizens, Experts, and the Environment: The Politics of Local Knowledge*. Durham: Duke University Press.

Stop the Spray. Access at http://www.stopthespray.org.

The argument that our social environments can increase or decrease our risk of illness and injury has a weak and a strong version. The weak version is that lack of access to medical care puts the poor at increased risk. This falls into the framework of contemporary health care reform proposals: if we can just deliver more preventive medicine and turn more poor people into patients we can decrease their risks.

The strong argument, which we advocate, is that social environments cause illness and injury directly. For example, every European country has some form of universal and often free access to medical care. Nevertheless, inequality of social status in these countries is associated with the risk of illness and injury.

The strong argument is that the most effective way to reduce risks of illness and injury is to change the social environment—which includes but is not limited to free access to medical care. The long history of research and practice that supports this strong argument focuses principally on the pernicious effects of inequity between social classes. The principal physiological mechanism for those effects is through the stress response.[1]

In general, the strong argument in favor of change in social environments as the best strategy for health promotion and risk prevention is based on what populations rather than individuals do. The objective of population-based strategies is to change what people encounter so that more of them make decisions that promote health and reduce risk. This is in contrast to strategies that attempt to directly affect each person's behavior.[2]

A rather dramatic example is the critical shortage of organs available for transplants in the United States. There is wide disparity in the percentage of people who are organ donors among nations and even among the individual United States. In the United States, about 28% of people choose to make their organs available for transplant should they die. In France, it's 99.9%.[3]

The difference is not some fabulously effective promotional campaign by the French. Instead, it is something quite simple. In France, when you get a driver's license or sign a medical release, you must choose not to be a donor. That is, you must decide to opt out. In the US, you must choose to be a donor—that is, you must opt in.

The simple and effective opt out public policy plays on a simple and effective rule of thumb shared by most people: if there's a default, do nothing about it. A simple difference in policy creates a simple difference in the social environment for individual choice, a different environmental cue that results in a significant social result and a significant medical effect for individuals who need an organ replaced.

The idea that social conditions affect health, illness, and injury is as old as the public health movement.[4] Concern for such issues remains alive today in public health organizations such as the American Public Health Association (APHA) and the National Association of County and City Health Officers (NACCHO).[5] However, the actual practice of public health is largely medicalized and functionally an extension of the medical system. That's because early in the 20th Century medical institutions (principally the American Medical Association) won a political war against public health institutions.[6]

In the last two decades, research has slowly increased in showing that social conditions, in particular disparities in social status, are strongly associated with the risk of illness and injury. It is a simple idea: if a person's social status is high, his or her risk of illness is less than someone with a lower status. Examples include increased risk of heart disease, cancer, diabetes and related metabolic disorders, work-related physical injury, infectious disease, lung disease, and, in children, developmental disabilities. The field has now acquired the label *social epidemiology*.[7]

The social determinants of illness and injury are also social and environmental justice issues. People of lower social status have fewer resources with which to resist, for example, the siting of a pollution-emitting power plant close to their neighborhood. That pollution increases the risk of a wide variety of illnesses. Whatever the economic virtues of an unequal distribution of wealth and income, unequal risks of illness and injury are not among them.

To repeat a point we've made before, the research on the social determinants of health is, like health care itself, not about health but about disease and diagnosis. When we think of social environments that promote health, we need to think about more than fewer cases of cancer. We need to think of social environments where people thrive.

Social capital is a dominant concept in the study of how to improve health and happiness.[8] The phrase itself is unfortunate for associating the essentially quantitative economic phenomenon of capital as an asset that yields an income stream with an essentially qualitative phenomenon: not just community life free of trouble for its members but community life to which people aspire. In spite of its faults,[9] social capital points to community life that is, like a healthy body, resilient to trouble and fertile ground for good living.

Think of society as divided into three parts: government, commerce, and civil society. Social capital is what gives civil society the power to resist the encroachment of the other two parts as well as organize the popular will in opposition to them. In research, the strength of social capital is measured indirectly—for example, by the number of relationships people have in a social network or by the percent of people involved in volunteer work. In real life, social capital is qualitative: the willingness of people to provide aid to others or come together for a common purpose.

There have been a considerable number of studies about the relationship between community connectedness and the risk of illness and injury. But only a few have studied the obvious core of social capital: the capacity of a community to organize itself effectively.[10]

Like personal health, the health of a community is its capacity for resilience, renewal, growth, and balance, its capacity to sustain its way of life.

The articles in this section illustrate how social environments affect health, illness, and injury. In the first, "Overworked, Sick, and Injured," we discuss how the conditions of work affect us and who is most at risk. Not surprisingly, risk falls along class lines.

In the second article, "Obesity, a Social Disease," we discuss research showing how connections between people affect health—in this case, weight gain. The research we discuss shows how weight gain "moved" through a population based on personal connections— that is, social networks.

The final article is "An Unhealthy Future." In it we discuss how abandoning the social safety net promises to increase illness in the future. We describe the effect of social inequity on stress and subsequently on health. We also describe how the effect strikes children and remains with them into and through adulthood and old age.

There is a physiological and political vicious cycle is promoted by stress-induced incapacity. Based on an analysis of political language, the cognitive linguist George Lakoff characterizes the political cultures of left and right as nurturing in contrast to hierarchical.[11] That left political cultures are better from the standpoint of risks of illness and injury is supported by the work of Vicente Navarro and his colleagues.[12] They found that nations with long traditions of socialist and social democratic governance—that is, nurturing governments—had better health as measured by infant mortality and life expectancy at birth.[13]

It's possible for governments to create social environments that reduce the risk of illness and injury through hierarchy, by submission to experts, and by the training of good patients. That is the approach that is institutionalized in our health care system.

What we've learned from social epidemiology is that this is not the best alternative for health care worthy of the name. In order to help us avoid the incapacity of illness and injury, as well as build our capacity to sustain a good way of life, the political economy and culture of health must have three characteristics.

First, it must have care (nurturing) as its center of gravity. Second, it must honor personal and local knowledge.[14] Third, it must be based on the three principles we've described: each person has a unique biology, bodies work as ecology, and for health and healing, do the simplest things first.

Notes

[1] For example, see Nancy Adler, et al. eds (1999) *Socioeconomic Status and Health in Industrial Nations: Social, Psychological, and Biological Pathways.*

[2] See Geoffrey Rose (1992) *The Strategy of Preventive Medicine.*

[3] Eric J. Johnson and Daniel Goldstein (2003) "Do Defaults Save Lives?"

[4] George Rosen (1993) *A History of Public Health.*

[5] The American Public Health Association http://www.apha.org/ and its *Journal of Public Health*; the National Association of County and City Health Officials http://www.naccho.org/ and its *Public Health Dispatch.*

[6] See the description in Paul Starr (1982) *The Social Transformation of American Medicine.*

[7] Some basic sources are the *Journal of Epidemiology and Social Health*, *International Journal of Health Services*, Richard Hofrichter ed (2003) *Health and Social Justice: Politics, Ideology, and Inequity in the Distribution of Disease*, Vicente Navarro ed (2002) *The Political Economy of Social Inequalities: Consequences for Health and Quality of Life*, Michael Marmot and Richard G. Wilkinson eds (2006) *Social Determinants of Health*, and "Unnatural Causes: Is Inequality Making Us Sick?"(2008) "Unnatural Causes: Is Inequality Making Us Sick?." Also see Lisa F. Berkman and Ichiro Kawachi eds (2000) *Social Epidemiology*, Ichiro Kawachi, et al. eds (1999) *The Society and Population Health Reader: Income Inequality and Health*, and Alvin R. Tarlov and Robert F. St. Peter eds (2000) *The Society and Population Health Reader: A State and Community Perspective.*

[8] The work of Robert Putnam brought attention to the subject in Robert D. Putnam (2000) *Bowling Alone: The Collapse and Revival of American Community* and Robert D. Putnam, et al. (2003) *Better Together: Restoring the American Community.*

[9] See Simon Szreter and Michael Woolcock (2004) "Health by Association? Social Capital, Social Theory, and the Political Economy of Public Health," Ben Fine (2000) *Social Capital Versus Social Theory: Political Economy and Social Science at the Turn of the Millennium*, and Ichiro Kawachi (2006) "Commentary: Social Capital and Health: Making the Connections One Step at a

Time."

[10] For example, Meredith Minkler ed (2002) *Community Organizing and Community Building for Health* and the work of the Prevention Institute http://www.preventioninstitute.org/ and the Sustainable Health Institute http://www.sustainablehealthinstitute.org/.

[11] George Lakoff (1996) *Moral Politics: What Conservatives Know That Liberals Don't* and more recently George Lakoff (2008) *The Political Mind: Why You Can't Understand 21st-Century American Politics with an 18th-Century Brain.* Lakoff uses the conceptual pair liberal-conservative and contrasts them using the metaphor of a family: the nurturing parent (liberal) versus strict father (conservative) the framing political culture.

[12] Vicente Navarro, et al. (2006) "Politics and Health Outcomes."

[13] Although a grim measure of medical and health care, infant mortality and life expectancy at birth are generally regarded as an accurate indicator of the overall condition of care.

OVERWORKED, SICK, AND INJURED

If you work evening or night shifts, you're at greater risk of stress-related illnesses such as heart attacks and diabetes. Shift workers are also more likely to get injured on the job—at almost twice the rate of day workers. On top of that, shift workers who return to work after they've been treated and given a so-called clean bill of health by their physician are not only more likely to be injured again but they're also more likely to be fired.

Shift work isn't healthy, financially as well as physically. Financially there are the direct costs of medical care and the indirect costs from lost income and lowered productivity.

Who are the people suffering from shift work? For the most part, they're the working class. A study by Allard Dembe and his colleagues found that almost 80% of workers who reported a work-related injury or illness were manual, clerical, or service workers. The remaining 20% were professionals or managers, a majority of whom are employees not independent business owners.

The Injured Class

On average, people who experience work-related injury or illness have an income that is only a little over twice the official poverty line. They tend to be single income households. They're young, averaging 31 years of age. And they have only a high school education. Since these are averages, its likely that more than half are younger that 31. It's also likely that a disproportionate number earn at or even below the official poverty line.

In other words, they are people who are just getting by. They really need their jobs. Surprisingly, African-Americans and Latinos are not over-represented in this class of shift workers. At least suffering from shift work seems to be egalitarian.

There's good reason to believe that these statistics misrepresent the degree of injury and illness suffered by people who are struggling. The statistics are based on people reporting illness and injury. A well-educated professional is far more likely to take time off, go to the doctor, and take advantage of the existing workers compensation system than is a minimum wage worker who lives from paycheck to paycheck.

Shift Work Biology

Why do these people suffer from shift work and overtime? Biologically, shift work disrupts circadian rhythms, the ticking of the biological clock that tells you it's time to sleep when instead you're running a drill press.

Socially, shift workers suffer because the needs of industry trump the health and safety of workers. Although not the Satanic mills of Charles Dickens's novels, current industrial practices still count workers as fodder. With the fear of losing steady work, people within sight of poverty have little choice but to take the jobs they can get and, if injured, get back to work as quickly as possible. Too often, they avoid treatment altogether out of fear of losing income or their job.

The pressure to stay on the job and to get back to work as quickly as possible creates its own cascade of stress and with it the risk of illness.

This is bad news. But it's not the worst. People who work long hours are at consistently greater risk of injury and illness than shift workers.

Long Hours are Worse

Biologically, long hours disrupt the circadian clock not by confusing your body because you're active when it thinks you should be sleeping, but because you're active when you should be resting. Yes, rest and relaxation should be part of your day. It's healthy.

Over the course of the day, stress hormones regulate your cycle of activity and rest. Stress hormones (in particular cortisol) enable you to be alert and energetic, but they take their toll on your tissues. Not only during sleep but also during waking hours, your body needs time to recover from the damaging effects of ordinary levels of stress. That's why people typically feel a nap coming on mid-afternoon and why normal cortisol levels decline during the evening.

Socially, long hours have two sources. One is the use of overtime as a substitute for hiring additional workers. This is a long-standing and time-honored way for companies to minimize costs: making two existing employees work overtime is cheaper than hiring a third employee. That's true for wage, salaried, and independent workers.

In addition, for salaried and independent workers industry has nurtured a butch work culture in which you are expected to put in 60 hours per week. Anything less and you're napping on the job—which actually would be a good idea.

If you pause, you've lost. Despite your white collar, you're still fodder.

Protection

Simplest things first: don't work the swing shift or the night shift; work as little overtime as possible; don't succumb to white collar workaholicism. When you can't avoid this particular toxic exposure, take remedial measures to protect yourself.

<u>Maintain a Consistent Sleep Schedule</u> Your body will try to take care of you by adjusting its rhythms to your schedule. So on your days off, go to bed and get up at about the same time you do during the work week.

Taking naps is a good idea because you can catch up on sleep. Sometimes your schedule is disrupted, such as when you go on vacation and instead of being active at night you're active during the day. As described under "Shift forward" below, allow your biology to shift to your new "time zone."

Develop Healthy Sleep Habits   Your circadian clock is sensitive to light, so make sure where you sleep is completely dark. Use a sleep mask and earplugs if you have to. Develop routines that tell your body to get ready for sleep, especially if you sleep after you come home from work. Don't take sleep drugs. If you have difficulty getting to sleep, there are a number of gentle methods that include nutrient, homeopathic, and flower essence remedies (see "A Good Night's Sleep" on page 169).

No Stimulants   Artificially making yourself alert with a stimulant only disrupts your biology further. It simply adds another stressor to an already stressful situation. Also avoid "energy" foods and drinks. They're active ingredient is sugar (or starch that becomes sugar). These foods also add to your biological stress. The best thing for you to do when you get drowsy is take a catnap or meditate. If you can't do that, do something vigorous (such as taking a brisk walk) that stimulates your body.

Shift Forward   If you work rotating shifts or have to fit activities around your work schedule, rotate clockwise. For example, if you're rotating from a night shift to a day shift, don't start the next day. Instead, start the day after. The idea is like what you do to avoid jetlag, essentially allowing your body to catch up to your new time zone.

Sleep and rest are good for us. Shift work, overtime, and long work hours take a tremendous toll on our biology. We deserve a culture, and especially a culture of work, that honors rather than ignores our biology.

The News

Nagourney, Eric. 2008. Safety: Nonstandard Work Shifts May Hinder Recovery. *New York Times*. January 29, 2008.

The Research

Caruso, Claire C. et al. 2004. *Overtime and Extended Work Shifts: Recent Findings on Illnesses, Injuries, and Health Behaviors*. National Institute for Occupational Safety and Health. Report 2004-143 (April 2004).

Dembe, Allard E. et al. 2007. Associations Between Employees' Work Schedules and the Vocational Consequences of Workplace Injuries. *Journal of Occupational Rehabilitation*. 17:641-51. DOI: 10.1007/s10926-007-9098-8.

Harrington, J Malcolm. 2001. Health Effects of Shift Work and Extended Hours of Work. *Occupational and Environmental Medicine*. January 2001 (58:1):68ff.

Resources

Your Own Health And Fitness. Resources on Mind, Mood, and Stress. Access at http://www.yourownhealthandfitness.org/topicsMindMood.php.

OBESITY, A SOCIAL DISEASE

Being fat has always invited scorn. It is the outward sign of personal deficit, most commonly sloth and gluttony. In the last decade it has become the whipping boy for a wide variety of illnesses, most prominently diabetes. The message has been clear: you're sick because you're fat because you can't control yourself.

With the medicalization of fatness under the sign of obesity, polite neutrality envelops discussions of obesity science in the mainstream media. Occasionally the older attitude peeks through. That's what happened when a study by Nicholas Christakis and his colleagues of the social determinants of fatness was published in the *New England Journal of Medicine*. The *New York Times* headline was "Find Yourself Packing It On? Blame Friends."

Why "blame?" If you're fat, did you do something bad?

This is yet another example of how mainstream media utterly fails to understand and accurately report science. It was an opportunity for the media to make the social determinants of health a prominent part of our common understanding. Instead, the media made the story about how wrong fat people must be.

Catching Body Fat

The *New York Times* article opens by describing the Christakis study as showing how obesity is transmitted from one person to another like a virus. Other articles used "contagious" in their headlines and descriptions of the study in a way similar to the *Times* article. Using "contagious" to explain increased fatness conjures solutions such as immunization and quarantine.

The Christakis study never uses the word "contagious" nor does it represent the rise in obesity as in any way akin to an infectious disease. Nor does the study discuss solutions taken from the conventional strategies for preventing and treating infectious disease.

Instead, these researchers point to social relationships and processes as causing the rise in body fat. For solutions, they point to those same processes.

The Christakis study uses data from the famous (and still continuing) Framingham Heart Study begun in 1948. The study uses information about relationships among participants to reveal how those relationships might affect weight gain. The data necessary to do this type of analysis was only available beginning in 1971 so the study covers the 32 years from 1971 to 2003.

Social ties of friendship, family, and neighbor were examined. Strength of friendships were evaluated by classifying them as one of three types, in order of strength from the perspective of a single person:

- mutual friend (two people identify each other as friends),
- person-perceived friend (a person identifies another as a friend but the other does not), and
- other-perceived friend (a person doesn't identify another as a friend but the other does).

These social ties were analyzed statistically for the probability that a person's body mass index (BMI) increased beyond the officially defined limit for obesity when their friend's BMI did the same. BMI is the standard measure for obesity and is a ratio of a person's weight (in kilograms) to their height (in meters squared).

The strongest effect happened between mutual friends—if a friend gained weight, the person's risk of gaining weight increased 171%. However, the association showed a wide range of variation—from modest (59% increase) to very strong (326% increase). Person-perceived friendships were next strongest (57% increase). Other-perceived friendships had no effect. Both had a wide range of variation.

Same-sex friendships of any of the 3 types had an effect similar in strength to person-perceived friendships. Opposite-sex friendships had no effect, although showed a wide range of variation from moderately negative (a person was likely to lose weight if the other gained) to moderately positive (both gained weight).

There was no effect shown between neighbors, although it varied widely in a way similar to opposite-sex friendships (from moderately negative to moderately positive).

Spouses and siblings had positive effects on BMI increase. Same-sex siblings had a slightly more powerful effect than opposite-sex siblings. What was distinct about these relationships as compared to friendships and neighbors is that variation was quite small. What that means is that although friends can have a more powerful effect on weight gain, family members, whether by marriage or birth, have a much more consistent effect.

Conclusions and Speculations

The Christakis researchers looked at three possible explanations for what they found.

First, people associate with others like him- or herself—birds of a feather flock together. The researchers rejected this explanation because their results showed a clear sequence—weight gain followed friendship not the other way around.

Second, friends share common experiences or exposures that lead to weight gain. The researchers rejected this explanation not only because weight gain was "passed" from friend to friend sequentially but also because neighbors had no effect and geographic distance did not affect the strength of the effect between friends—suggesting shared environmental exposures had no effect.

Third, a friend influences a person in a way that permits or induces weight gain. This is the explanation the Christakis researchers say their study supports. It's supported by the sequential emergence of weight. It's also supported by the strength of different relationships: mutual friendships are more powerful than one-sided friendships and family relationships.

The researchers speculate on two kinds of influence. One affects a person's values regarding weight gain. The other affects a person's preferences—for example, by affecting acceptable food choices.

Social Solutions

It's unfortunate that the study ends on speculation about what should be the most interesting aspect of their work: how to change a social network so it promotes health. In their concluding paragraph they express the hope to "harness this same force to slow the spread of obesity."

An obvious place to start is to turn the study on its head. The study should have asked whether weight loss moved as readily through the social network as weight gain.

The study begs the question about weight gain. It shows that weight gain moves through a social network, but it doesn't show how it gets started.

A weakness of the study is how it measures "obesity." It simply looks at whether someone's BMI rises above 30, the official boundary for the diagnosis Obesity. That's someone who stands 5'7" and weighs 191 pounds. What if the line was at 35 (the boundary for Clinical Obesity) or at 25 (the boundary for Overweight)?

One of the most significant studies on the relationship of BMI to health found that the people with the lowest mortality were Overweight (BMI 25 to 30). People classified as Obese (BMI 30 to 35) had about the same risk of dying as those classified as Normal (BMI 18 to 25). And the mortality risk for both was only slightly greater than for Overweight, the classification least at risk.

The study and the media make the same incorrect assumption: excess body weight is a disease outright. In fact, it's a symptom of metabolic imbalance. Nevertheless, the study's framework is a useful one: what are the social mechanisms that create metabolic imbalance whose symptom is excess body weight?

The researchers are looking for the right solutions in the social network that gives life to the symptom. What social ties do we need to sustain our health?

The mission of the Sustainable Health Institute is to support people in answering that question.

The News

Chang, Alicia. 2007. Study: Obesity Is 'Socially Contagious.' *San Francisco Chronicle.* July 25, 2007.

Gellene, Denise. 2007. Obesity is 'Contagious,' Study Finds. *Los Angeles Times.* July 26, 2007.

Kolata, Gina. 2007. Find Yourself Packing It On? Blame Friends. *New York Times.* July 26, 2007.

The Research

Christakis, Nicholas A. et al. 2007. The Spread of Obesity in a Large Social Network over 32 Years. *New England Journal of Medicine.* July 26, 2007 (357:): 370-79.

Resources

California Newsreel. 2008. *Unnatural Causes: Is Inequality Making Us Sick?* Access at http://www.unnaturalcauses.org.

Sustainable Health Institute. Access at http://www.sustainablehealthinsitute.org/.

Your Own Health And Fitness. Resources on Diabetes, Insulin Resistance, Metabolic Syndrome, and Obesity. Access at http://www.yourownhealthandfitness.org/topicsDiabetes.php.

AN UNHEALTHY FUTURE

People in the United States can look forward to a future of ill health. This is not because the medical treatment system, euphemistically yet universally referred to as the health care system, is failing in an epidemic of overdiagnosis and overtreatment.

We can expect an unhealthy future because our political culture has, for quite some time now, entirely abandoned caring for those least capable of caring for themselves. Mostly children.

In 2007 the McClatchy Newspapers published an analysis of recent census data on poverty here in the land of opportunity. Poverty is increasing. In fact, it's been increasing for almost three decades. Despite economic growth and increased worker productivity, the fruits of that growth have been harvested almost exclusively by the owning classes.

Meanwhile, the number of people in severe poverty (people with half the income of the official poverty level) has increased steadily. And the number of people not in poverty with an income greater than twice the poverty level has steadily declined.

Goodbye Welfare, Hello Self-Esteem

What's being done to alleviate this suffering?

Perhaps you remember the Welfare Reform Act of 1996, championed by then-President Bill Clinton and happily passed by a Republican Congress. Its ostensible purpose was to reduce welfare costs and get people into the workforce where they could build their self-esteem on a minimum wage that becomes smaller each year in real buying power.

The Associated Press reported on how this happy scheme is working. It's failing. Although cash payments have declined, spending on other programs such as Medicaid and Food Stamps have more than compensated so that total spending is higher than the old welfare system would have been. What's more, that spending would explode if all the people who are eligible participated. One study estimates that only 10% of eligible people apply for these supplemental programs.

As to entering the happy world of the workforce, "struggle" is as good as it gets. "Grim" and "stuck" are more accurate descriptions of the descent into poverty experienced by, mostly, single mothers and their children.

The economics are quite plain: tax dollars are subsidizing businesses in yet another way by creating an underclass forced to work for dirt. Instead of enforcing a living wage, people (again, mostly single mothers) are forced to struggle with a combination of low wages at jobs without benefits and little security while various government programs subsidize their food, shelter, and medical care.

Stress and Struggle

There are some obvious effects on health. For example, being forced to choose between medical care and some necessity such as rent and heat.

There are less obvious and much longer term effects from this abandonment. There's a well-documented relationship between income security and health. In a nutshell, the stress of insecurity promotes inflammation that in turn promotes illness.

It goes beyond that. Children who experience extreme stress are more likely to have worse health as adults regardless of the stressors they experience as adults. Recent research has identified the process that causes this.

A stressful experience acts through your sympathetic nervous system (SNS)—responsible for most homeostatic processes such as the beating of your heart. Sympathetic nerves originate in your spinal cord. Your SNS communicates directly with your adrenal glands (stress response) and your lymph glands (immune response). The communication is in both directions, both from and back to the SNS.

Your SNS is responsible for the flight-fight-freeze reaction to threatening and stressful situations. It stimulates your adrenal glands to produce stress hormones that promote inflammation. The biological sense of this is that, when under attack, your body wants to be mobilized in case of injury. Inflammation recruits the body's immune defenses.

The SNS also directly stimulates lymph glands to produce inflammatory biochemicals.

Pro-inflammatory biochemicals from both sources stimulate the brain to release hormones that eventually produce glucocorticoids, cortisol being the most widely known. These biochemicals gradually turn off the inflammatory response.

This is a very nice feedback loop. The nervous system gets stimulated by a stressor and stimulates the endocrine system and immune system. The stress hormones from the endocrine system stimulate the immune system too. The stimulated immune system then signals the brain. This time the nervous system signals the endocrine system to wind down the stress response.

As this unfolds, the brain is paying attention to what's happening. The person feels emotional shifts as their stress response develops and declines.

However, extreme chronic stress such as abuse in early life can permanently disrupt this adaptive feedback loop. The SNS and endocrine systems remain on alert with glucocorticoids that permanently downregulate the immune system and emotional state.

Abandoning Children

The best predictors of child abuse and neglect are, in order, poverty, alcohol and drug abuse, and a family history of abuse. It is interesting to note that white children are more likely to be abused or neglected than African-American or Hispanic children.

Our society's abandonment of children and their mothers to poverty is cursing their future. And their numbers are growing.

The old welfare program was called Aid to Families with Dependent Children. The idea was that children, particularly preschoolers, should have a full-time parent at home with them. Typically, that meant the child's mother. The science supports that as very desirable for everyone.

All gone now. And by and large due to the people who espouse family values, people whose motto seems to be "Life is sacred before birth. After that, you're on your own."

The most obvious place to start is in the prevention of abuse and neglect in the first place. Funding social services that promote the nurturance of children is a way to start—resources to heal the abuser and protect the child. More fundamentally, economic security for families would go even further in preventing abuse. In addition to the positive health effect from reducing abuse, economic security would have a positive health effect for everyone.

Children who have already been abused and neglected need treatment. Recovery is never simple, especially because the mistreatment can be difficult to identify. The objective is to reset the child's emotional life as well as to reset her or his immune system, sympathetic nervous system, and endocrine system.

As adults, recovery becomes even more difficult because the abused child has had time to develop adaptive mechanisms. Often, the adaptations are harmful. Working through them is difficult precisely because they become embedded in the child's and the adult's life in a tangle of emotional, hormonal, nervous system, and immune responses.

The News

Associated Press. 2007. Welfare State Growing Despite Overhauls. *New York Times*. February 26, 2007.

Pugh, Tony. 2007. US Economy Leaving Record Numbers in Severe Poverty. *McClatchy Newspapers*. February 22, 2007. Posted online at http://www.realcities.com/mld/krwashington/news/nation/16760690.htm.

The Research

Danese, Andrea et al. 2007. Childhood Maltreatment Predicts Adult Inflammation in a Life-course Study. *Proceedings of the National Academy of Science*. January 23, 2007 (104:4): 1319-24. DOI:10.1073/pnas.0610362104.

Glaser, Ronald and Janice Kiecolt-Glaser. 2005. Stress-induced Immune Dysfunction: Implications for Health. *Nature Reviews Immunology*. March 2005 (5): 243-51. DOI:10.1038/nri1571.

Woolf, Steven. 2006. The Rising Prevalence of Severe Poverty in America. *American Journal of Preventive Medicine*. 2006 (31:4): 332-41. DOI: 10.1016/j.amepre.2006.06022.

Resources

McEwen, Bruce. 2004. *The End of Stress as We Know It*. New York: Dana Press.

The ChildTrauma Academy. Access at http://childtraumaacademy.org/

Navarro, Vicente et al. 2006. Politics and Health Outcomes. *The Lancet*. September 14, 2006. DOI:10.1016/S0140-6736(06)69341-0.

Your Own Health And Fitness, Resources on Hormones. Access at http://www.yourownhealthandfitness.org/topicsHormones.php.

Your Own Health And Fitness, Resources on Immunity. Access at http://www.yourownhealthandfitness.org/topicsImmunity.php.

Your Own Health And Fitness, Resources on Mind, Mood, and Stress. Access at http://www.yourownhealthandfitness.org/topicsMindMood.php.

Your Own Health And Fitness, Resources on Politics, Advocacy, Prevention, and Social Health. Access at http://www.yourownhealthandfitness.org/topicsPolitics.php.

One of the great revolutions in Western medical science was the discovery that an exposure (such as industrial chemicals)[1] or an event (such as suffering abuse as a child)[2] can lead to illness in the distant future. More recently, researchers have discovered relationships between exposures and illness that are transgenerational where an exposure affects the health of unborn children and grandchildren.[3]

What was revolutionary is that by eliminating an exposure or event, the threat of illness is greatly reduced. Knowing the exposures that put people at risk enables individuals and communities to put a stick in the wheel that turns from exposure to illness. Knowledge of this kind is the very foundation of public health. It is also at the very foundation of decisions that health conscious people make—people who pay attention to what they eat, stay physically fit, minimize their exposures to toxins, and stay informed about health issues.

It is a very good thing.

However, in the hands of the medical institutions that dominate our health care system, the prevention revolution has become a practice focused on the characteristics of patients in what we call *risk factor medicine*.[4] Instead of focusing on a person's exposure to environmental pollution and the like, risk factor medicine focuses on personal characteristics such as serum cholesterol, blood pressure, and body weight. Risk factors include what are characterized as personal or lifestyle choices such as smoking, drinking alcohol, or eating saturated fats.

Risk factor medicine lends itself to the popular sport of blaming the victim: people get sick because they make bad choices. This is not a sport restricted to conventional medicine.

Nevertheless, we are in fact surrounded by exposures that put us at risk of illness and injury—whether from bad environments or bad choices. Each day we make choices to avoid (or not avoid) those exposures—at least the ones we know about. As health conscious people know, doing that could turn into a fulltime job. Because time is scarce, we often use our intuition and rules of thumb. Some common strategies include following the experience of friends and family, health professionals, and people identified as health experts. On our own, we draw our own conclusions from what we read or hear in the media (mainstream or alternative), advertising and other promotional materials created by businesses, and advertising and other promotional materials created by health institutions and social service organizations.

This is a tricky business. An ocean of information exists on the association of exposures with risks of illness and injury. Yet another ocean of information exists on what to do about those exposures. How does someone sift through it? Would he want to?

A good place to start is in knowing how likely each person is of suffering a specific illness so that he can take appropriate action. Is he worried about cancer? A heart attack? Physical injury? Mental illness?

A group of researchers at the Veterans Administration did just that. They created a risk chart and published it in the *Journal of the National Cancer Institute.*[5] The researchers used a consistent method to compare the likelihood that someone would die from one of the top dozen causes of death. Those probabilities were organized by age, sex, and smoking status.

Based on that list, doctors and patients can identify what a patient should be worried about. In a separate editorial, the important issue of how best to communicate this kind of science to civilians was discussed.[6]

A principal motivation in publishing these charts was to set some realistic expectations among both doctors and patients about the actual risks of illness and injury. In particular, it seems to be an attempt to reduce the perpetual panic about cancer. It is more generally concerned with counteracting the increasing pattern of overdiagnosis and overtreatment among both doctors and patients immersed in a medical atmosphere of panic and fear.[7]

However, although the study is a noble effort, the result is ultimately disappointing. Three things stand out. First, the charts don't tell us about the relationship between exposures and risks but instead tell us the likely cause of death for someone of a particular age, gender, and smoking status. That's only part of the picture because, second, the charts are about dying, not suffering, death, not illness and injury. Third, the charts are about diagnoses and not about the exposures that start the wheel of suffering and death turning.

It is of interest to know that, for example, a man at any age is more likely to die in an accident than from prostate cancer. It's also of interest that dying of the flu doesn't even register as a likely cause of death—something to keep in mind when hysteria over getting vaccinated breaks out in the fall. The big news—although it shouldn't be news at all—is that being a smoker makes it much more likely that someone will die of a heart attack, stroke, lung cancer, pneumonia, emphysema, or chronic bronchitis at any age, whether man or woman.

So if you smoke, stop it. It's bad for you.

What also emerges from the article is that, although the risk charts will tell us what might kill us, the charts don't tell us how much we'll suffer until we die of whatever ultimately kills us. On the face of it, that seems an easy thing to do, what with the current focus on prevention in health science. But the study's risk chart casts doubt on this, too.

Despite decades of spending on research of heart disease and cancer and their treatment, they're still the two things most likely to kill us. You might think, "Well, you have to die from something." How about old age? It's still a legitimate entry on a death certificate.

The failure in both the research and treatment of heart disease and cancer is the failure to examine and take action on them as environmentally caused.[8] Instead, risk factor medicine for heart disease has focused research and treatment on driving serum cholesterol to dangerously low levels with toxic side effects.[9] And risk factor medicine has focused cancer research and treatment on aggressive and dangerous screening practices followed by regimens of surgery, radiation, and chemotherapy—cut, burn, and poison—with all their ill effects.[10]

So don't expose yourself to environmental pollutants. They're bad for you.

A chart that tells someone what's likely to kill him isn't very helpful. He can look at his family history and make a pretty good guess. What he probably really wants to know is what puts him at risk of suffering.

For example, it would be helpful to have a risk chart that compares the suffering from treatments using pharmaceuticals to the suffering from treatments using nutrients. It would be helpful to have a risk chart for cancer therapy that compares the suffering from standard cut, burn, and poison strategies to the suffering of alternative, non-invasive therapies. Better yet, it would be useful to have a risk chart about chronic diseases that compares the risks from different ways of life—where you live and how you live. We don't mean by this the promotional books, plans, and programs sold to consumers as guides to vibrant (or equivalent superlative) health. Instead we mean some good, solid epidemiology on good places and good ways to live. The South Beach Diet and the Mediterranean Diet don't count: they're diet plans, not ways of life.

It's unlikely that such a chart will ever exist. However, each of us does things every day to find or create environments that help us avoid illness and injury. We also do things that improve our health—things that build our biological capacity for resilience and successful adaptation. Sometimes that involves careful study of an issue. Always it involves using our best judgment and what makes sense. We advocate three princples.
- Do what supports your unique biology.
- Do what supports your body's balance, it's unique ecology.
- Do the simplest things first.

The first article in this section, "Avian Flu Roundup," looks at a classic case of prevention: vaccination against an infectious disease. When the article was written, a near-panic had been whipped up by public health officials over an allegedly pending pandemic that never materialized. This article challenges the assumptions on which not only the avian flu panic was based but the annual panic over routine flu vaccination.

The next two articles, "Too Few Mammograms" and "In Your Prostate," criticize what passes for cancer prevention in conventional medicine.

The final article, "Antioxidant Myths," examines the bias in conventional research against the use of antioxidants for protection and prevention. The article also examines how that bias is carried over into the mass media by journalists unable to critically evaluate the science.

Notes

[1] For example, Dario Consonni, et al. (2008) "Mortality in a Population Exposed to Dioxin after the Seveso, Italy, Accident in 1976: 25 Years of Follow-up."

[2] For example, Ronald Glaser and Janet Kiecolt-Glaser (2005) "Stress-induced Immune Dysfunction: Implications for Health."

[3] For example, Agnes Smink, et al. (2008) "Exposure to Hexachlorobenzene during Pregnancy Increases the Risk of Overweight in Children Aged 6 Years."

[4] Layna Berman and Jeffry Fawcett (2005) "Risk Factor Medicine."

[5] Steven Woloshin, et al. (2008a) "The Risk of Death by Age, Sex, and Smoking Status in the United States: Putting Health Risks in Context." The work has now been expanded into a book targeted to health care consumers: Steven Woloshin, et al. (2008b) *Know Your Chances: Understanding Health Statistics.*

[6] Michael J. Thun, et al. (2008) "Risky Business: Tools to Improve Risk Communication in a Doctor's Office."

[7] H. Gilbert Welch, et al. (2007) "What's Making Us Sick Is an Epidemic of Diagnoses." See also Layna Berman and Jeffry Fawcett (2007a) "Overdiagnosis and Overtreatment Part 1," Layna Berman and Jeffry Fawcett (2007b) "Overdiagnosis and Overtreatment Part 2."

[8] For example, on heart disease see Malcolm Kendrick (2007) *The Great Cholesterol Con: The Truth about What Really Causes Heart Disease and How to Avoid It* and on cancer see the Cancer Prevention Coalition, access at http://www.preventcancer.org.

[9] For example, International Network of Cholesterol Skeptics, access at http://www.thincs.org, and Duane Graveline (2004) *Lipitor, Thief of Memory: Statin Drugs and the Misguided War on Cholesterol.*

[10] For example, Devra Davis (2007) *The Secret History of the War on Cancer* and Samuel Epstein (1998) *The Politics of Cancer Revisited.*

AVIAN FLU ROUNDUP

Headlines are now reporting the seemingly inexorable march of the "deadly avian flu" toward us: first Asia, then the Middle East, Eastern Europe, and now Western Europe. The Third World is not spared: cases in Egypt and Nigeria have been reported.

But the reporting has blurred the distinction between infections in birds and infections in humans. Spread of the disease is reported, but it is essentially the inevitable consequence of bird migration.

When people die from the H5N1 "deadly" avian flu strain, little care is taken to inform you that few people have actually died and that those who died were exposed because they handled infected birds. The spread of the disease has thus far been from bird to bird and from bird to human. What has national and international public health officials wringing their hands is the mutation that will cause human-to-human transmission.

Despite the attention paid to the H5N1 flu virus, there's scant discussion of the actual risks.

How Dangerous is the Bird Flu?

While "deadly" has been repeatedly attached to it, until recently no one had asked how deadly the H5N1 strain of avian flu actually is.

"Deadly" got attached because about half of the small number of people, mostly in Asia, who have been diagnosed with the H5N1 virus have died. These were people who made it to a hospital or clinic in a city. This doesn't tell us much about what's going on in the countryside. That's important because so far all the known cases have occurred because a human was infected by a bird. Most of that contact happens in the countryside.

In January 2006, researchers from the Karolinska Institute in Stockholm published a paper that suggests that the avian flu might not be as scary as it's advertised. These researchers have been working on health issues in a province in Vietnam for over seven years. During the spring of 2004 they collected information about the incidence of what they called "flu-like symptoms" and exposure to sick birds. So far, it's the best estimate of the avian flu's effects on an entire population.

Only about 18% of the people exposed to domestic poultry developed "flu-like symptoms"—which is not, as the researchers take pains to point out, the same as being diagnosed with H5N1. In addition, the birds were not diagnosed with H5N1—they were simply sick birds. However, these are the conditions that give rise to avian flu in a country that has had one of the highest number of bird flu deaths. Significantly, no deaths were reported in this study.

The researchers speculate that infection by H5N1 in Vietnam and likely elsewhere is more common than supposed and that its effects are not nearly as "deadly" as we've been told. Another way to say this is that many more people than we know have been infected and survived because their immune systems worked.

H5N1 Flu is Hard to Catch

Flu viruses are spread through the respiratory system. Basically, you breath in some viruses, they latch onto cells that line your nose and throat, then spread to your lungs.

Viruses attach to specific molecules on the surface of cells. Each of these tissues has a different set of surface molecules. These in turn differ between humans and birds.

It turns out that H5N1 infects birds because bird upper respiratory cells have the right kind of surface molecules. Human nose and throat cells don't have the right molecules for H5N1 to latch onto. So it's hard to get infected.

However, human lung cells do have the right surface molecules. Which is a reason why once someone is infected it's serious business.

What the researchers who discovered all this worry about is whether H5N1 will mutate so that it attaches to human nose and throat cells. With this type of adaptation, the virus can move more easily from human to human. But after over 5 years of monitoring this virus, there's been no sign of that mutation.

This is not to say that there is no threat. However, the threat has less to do with the alleged deadliness of the virus and much more to do with how we support our immunity.

And what makes for a healthy immune system? One clue is in the research paper from the Karolinska Institute. In classifying people from very poor to very rich, the researchers found that the poorest were almost 2½ times as likely to get sick as the very rich, with a nice gradient in between—the better your circumstances, the better your chances of avoiding the flu.

This isn't news to many people. Researchers who study the social causes of sickness and health have observed that in Europe during the late 19th Century and in developing countries in the 20th Century, it is not the miracles of modern medicine that turn health statistics around; it's the rise in economic security.

This is not a topic of polite conversation in the halls of government. And yet we all know it to be true. Security from disease is bound to security from want. The flu doesn't just happen to us individually. It happens to us all, whether we're exposed, infected, get sick, or die. The flu runs through a population. Some are safer than others because their lives are safer.

The Panic

Why is "deadly" persistently associated with H5N1? What's gained by fomenting panic?

One reason is that government agencies want people to be aware and prepared. In response to the blistering criticisms of the US in the wake of Hurricanes Katrina and Rita, we've seen a flurry of activity intended to convince us that disaster preparedness agencies are paying attention and taking action.

When the threat of H5N1 was first taken seriously by these agencies, there was big talk about developing vaccines and conducting widespread immunizations. Reluctant vaccine manufacturers were enticed by relief from any legal responsibility for injuries that might result from fast-tracking vaccine production.

But that hasn't happened. So the fallback position was the plan to kick production of anti-viral drugs (especially Tamaflu) into high gear. And that hasn't happened.

Now the discussion has shifted to preparing to care for all the victims of the flu pandemic. And on the heals of that discussion is the one about how clinical facilities will be overwhelmed.

Continuous news coverage about the "deadly" flu that is imminent stokes the fires of panic. Protection is not available, heightening the sense of panic. Finally, the institutions we'll need to care for us when disaster hits won't be able to handle it, adding yet more fuel to the sense of panic.

This does not lead to a greater sense of safety. Quite the opposite is true.

Fear is a very useful emotion: it enables you to focus on immediate causes of danger and how to escape. But a general atmosphere of fear is not helpful. In fact, it's counterproductive.

In an interview on *Your Own Health And Fitness*, Ana-Marie Jones of Collaborating Agencies Responding to Disasters (CARD) describes her strategy: preparing for success makes communities resilient when faced with disasters. But people who live with hope and a sense of their own power are more difficult to govern than people who live in fear.

Real Protection

The flu spreads in a community through exposure and infection. The people at the highest risk are the elderly and people with compromised immune systems.

A review of studies about how well vaccinating old people worked to prevent the flu found that old people in institutions were helped, but those living independently in the community were not. This suggests that the important thing is not vaccination but exposure: the risk of exposure is much greater in institutions. It also suggests that healthy old people able to live on their own have more resilient immune systems than institutionalized old people.

In general, the best protection is a healthy immune system. Support it with supplements such as vitamin C, immune boosters such as colostrum, homeopathic remedies such as occillococcinum, and anti-viral herbs such as black elderberry. For more, see "Flu Vaccines" in PHO #6.

You can also reduce your own exposure and reduce how much you expose other people with two simple things.

Researchers have shown that viruses are completely removed with 10 seconds of hand washing with soap and water. Soap binds easily to a virus's outer shell, especially a flu virus. Hand washing is particularly important after handling cash or other materials that can carry viruses.

Researchers have also found that hydrating your sinuses with an aerosol spray of 0.9% saline solution (water and a little salt) dramatically reduces the viral load when you sneeze or even when you just exhale. If you're infected, that reduces the chance that you'll infect others.

Resources

Anonymous. 2006. Why Humans Don't Easily Catch Bird Flu. *New Scientist.* March 22, 2006: 21.

Birn, Anne-Emanuelle. 2005. Gates's Grandest Challenge: Transcending Technology as Public Health Ideology. *The Lancet.* August 6, 2005 (366):514-9.

Collaborating Agencies Responding to Disasters. Access at http://www.first-victims.org.

Edwards, David et al. 2004. Inhaling to Mitigate Exhaled Bioaerosols. *Proceedings of the National Academy of Science.* December 14, 2004 (101:50): 17383-8. DOI:10.1073/pnas.0408159101.

Jefferson, Tom et al. 2005. Efficacy and Effectiveness of Influenza Vaccines in Elderly People. *The Lancet.* October 1, 2005 (366): 1165-74. DOI:10.1016/50140-6736(05).

Jones, Ana-Marie. 2005. Avian Flu: What to Do. *Your Own Health And Fit-*

ness. Broadcast November 15, 2005.

Sickbert-Bennett, Emily et al. 2005. Comparative Efficacy of Hand Hygiene Agents in the Reduction of Bacteria and Viruses. *American Journal of Infection Control.* March 2005 (33: 2): 67-77. DOI:10.1016/j.ajic.2004.08.05.

Tenpenny, Sherri. 2005. Eliminating Bird Flu Fears: 10 Facts You Need To Know. *Red Flags.* November 2, 2005. Access at http://www.readflagsdaily. com.

Thorson, Anna et al. 2005. Is Exposure to Sick or Dead Poultry Associated With Flulike Illness? *Archives of Internal Medicine.* January 9, 2006 (166): 119-23.

❧

TOO FEW MAMMOGRAMS

Dr. James Michaelson lamented, "If we could pay more attention to the management side of screening, we could really make the experience better and save a lot of lives." Dr. Michaelson led a team of Harvard Medical School researchers in a study of over 72,000 women who had mammograms at Massachusetts General Hospital. The study found that few women returned for follow-up mammograms.

The study results were also of concern to the American Cancer Society (ACS). Dr. Herman Kattlove of the ACS commented that "[w]e have a problem in mammography in this country—the message still hasn't gotten out that mammography will save lives." Drs. Michaelson and Kattlove must have missed the report from the prestigious Cochrane Collaboration that found screening for breast cancer using mammography saved no more lives than palpation (physical examination).

The Cochrane Collaboration Report

Published in 2001 through the Cochrane Collaboration, Screening for Breast Cancer with Mammography evaluated all studies of the relationship between mammographic screening and breast cancer mortality.

The authors, Dr. Ole Olsen and Dr. Peter Gøtzsche, had conducted a similar study in 2000 at the request of the Danish government to determine the effectiveness of mammography. For the Cochrane study, Olsen and Gøtzsche conducted a search of thousands of studies concerning breast-cancer screening trials. Nine studies met their selection criteria, intended to ensure that study data could be compared.

Of the nine, only five were conducted in a way that allowed their results to be compared meaningfully. Two of the five had medium-quality data (bias that could be easily corrected). Three had poor-quality data (significant bias was suspected that could not be corrected).

An example of bias is how the deaths of women in the study were classified. Research indicates that after a woman is treated for breast cancer, her death is less likely to be classified as due to breast cancer. Presumably, this happens because treatment signifies "cured," so the pathologist looks at other causes first. In the studies that Olsen and Gøtzsche examined, women who received mammograms were far more likely to be treated than women screened by palpation. As a consequence, a mammogrammed woman who died from breast cancer was more likely to have her death misclassified as something else because she was more likely to have been treated. This biases the results, so that studies showing a benefit actually undercount the number of breast cancer deaths among mammogrammed women.

Mammograms and Breast Cancer

The results of the two medium-quality studies showed no relationship between mammographic screening and breast cancer deaths after 7 years and after 13 years. The three poor-quality (biased) studies showed a significant reduction in breast cancer deaths for women who had mammograms.

In the two least-biased (medium-quality) studies, for women under 50, the risk of dying from breast cancer after 7 years was actually greater for women who had mammograms. Otherwise, mammograms had no effect at 13 years for under-50 women, nor for over-50 women at either 7 years or 13 years.

Using all the studies that included data on death from all causes, Olsen and Gøtzsche found that deaths from all cancers and from all causes were identical between women screened using mammogram versus palpation. This is an important observation. It says that, regardless of any ambiguity in mortality from breast cancer, mammograms don't seem to save lives in the broadest sense. Olsen and Gøtzsche acknowledge, however, that their observation is only suggestive. A larger study would be required to yield statistically valid results.

Saving Lives?

The breast cancer orthodoxy promoted by the ACS and the National Cancer Institute (NCI) is that breast cancer mortality has been dropping over the last 20 years because of early detection through mammographic screening. As John Lee, MD and David Zava, PhD point out in What Your Doctor May Not Tell You About Breast Cancer, it's a statistical trick.

First, in the conventional statistics, the death clock starts from the time of detection. On average, mammograms detect cancers a year earlier than palpation. So a cancer discovered by palpation has been growing for a year. If death rates are adjusted for that year, then the breast cancer death rates are identical. In other words, early detection makes no difference for breast cancer survival.

Second, the rise in survival rates are a result of detecting a ductal carcinoma in situ (DCIS). Only 1 out of 100 of DCIS detected develop into malignancies. If these are removed from the statistics, the rate of breast cancer deaths is increasing, not decreasing.

The Risks

Radiation Risk   Although the level of radiation exposure in a mammogram has decreased significantly over the last 10 years, radiation is both cumulative and has no safe lower limit. The more radiation your body takes, the greater your risk, which includes not only cancer but heart disease.

False Positives and False Negatives   When a mammogram detects a lump, it's common for it to be biopsied. A pathologist will look at the tissue sample and determine whether it is malignant. "False positive" means that the pathologist diagnosed the tissue as cancer when it was not. "False negative" means that the pathologist did not diagnose cancer, but in fact the tissue was cancerous. When highly experienced pathologists were given biopsied tissue identified by palpation, their diagnoses were almost 100% in agreement. The chances of a false positive or false negative on these biopsies was small. When these same pathologists were given tissue identified by mammogram, their diagnoses were dramatically inconsistent. The chances of a false positive or false negative was much greater.

Proliferation   As early as 1928, scientists were concerned that compressing a malignant tumor could dislodge a cancer cell, rupture blood vessels, and spread the cancer.

Overdiagnosis and Overtreatment   Even though the majority (8 out of 10) of DCIS tissue discovered by mammography never "goes bad," once identified, there's incredible pressure to perform biopsies and undertake treatment (lumpectomy plus radiation or mastectomy plus chemotherapy). As Olsen and Gøtzsche report, mammogrammed women were diagnosed and treated a third more often than palpated women: with mammograms, your chance of survival might not be greater, but your chance of being diagnosed and treated is.

Pain and Suffering   Squashing your breast for a mammogram is at best uncomfortable. Usually, it hurts. Overtreatment from a premature and false positive biopsy is traumatic, physically and emotionally.

Delays   Mammography facilities have decreased over the past 10 years. The NCI projects fewer radiologists specializing in mammography. In many areas of the country, women have to wait up to 5 months for routine mammograms.

Between Mammograms   The current ACS and NCI recommendation is for annual mammograms. However, the most dangerous cancers will not wait around for a year. They are dangerous precisely because they grow rapidly: in the year between mammograms, an aggressive breast cancer can triple in size.

The Safe Alternative

BSE   Each month, perform a breast self-examination (BSE). That is, palpate your breasts.

CBE   Have an annual clinical breast examination (CBE) performed by a nurse trained in CBE. And have her evaluate your BSE technique.

In their 2001 article "Dangers and Unreliability of Mammography: Breast Examination is a Safe, Effective, and Practical Alternative," Dr. Samuel Epstein (author of The Politics of Cancer Revisited) and his co-authors cite the Canadian National Breast Screening Study (one of Olsen's and Gøtzsche's least biased studies): "the addition of mammography screening to physical examination has no impact on breast cancer mortality."

Meanwhile, the Institute of Medicine (IOM), one of the National Institutes of Health, released Saving Women's Lives: Strategies for Improving Breast Cancer Detection and Diagnosis in early 2004. The study describes improvements to mammographic technology and procedures along with new technologies, such as ultrasound, thermography, and MRI (magnetic resonance imaging).

You might have heard that some of these technologies are better alternatives to mammography. Ultrasound is one that is readily available. Yet the issue is not discovering a technology that will encourage women to subject themselves to screening. The issue is that early discovery by any of these technologies does not improve survival when compared to BSE and CBE.

Drs. Michaelson and Kattlove fret over the inadequate return rate of women for follow-up mammograms, especially poor women. In contrast, Dr. Epstein suggests devoting mammography resources to BSE and CBE training, especially among women in underserved communities.

As PHO went to press, research was reported on the success of MRI in detecting growths earlier than mammography. It's also ten times as expensive. MRI advocates point to its use on women at high risk.

But we already know what those risks are: a specific gene or a sister or mother with breast cancer before 50. To really do something about saving these women's lives, they should get better prevention following Dr. Lee's and Dr. Zava's book.

Big Box Medicine thinks that you need more technology to protect you from breast cancer. But the evidence strongly suggests you just need support so you can pay attention to what your body is telling you.

Resources

American Cancer Society, Women Skip Lifesaving Mammograms. Access at http://www.cancer.org/docroot/NWS/content/NWS_1_1x_Women_Skip_ Lifesaving_Mammograms.asp.

Blanchard, Karen, et al. 2004. Mammographic Screening: Patterns of Use and Estimated Impact on Breast Carcinoma Survival. *Cancer.* August 1, 2004. 101(3): 495-507.

Epstein, Samuel S, Rosalie Bertell, and Barbara Seaman. 2001. Dangers and Unreliability of Mammography: Breast Examination is a Safe, Effective, and Practical Alternative. *International Journal of Health Services.* 31(3):605-615.

Lee, John, MD and David Zava, PhD. 2002. *What Your Doctor May Not Tell You About Breast Cancer.* New York: Warner Books.

Olsen, Ole and Peter C. Gøtzsche. 2001. Screening for Breast Cancer with Mammography. *Cochrane Database of Systematic Reviews.* 4: CD001877.

Welch, H. Gilbert. 2004. *Should I Be Tested for Cancer?* Berkeley: University of California Press.

IN YOUR PROSTATE

In *Should I Be Tested for Cancer?*, H. Gilbert Welch, MD writes that "over the last quarter century more than a million men have been diagnosed with prostate cancer who would not have received this diagnosis in the early 1970s."

This dramatic increase is not evidence of a prostate cancer epidemic. It is the result of early detection from the introduction of the PSA test.

As one would expect, with the dramatic increase in the number of prostate cancer diagnoses has come an increase in treatments: radiation and surgery.

In response to news of renewed interest in the PSA test, Dr. Mark Jordan, chief of urology at the University of Medicine and Dentistry of New Jersey, observed, "We're not even sure if prostate cancer surgery prolongs life."

The news reported that a dramatic increase in a man's PSA level could mean cancer is running amok in his prostate gland. Such a man is likely to have biopsies of his prostate. If his biopsies are suspicious, he's likely to have his prostate irradiated or removed.

The Resurrection of the PSA Test

PSA screening has waned over the last decade. With it has come a decline in the number of diagnoses, biopsies, and surgeries.

When first introduced, the PSA was a great improvement for screening men for prostate cancer. Before the PSA, screening was performed by a digital rectal exam (DRE), which is just what it sounds like: a physician dons a surgical glove, liberally applies K-Y Jelly, inserts a finger in your rectum, and physically feels your prostate gland.

The PSA not only relieved men from the discomfort of a DRE, it detected suspicious prostate activity earlier than a DRE. In respect to early detection, the PSA is akin to mammography.

After 20 years of enthusiastic use, however, research showed that men's PSA levels varied widely. As a result, a "high" reading turned out not to mean very much.

With the new research showing that men with accelerated PSA levels are at greater risk of having cancer, the PSA is back in business.

Overdiagnosed and Overtreated

PSA stands for "prostate specific antigen," a misleading name: PSA is produced in the prostate and in breast tissue. PSA works in the prostate to counteract the effect of angiogenesis, the growth of blood vessels. Cancer cells cause angiogenesis so they can be fed. In response, your prostate increases PSA levels to cut off the cancer's blood supply.

But your prostate doesn't say, "Yikes! Cancer! Get some PSA over here!" Instead, it pumps out PSA in response to cell crowding, which can be the result of bigger cells or more cells. When not cancerous, this is referred to as BPH: interchangeably benign prostate hypertrophy (bigger cells) or benign prostate hyperplasia (more cells). Frequently, BPH accounts for prostate enlargement.

PSA levels also increase from pressure, which is why your doctor is supposed to draw the blood for the PSA before he or she K-Y Jellys your rectum.

So a high PSA level or a dramatic increase in PSA is a signal of cell crowding. But too often it's used directly as a signal of cancer. Typically, a biopsy will be performed to confirm this preliminary diagnosis.

The procedure for a prostate biopsy consists of inserting a thumb-sized probe equipped with a camera at its tip in (you guessed it) your rectum. When the probe reaches your prostate, a needle comes out of the probe, passes through your rectum wall and into your prostate. The needle then extracts some cells. Typically, five samples in all are taken and sent off to the lab.

About half of the men biopsied experience some kind of complication, usually blood in their urine. In 2 out of 100 cases, the complication is serious enough to require hospitalization. If some of the cells sampled are identified by the pathologist as cancer, treatment will typically consist of irradiating the prostate or removing it. Because cells are taken from a limited number of locations, even negative readings can lead to a perpetual cycle of testing and biopsy: the cancer isn't where the first sample was taken, but it might be somewhere else in the prostate.

The result is overdiagnosis and overtreatment.

A scary PSA level or PSA acceleration is likely to lead to a diagnosis of prostate cancer and subsequent treatment. Yet even with the early detection system that PSAs provide, the number of men who survive after treatment remains the same. As we discuss in our article on mammography, what early detection through PSA screening produces is more diagnosed cases and more men treated with radiation and surgery.

Hormone Imbalance

In his monograph *Hormone Balance for Men*, John Lee, MD describes a different approach.

Prostate cancers are very slow going. In men over 65, a prostate tumor typically doubles in size every five years. For a woman, by comparison, a breast tumor can double in four months.

The way in which a normal prostate cell becomes a cancer cell is the same as the way in which a breast cell turns into a cancer cell. And that is due to what Dr. Lee calls estrogen dominance.

Estrogen? In men? Yes. Estrogen plays a key role in, among other things, maintaining healthy brain function in both men and women.

Estrogen dominance does not refer to an absolute level of estrogen, but to the ratio of estrogen to progesterone and testosterone. As a man ages, his testosterone and progesterone decline and his estrogen rises. Symptoms of estrogen dominance include excess weight, urinary problems, anxiety, insomnia, and prostate enlargement.

When not balanced by sufficient testosterone and progesterone, estrogen creates a byproduct that destroys some of the building blocks of DNA. This damage leads directly to cancer of the breast and uterus in women, and to prostate cancer in men.

Testosterone Gets a Bad Rap

Dr. Charles Huggins received a Nobel prize for his work on the prostate: testosterone seemed to be the culprit. His conclusion was based on his observation that castration slowed down prostate cancer growth. However, testes also produce estrogen.

So the concept that testosterone promotes prostate cancer is ill-founded. Supplementation with bio-identical testosterone balances estrogen, resolves BPH (prostate enlargement), and helps prevent and treat prostate cancer.

Bringing a man's testosterone level in balance with estrogen might increase PSA levels. Conventional wisdom might regard this as a sign that a cancer is getting worse. In fact, it's a sign of health: more PSA means that your body is working to cut off the blood supply to crowded cells, both BPH and cancer.

The right balance of testosterone not only protects your prostate, but it also protects your heart.

The third component in this balancing act is progesterone. As it does for women, progesterone balances the effects of estrogen. Progesterone also neutralizes the conversion of testosterone into DHT (dihydrotestosterone) which is responsible for male pattern balding and the increase of prostate cells.

Restoring Balance

Are your estrogen, testosterone, and progesterone in balance? The most accurate measure is through a saliva test or a blood test for free hormones. These measure the hormones available to your tissues and organs. Typically, doctors test total levels, which do not measure what's actually available to your body.

You might have to educate your doctor about the value of saliva tests and free hormone tests. One resource is *What Your Doctor May Not Tell You About Breast Cancer* by John Lee, MD and David Zava, PhD. Information is also available at the ZRT Laboratory Web site www.SalivaTest.com.

When taking hormone supplements, make sure you use bio-identical testosterone and progesterone. Patented versions that are not bio-identical are not only ineffective, but also patented (methyl) testosterone is associated with increased cancer risk.

If scary things happen with your PSA tests or from a DRE, before leaping into biopsies and radical treatments, look first at getting your hormones into balance.

PSA screening in Sweden is uncommon, as are radical treatments. Physicians and patients watch and wait. After this practice became common, prostate cancer deaths declined.

Resources

Lee, John, MD. 2003. *Hormone Balance for Men: What Your Doctor May Not Tell You about Prostate Health and Natural Hormone Supplementation.* Available from www.JohnLeeMD.com.

Lee, John, MD and David Zava, PhD. 2002. *What Your Doctor May Not Tell You About Breast Cancer.* New York: Warner.

Welch, H. Gilbert, MD. 2004. *Should I Be Tested for Cancer?* Berkeley: University of California.

ZRT Laboratory. http://www.zrtlab.com.

ANTIOXIDANT MYTHS

A good example of bad science journalism appeared in the August 5, 2006 issue of the *New Scientist*. There's a teaser on the magazine's cover for the article: "The Antioxidant Myth: How we fell for a medical fairy tale."

The bulk of the article is devoted to describing research that alleges no benefit from taking antioxidant supplements. The gist of the article is this: populations with diets of antioxidant-rich foods have less disease; tests in the lab on cell cultures show that antioxidants reduce harmful free radicals; yet when clinical trials are conducted with antioxidant supplements, the outcomes are disappointing.

It's not until the end of the article that a dissenting voice is heard. A representative from the Council for Responsible Nutrition points out that antioxidants don't work like drugs, that antioxidants work together. The article lingers not on this topic, but does take the time to note that the Council is the trade organization for supplement manufacturers. You, the reader, are smart enough to know what that means: dismiss what they've said because it's obviously biased.

Biased Science Journalism

Why is this bad science journalism?

The Council's view is shared by a wide range of researchers and practitioners. Those researchers and practitioners have a good deal to say about the benefits of antioxidant supplements, the study's that show a positive effect, and the weaknesses of the study's that show no effect or harm.

Why wasn't someone from, for instance, the Linus Pauling Institute interviewed and quoted? Because it wouldn't give the odor of bias provided by a quote from a trade association.

Speaking of odor, the author, Lisa Melton, identifies herself as "science writer in residence at the Novartis Foundation in London." Novartis is a leading pharmaceutical company. Pharmaceutical companies and the science that blossoms from them belittle vitamins and minerals—at least unpatented vitamins and minerals.

The shameful thing about this article and the editorial that covers it, what makes it bad science journalism, is its gross bias and condescension.

A major criticism of antioxidant clinical trials is their faulty design, a fact alluded to by the representative from the Council for Responsible Nutrition. In addition to the very important issue regarding how antioxidants work together, these experiments often ignore the test subject's unique metabolism and nutrient status. Practitioners and civilians who successfully use antioxidants and other supplements know this. Antioxidant clinical trials have also been sloppy about what form of antioxidant the researchers use.

The bias of the *New Scientist*'s editors shows up in how they frame their favorable comment on the article. They describe receiving supplements from a PR firm and how, by golly, they weren't going to fall for that nonsense. The article itself bemoans the alleged fact that, despite all of the great science showing antioxidant supplements don't do anything, people will continue to take them. We're just a gullible bunch of yahoos towed around by the promise of health made by unscrupulous sellers of potions and nostrums. We're just too stupid to realize when we're being conned.

The objective, scientific folks at *New Scientist*, on the other hand, have a firm grasp of the evidence, have decided that antioxidants don't work, and believe that you're a fool to think otherwise.

Fairy Tales Can Come True

If Lisa Melton, the "science writer in residence at the Novartis Foundation," had taken the trouble to investigate *all* of the research available on the benefits of antioxidants, she would have written a very different article.

Vitamin E takes a drubbing in the article. A big deal is made in the article about a study (actually, a review of 19 clinical studies) that found that vitamin E did nothing at low doses and harm at high doses when administered to heart patients. We commented on the weaknesses of this same study in "Antioxidant Follies" (PHO #4).

That study looked at people who were already sick. Yet the article is supposedly about how antioxidants don't work to *prevent* illness. Unmentioned are the five large observational studies cited by the Linus Pauling Institute that showed a significant beneficial preventive effect from vitamin E, whether through diet or supplements.

But the article only wants to look at clinical trials, the so-called "gold standard" for evidence. We discussed this issue in "Nutrient Supplements Are Good for You" (on page 85) with regard to another flawed review, this one of multi-vitamins. One of the great failings of clinical trials is that they do not account for the social class or other stressor status of the study participants. Stress causes oxidative stress, which increases the need for antioxidants. Observational studies such as those that showed a benefit will tend to find this stress-based effect if they observe people from a genuine cross-section of social classes.

Antioxidant Network

Lester Packer has been one of the leading researchers in the health effects of oxidative stress and antioxidants. He describes the interdependence of the principal antioxidants, calling it the *antioxidant network*.

The five principal antioxidants in the network are vitamin C, vitamin E, lipoic acid, coenzyme Q10 (CoQ10), and glutathione. While each has a unique role to play in protecting against oxidative stress, each one supports the others by helping to regenerate them.

For example, a molecule of vitamin E neutralizes a free radical by absorbing the heightened energy that makes free radicals so reactive. The vitamin E molecule then becomes a weak free radical itself. A molecule of vitamin C absorbs that energy to restore the vitamin E molecule to its antioxidant vigor. A glutathione molecule then restores the vitamin C molecule.

Don't we eventually run out of molecules to absorb free radical extra energy? First, each antioxidant action is like a cushion that reduces the excess energy. Second, we have the capacity to synthesize new antioxidant molecules and obtain the others from food.

Lipoic acid, glutathione, and CoQ10 are synthesized in your body. Glutathione, for example, is synthesized from the amino acid methionine, an amino acid found only in animal protein. However, we can't synthesize vitamin C or vitamin E and must get what we need from food or supplements.

Most conventional research does not take these interactions into account in their design. Instead they are designed using antioxidants as though they were a pharmaceutical: one pill at a time with no consideration of the study participants' individual antioxidant or oxidative stress status. Its biased research by design, whether intentional or not.

The Enlightenment philosopher Spinoza observed that, because we are finite creatures, we of necessity view the world from a perspective. He thought we should strive to understand that perspective so that we are not its captives. *New Scientist* is not alone in allowing its perspective to degenerate into bias. The problem is that they don't think they have a perspective. They have science, so they can't be biased. They should know better. That antioxidants don't work is the real antioxidant myth.

The News

Melton, Lisa. 2006. The Antioxidant Myth. *New Scientist*. August 5, 2006.

The Research

Kregel, Kevin and Hannah Zhang. 2007. An Integrated View of Oxidative Stress in Aging: Basic Mechanisms, Functional Effects, and Pathological Considerations. *American Journal of Physiology - Regulatory, Integrative and Comparative Physiology.* 292 (January 2007): R18-36.

Miller, Edgar, et al. 2005. Meta-Analysis: High-Dosage Vitamin E Supplementation May Increase All-Cause Mortality. *Annals of Internal Medicine*, 142(1), January 4, 2005..

Resources

Fawcett, Jeffry, 2005. Antioxidant Follies. *Progressive Health Observer.* 4 (December 2004/January 2005): 1ff.

Higdon, Jane. 2003. *An Evidence-Based Approach to Vitamins and Minerals.* New York: Thieme.

Linus Pauling Institute, Micronutrient Information Center. Access at http://lpi.oregonstate.edu/infocenter/.

Packer, Lester. 1999. *The Antioxidant Miracle.* New York: John Wiley and Sons.

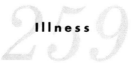
Teresa, an 88-year old woman living in the Bronx, suffered from anxiety and confusion. Her doctor put her on Risperdal, an antipsychotic drug. Subsequently she had trouble walking. Her daughter Ramona took her to another doctor who discovered that Teresa had low thyroid. Ramona moved her mother into a nursing home believing that Teresa would be better served in a controlled environment.

In the nursing home, screams erupted from Teresa, she drooled, she twitched. The psychiatrist who served the nursing home took her off Risperdal—its side effects include those from which Teresa suffered. However, the psychiatrist then put Teresa on 2 other antipsychotic drugs plus a sedative.

Teresa's condition deteriorated. Only when Ramona took her mother to a third doctor who took her off all the drugs did Teresa's condition improve.[1]

The failure of the first two doctors' heroic interventions illustrates how the medical system is prone to overdiagnosis and overtreatment. But there is a deeper lesson to learn from this story.

Teresa was suffering from anxiety and confusion. The doctors used drugs to make those symptoms go away. In doing that, they elicited yet more suffering. From Teresa's and Ramona's point of view, the treatments were the cause of the suffering. From the doctor's point of view, the drugs were the cures for that suffering.

The difference is fundamental and huge. It is an intractable characteristic of the medical system. It illustrates a distinction made by medical historian Robert Aronowitz in his book *Making Sense of Illness*:[2] the distinction between *individual illness* and *specific disease*.

> Historians of medicine have labeled as "ontological" the view that diseases are specific entities that unfold in characteristic ways in the typical person. In this framework, diseases exist in some platonic sense outside their manifestations in a particular individual. The other compelling account of illness, the "physiological" or "holistic," stresses the individual and his or her adaptation, both psychological and physical, to a changing environment. In this framework, illness exists only in individuals. These ideal-typical notions have been in a state of dynamic tension since antiquity.[3]

We can see this tension in a home reference such as *Smart Medi-*

cine for Healthier Living[4] that presents holistic practices alongside conventional practices. It's very organization reflects the tension between individual illness and specific disease: some entries are what someone might suffer from (for example, anxiety and confusion) while other entries are diagnoses (for example, hypothyroidism).

Health care institutions operate principally within the specific disease framework. That framework has been at the core of the dominant institutions of medical science and practice and health policy for the last century. In particular, it gained dominance as medical science and practice shifted from acute to chronic illness.

As we discussed "Protection and Prevention," health science and medical practice over the last century have shifted from the treatment of acute disease to the prevention of acute and chronic disease. In addition, the dominance of the specific disease framework has conjured diseases out of symptoms.

Teresa's story is an example. The first article in this section, "Aging as a Diagnosis" is another. It describes how degeneration with age is assumed and that a characteristic of degeneration (frailty) is worthy of elevation to the status of a diagnosis—in other words, it's a specific disease. Functionally, this turns attention away from what the sufferer can do for herself and toward what health professionals can do to her.

This is a characteristic of how suffering is dealt with in medical institutions. Things that can be done to or for patients[4] are many and varied. Things that can be done to support a sufferer in discovering and doing the simplest things for herself are few and far between.

In the second article, "Hypertension All Around," we discuss a classic example of how symptoms are turned into a disease. It describes how standards are set so that the largest number of people receives medical treatment. The rationale is that high blood pressure is a risk factor for heart attacks, strokes, and kidney disease. Not only does the rationale make little sense, the treatment of hypertension focuses exclusively on eliminating the symptom.

Blood pressure medications are famous for their side effects, in particular the nutrient deficiencies they cause. As with Teresa, people on blood pressure drugs often suffer. Just as often, multiple drugs are used to treat the side effects that result from the preceding round drugs.

This raises an interesting question: should drugs be considered diseases? After all, an infectious disease is an abnormal functioning of the body that shows up as a characteristic set of symptoms that are caused by a biologically active agent. Drugs certainly count as biologically active agents.

"Blood Sugar Derangement" is the third article in this section. In it we discuss the risks faced by people diagnosed with type 2 diabetes, specifically from the very medications prescribed to treat them. We also discuss the notion that diabetes isn't properly a disease and that the blood sugar derangement that results in a diagnosis would be better treated as the consequence of the actual cause: stress.

The fourth article, "Fat and Death," examines the so-called obesity epidemic. While some forms of excess body weight are a consequence of diseases and imbalances, the increase of body weight in the population is not a disease. It's a symptom of metabolic disruptions largely caused by environmental exposures. Instead, research and media bias have turned it into another opportunity to chastise people for gluttony and sloth.

The last article, "Health Inequity and Toxic Load," discusses a comparison between the medical status of citizens of the United States and Britain. We discuss how both social inequity and toxic load explain the better medical status of Britons.

Social inequity and toxic exposures have no place in the specific disease framework as it is currently institutionalized. Although medical treatments and standards of care for the effects of inequity and toxic exposure exist. But alleviation of disparities among social classes and exposures to toxins are nowhere to be found among those treatments and standards.

The point here is not that the specific disease framework is wrong and the individual illness framework is right. It is that the one defines the institutions of medicine and health to the exclusion of the other. For the individual person, like Teresa, it is the grasp of their individual illness that must guide her actions. The experts on specific diseases are handy, but they must always serve the alleviation of suffering not the curing of disease.

Notes

1   Laurie Tarkan (2008) "Doctors Say Medication Is Overused in Dementia."
2   Robert Aronowitz (1998) *Making Sense of Illness: Science, Society, and Disease.*
3   Ibid page 8.
4   Janet Zand, et al. (1999) *Smart Medicine for Healthier Living: A Practical A-to-Z Reference to Natural and Conventional Treatments for Adults.*
5   "Patient" like "consumer" and "citizen" are social roles that an individual, biologically and historically unique person assumes in response to environmental cues or is forced to assume in a particular institutional environment—such as a doctor's office.

AGING AS A DIAGNOSIS

Frailty from aging is about to be christened as an official diagnosis. An article in the *Boston Globe* describes how researchers are providing hope for a condition that seemed hopeless—at least according to this article's version of reality.

Frailty as a diagnosis is likely to have a life like metabolic syndrome: a collection of symptoms that leads to treatment with drugs. Like metabolic syndrome, you will be officially frail if you experience three of five symptoms: weight loss, decreased daily activity, muscle weakness, exhaustion, and slow walking speed. If you have two, then you'll be at risk of being frail (although not *officially* frail).

How odd.

But that's how the conventional thought process works: we have to have a diagnosis so we can do something. And the "something" is usually pharmaceuticals or invasive surgery.

Although the endpoint for the article describes how the pharmaceutical giant Merck is developing drugs to combat muscle weakness and how ACE inhibitors are being studied for the same purpose, a good deal of space in the middle of the article is devoted to a method that is already known to work: exercise. The NIH is even throwing research money at the study of how exercise affects frailty.

Another Made-up Disease

The *Globe* article quotes one researcher as identifying the root causes of frailty as low hormones, malnutrition, anemia, and chronic inflammation. Another researcher describes muscle weakness as the result of malnutrition caused by a "vicious cycle" of illness, medication, and environmental assaults. And other researchers are described as firing up experiments with testosterone in men as a way to restore strength. (Why aren't they studying the effects of testosterone in women?)

Oh, but here's the trick. The researchers are concerned about testosterone causing blood clots. That's a dead giveaway that they're testing patented testosterone not bioidentical testosterone.

Patented testosterone does not match the hormone produced by your body. It doesn't work. It's been known for a long time that it causes problems. On the other hand, we know that bioidentical testosterone works very well without side effects. But bioidentical testosterone won't be in these studies. This whole project seems to be one step forward and two steps back.

One of the most irksome things about the *Globe* article and the research projects it describes is the utter ignorance of researchers and practitioners who, for quite some time, have been looking at how to counter the effects of aging as we grow older.

Low hormones? We know how to deal with that using bioidentical hormone supplementation.

Malnutrition? We know how to provide a nutrient-rich diet that includes nutrient supplementation.

Anemia? Typically it's a product of malnutrition and hormone imbalance.

Chronic inflammation? Again solved by the right nutrients or by the proper treatment of an inflammatory condition such as diabetes or heart disease—both treatable with nutrients. And exercise. And hormone balance.

We don't need another made-up disease that doctors can throw drugs at. We already know when someone is frail. We don't need a diagnosis. We need to help each other age well—using the knowledge we already have about nutrient and hormone balance.

Growing Old and Aging

When frailty becomes an accepted diagnosis, it's likely that a national frailty association will be formed promoting concern for this new disease. A frailty epidemic might even be discovered.

What nonsense.

Frailty is a consequence of aging, that long slide into disability that ends with death. But aging is not an inevitable consequence of growing old. A very eloquent statement of this fact comes from an unlikely source: Don Hamilton's *Homeopathic Care for Cats and Dogs*. "The gradual deterioration that we associate with aging is really chronic disease. Healthy individuals remain relatively strong throughout their lives and deteriorate rapidly as they near death (p. 30)."

Aging is the body's incapacity to repair itself. A leading theory attributes the incapacity to oxidative stress. Recent research focuses attention on how oxidative stress affects mitochondria.

We discussed the mitochondrial theory of aging in "Healthy Mitochondria" (PHO #9). Mitochondria are small organelles in virtually every cell that produce all of your energy. It is an inherently oxidative process. This process is controlled by each mitochondrion's DNA, which is separate from the cell's DNA. Although mitochondrial DNA is very resilient (it can be 90% damaged and still do its job) it is also quite vulnerable.

Like the cell's DNA, mitochondrial DNA includes instructions for the enzymes that repair damage and "proofread" copies of DNA when a mitochondrion divides. Because it is much simpler than the cell's DNA, a mitochondrion's set of repair enzymes is also much simpler. While free radicals and reactive oxygen species damage both kinds of DNA, mitochondrial DNA can't recover as easily as the cell's DNA.

As we discussed in "Healthy Mitochondria," antioxidants in food and supplements help thwart oxidative stress. "Antioxidant Myths" on page 255 discusses antioxidants further.

Avoiding environmental stressors that cause oxidative stress in the first place is of equal importance to loading up with antioxidants. Air pollution (including tobacco smoke) and toxins are oxidative stressors. Exposures such as allergens and electromagnetic fields that cause inflammation promote oxidative stress.

The connection between damaged mitochondria and the degeneration of tissues that constitutes aging is mediated by inflammation. So in addition to antioxidants, aging is reduced by reducing inflammation. Jack Challem's *The Inflammation Syndrome* describes nutrient strategies for combating chronic inflammation. Hormone balance also affects inflammation and your body's capacity to repair itself and is described in the work of John Lee and David Zava as well as on the Educational Resources page of the ZRT Laboratory website.

The News
Dembner, Alice. 2006. Science Gaining on Elders' Frailty. *Boston Globe*. September 3, 2006.

Kolata, Gina. 2006. If You've Got a Pulse, You're Sick. *New York Times*. May 21, 2007.

The Research
Boockvar, Kenneth and Diane Meier. 2006. Palliative Care for Frail Older Adults. *JAMA*. November 8, 2006 (296:18): 2245-53.

Fried, Linda et al. 2001. Frailty in Older Adults: Evidence for a Phenotype. *The Journal of Gerontology*. 56: M146-57 (2001).

Kregel, Kevin and Hannah Zhang. 2007. An Integrated View of Oxidative Stress in Aging: Basic Mechanisms, Functional Effects, and Pathological Considerations. *Amercian Journal of Physiology - Regulatory, Integrative and Comparative Physiology*. 292 (January 2007): R18-36. COI: 10.1152/ajpregu.00327.2006.

Resources
Challem, Jack. 2003. *The Inflammation Syndrome*. New York: John Wiley and Sons.

Challem, Jack. 2004. Inflammation and Chronic Illness. *Your Own Health And Fitness*. Broadcast July 13, 2004.

Fawcett, Jeffry. 2006. Healthy Mitochondria. *Progressive Health Observer.* 9 (Winter 2006): 2ff.

Hamilton, Donald. 1999. *Homeopathic Care for Cats and Dogs.* Berkeley, CA: North Atlantic Books.

Lee, John, MD. 2003. *Hormone Balance for Men.* Available from www.John-LeeMD.com.

Lee, John, MD and David Zava, PhD. 2002. *What Your Doctor May Not Tell You About Breast Cancer.* New York: Warner.

Welch, H. Gilbert et al. 2007. What's Making Us Sick Is an Epidemic of Diagnosis. *New York Times.* January 2, 2007.

Your Own Health And Fitness, Resources on Aging. Access at http://www.yourownhealthandfitness.org/topicsAging.php.

Your Own Health And Fitness, Resources on Exercise and Musculoskeletal Health. Access at http://www.yourownhealthandfitness.org/topics-Hormones.php.

Your Own Health And Fitness, Resources on Hormones, Women's Health, and Men's Health. Access at http://www.yourownhealthandfitness.org/topicsHormones.php.

ZRT Laboratory, Hormone Education. Access at http://www.zrtlab.com/Page.aspx?nid=3.

HYPERTENSION ALL AROUND

Physician Paul Rosch, MD describes how in 1970 the standard for blood pressure in adults was 100 plus the person's age over 90. So if you were 50 years old, normal for you would be 150/90. He also notes that medical texts advised doctors to consider blood pressure in the context of treating the whole patient.

Not so today. Since 1977 six separate commissions created by the National Institutes of Health have established increasingly restrictive blood pressure standards and expanded drug treatments.

According to the latest standard set in 2003, a blood pressure of 120/80 is the upper end of normal regardless of age or gender. Blood pressure over 140/90 is classified as the disease of hypertension. And blood pressure in between is the almost-disease of prehypertension, a condition calling for treatment.

Recently, a new organization was formed to beat the drum for detecting and treating hypertension. The National Campaign to Control Hypertension (NCCH) warns that hypertension "contributes to hardening of the arteries (atherosclerosis), increases the risk of heart attack, stroke, and kidney failure."

Although NCCH is not a government agency, its concerns and advice are identical to those of the National Institutes of Health. NCCH is "supported by an unrestricted educational grant from Novartis Pharmaceutical Corporation." Novartis is a major supplier of hypertension drugs.

There's more to these standards than encouraging physicians to follow these diagnostic and treatment protocols. A physician who does not treat a patient diagnosed with hypertension might rightly fear censure by their medical board.

If you're diagnosed with hypertension or prehypertension, should you worry?

Blood Hydraulics

Blood pressure is measured in millimeters of mercury (mmHg). The reference is to the original measuring device that consisted of a calibrated tube of mercury. The column of mercury in the tube rose and fell in response to pressure pumped into a cuff around a patient's arm. The calibrations on the tube were more or less arbitrary, like the scale on thermometers. The column of mercury is gone, but the cuff remains—and the scale.

To take a blood pressure reading, the cuff is inflated then slowly deflated. A person or a machine detects when the sound of your heart beat starts and stops. Your *systolic* pressure (the high number) is when it starts. Your *diastolic* pressure (the low number) is when it stops.

A blood pressure of 120/80 means a systolic of 120 mmHg and a diastolic of 80 mmHg. The systolic pressure measures the pressure in your blood vessels when your heart pumps blood out, The diastolic when your heart pulls blood in.

The higher the number, the more effort it takes to move blood through your cardiovascular system. A high systolic means more effort to pump blood out. A high diastolic means more effort to pull in blood.

From a purely mechanical standpoint, there are three factors that can affect blood pressure:
• the strength of the heart in pushing and pulling blood (harder push or pull, higher pressure),
• the rigidity of the blood vessels (more rigid, higher pressure), and
• the viscosity ("thickness") of blood (greater viscosity, higher pressure).

As physician Malcolm Kendrick, MD points out, from this perspective the claim that hypertension "contributes" to heart attack, stroke, and kidney failure makes no sense at all. High blood pressure is a sign that one of these three factors is amiss. It's a symptom, not a disease.

But wait. Doesn't it make perfect sense that high blood pressure causes strokes? After all, a stroke blows out a blood vessel in the brain.

Actually, only about 10% of strokes are of this blown-blood-vessel type. The other 90% are from a blood clot or chunk of arterial plaque that blocks blood flow. High blood pressure isn't relevant here either—it's a symptom of what causes the blood to clot or plaque to form and get loose.

The Silent Killer

Its promoters like to call hypertension the "silent killer." They point to clinical trials that show an association between drug treatments for hypertension and reductions in heart attacks and strokes. But this ignores the direct effect these drugs have on the cardiovascular system. In fact, the cardiovascular effect is more likely the cause of reduced hypertension rather the other way around.

The condition of principal concern here is *essential hypertension*. Technically, that means high blood pressure the doctor can't attribute to some other condition.

The first salvo in treatment is to change the patient's diet (especially to reduce the use of salt), increase physical activity, and lose weight. Typically, these have no effect unless the patient's blood pressure is extreme.

And so the prescription of drugs follows, starting with *diuretics*. This class of drug is intended to flush water and with it salt out of the patient's system. Typically, diuretics don't work either. Thus begins the escalation in drug therapy, leading to multiple prescriptions, their side effects, and more drugs to deal with the side effects.

This state of things seems to be yet another example of overdiagnosis and overtreatment. And while hypertension as a disease is overdiagnosed and overtreated, the underlying cause is underdiagnosed and undertreated.

The Magic Number

Weightlifters can have a blood pressures of 400/250 while lifting. Less dramatically, blood pressure rises and falls in response to the body's needs. Chief among these is stress.

When your body is on alert, stress hormones send signals for your blood to move *pronto* to the where it's needed—such as when you go to the doctor.

One study found that one in four people have "whitecoat hypertension" their blood pressure goes up at the doctor's office. Another study of patients on multiple hypertension medications found that when they were admitted to a hospital and taken off the medications (either intentionally or unintentionally) their blood pressure dropped. When released from the hospital and in normal life and back on drugs, their blood pressure went up.

Blood pressure measurements are affected by time of day, room temperature, a full bladder, when you last ate, drank, or smoked, whether the measurement is taken standing, sitting, or lying down, and how long you've been in any of those positions.

There are two questions here. First, what's a good blood pressure *for you*? And second, if your blood pressure isn't good, what do you do about it?

Good Blood Pressure

A good blood pressure for you is not the magic number promoted by the NCCH and the health establishment. Nor is it the old rule-of-thumb of 100 plus your age over 90—although that standard is likely better than the current one-size-fits-all standard.

The place to start is your current health situation and your health history. That's the context for understanding your blood pressure as a symptom. This includes your age. As you age, it might simply take more pressure for your body to make sure blood reaches all your tissues.

We've already mentioned that both acute and chronic stress affect blood pressure through the action of adrenaline (acute stress) and cortisol (chronic stress). Here are some other major chronic conditions that affect blood pressure.

- Hypothyroidism is a major undiagnosed condition that can cause high blood pressure because thyroid counters the effect of cortisol.
- Hyperthyroidism also can cause high blood pressure by overstimulation.
- Diabetes and insulin resistance increase the viscosity of blood because red blood cells become stiffer and therefore more effort is needed to push them through narrow capillaries.
- Kidney disease can cause an imbalance in the production of renin, the hormone that regulates blood vessel rigidity.
- Atherosclerosis constricts blood vessels and can force the heart to work harder in pumping blood through.
- Heart disease weakens the diastolic pull of blood, forcing a harder systolic push.
- Sleep apnea and other disorders that increase the concentration of red blood cells and thus increase viscosity with a kind of red blood cell traffic jam.
- Clotting factors increase blood viscosity by making the red blood cells stick together more readily.

Since these are all inflammatory processes, an anti-inflammation diet reduces the underlying condition and lowers blood pressure. This includes foods and supplements rich in antioxidants. The most important of these are vitamin C and vitamin E, coenzyme Q10 (*CoQ10*), and lipoic acid. It also includes Omega 3 fatty acids from food and supplements.

Pass the Salt

You probably think that salt is bad for hypertension. In fact, few people respond to lowered salt (sodium) intake. Some physicians have patients switch from refined to unrefined salt with good results because unrefined salt has other, complementary minerals. Note that refined salt is what's typically used in processed foods, so read the label—or better still, avoid processed foods altogether.

The sodium in salt is balanced in your kidneys by potassium in regulating renin, the hormone that increases blood vessel rigidity and blood pressure. In other words, sodium intake needs to be balanced by potassium intake. Other minerals that can be out of balance with high blood pressure are calcium and magnesium: a magnesium/calcium supplement at bedtime often lowers blood pressure.

Finally, as the most muscular of muscles, the heart needs a good supply CoQ10 and *carnitine*. The heart muscle uses a huge amount of energy—one third of the heart's weight is *mitochondria*, the energy producing organelles in each cell.

The heart burns fatty acids exclusively for fuel. Carnitine is required to move long-chain fatty acids into the mitochondria. Not surprisingly, meat is the principal food source for carnitine, since meat is muscle.

Producing energy is an oxidative process. To counter oxidative damage caused by mitochondrial byproducts, the heart uses CoQ10. Around the age of 30, the body's production of CoQ10 starts to decline.

The pull that creates diastolic blood pressure is energetically much more demanding than the systolic push. Low CoQ10 and low carnitine can prevent the heart muscle from producing the energy needed for the diastolic pull of blood into the heart. This condition, called *diastolic dysfunction,* is often the first sign of heart failure. Diastolic dysfunction can be diagnosed with a simple, noninvasive procedure. Supplementation with CoQ10 and carnitine can often return the heart to normal functioning.

And just so we don't let an opportunity pass to criticize the use of statins, these drugs are notorious for depleting CoQ10 thereby increasing the risk of diastolic dysfunction and with it high blood pressure as a "side effect."

Resources

Berman, Layna. 2004. Heart Disease: Another Perspective. *Your Own Health And Fitness.* Broadcast April 27, 2004.

Challem, Jack. 2004. Inflammation and Chronic Disease. *Your Own Health And Fitness.* Broadcast July 13, 2004.

Kendrick, Malcolm. 2003. High Blood Pressure: It's a Symptom, not a Disease, Stupid! *Red Flags Weekly* . Access at www.redflagsdaily.com/kendrick/2003_jan09.php.

Langsjoen, Peter et al. 2003. Discussions: Jan 2003 About Hypertension. *The International Network of Cholesterol Science.* Access at www.thincs.org/discuss.Jan03.htm.

National Campaign to Control Hypertension. Access at http://www.controlhypertension.org.

Rosch, Paul J. 2003. The Emperor's New Clothes: Aggressive New Guidelines for "Prehypertension." *The Weston A. Price Foundation.* Access at www.westonaprice.org/moderndiseases/prehypertension.html.

BLOOD SUGAR DERANGEMENT

Two studies point to new health risks faced by diabetics. A Japanese study in the Archives of Internal Medicine found that diabetics have an increased risk of all types of cancer, but especially liver, pancreatic, and kidney cancer. And a study in the journal Critical Care found that diabetics are at greater risk of organ failure and of death from any cause.

The context for the Japanese study is the growing rate of diabetes in Japan and around the world. The context for the Critical Care study is the steady rise in body weight characterized as an obesity epidemic, also worldwide. These two studies will no doubt add new vigor to the aggressive treatment of diabetes.

The studies are flawed. Two flaws are of particular interest.

What's Wrong With the Studies

The first concerns what counts as "diabetic." Subjects in both studies were asked whether a doctor had told them they were diabetic or whether they had been prescribed drugs for blood sugar derangements. This tells us nothing about just how deranged each subject's blood sugars were—what the pros call glycemic control.

Are the naughty people whose blood sugars are wildly out of control at greater risk than the nice people who are only a little out of control? We don't know, although the assumption is that the naughtier someone is the more likely it is that he or she will be punished with misery and death.

The second weakness is that we know nothing about the drugs these people were taking. Loading up diabetics with drugs is standard practice.

First, there are the drugs for blood sugar control itself and then there are the drugs prescribed to prevent the health disasters that await diabetics. Most prominent among these are statin drugs intended to prevent heart attacks.

Statins are almost an automatic prescription because diabetics have a greater risk of heart attacks. It's also believed that the anti-inflammatory effect of statins is beneficial because diabetes is an inflammatory disease. And then there's likely to be blood pressure drugs thrown in for good measure.

What kind of toxic soup is being brewed with these mixtures? No one's asking. What we know from toxicology doesn't bode well: when combined, chemical pollutants often do more damage than the individual chemicals alone.

We don't even need to go as far as combined effects. We can start with the toxic effects of the individual drugs prescribed for diabetics.

Toxic Prescriptions

Sulfonylureas are a class of drug that has been around since the 1950s. In 2001 over 32 million prescriptions were written for one or another of the sulfonylureas. These drugs have a known and not insignificant risk of death associated with them. That risk was first observed in 1970.

In early 2006 a study in the Canadian Medical Association Journal (CMAJ) looked at this issue and found that, for example, deaths among people taking sulfonylureas exceeded deaths among people using other drugs by 28 deaths per thousand.

Doing a little math leads to a shocking result. Let's allow for the number of prescriptions to have grown from 32 million per year to 36 million this year. If each diabetic was written one prescription per month, 3 million people were written 12 prescriptions each year for a total of 36 million prescription during 2006. At a rate of 28 excess deaths per thousand, 84,000 people died in 2006 as a result of taking this drug.

It's known why this happens. Sulfonylureas stimulate insulin secretion by blocking potassium channels in pancreatic beta cells. This allows calcium to flow into the beta cells causing insulin to be released. But these drugs don't distinguish between beta cells and other cells—such as those of the heart and arteries. So while the drug stimulates insulin secretion, it also disrupts the heart's electrical signals.

This is not a side effect. It's how the drug works. Newer versions target only beta cells, yet the versions that do not discriminate remain the most widely prescribed.

Blood Sugar Control

Even before you're diagnosed as diabetic, these drugs still might be thrown at you. Pre-diabetes, metabolic syndrome, and excess body weight are all assumed to presage diabetes. Drugs might be prescribed to prevent things from getting worse.

Metformin is a drug commonly prescribed for these conditions where blood sugars are only a little out of control. The theory is that by bringing blood sugars under control, the patient's condition won't get worse.

Unfortunately, this doesn't seem to be true. The National Diabetes Center reviewed research on the effect of medication regimes on the progression of blood sugar control. They found that no matter how aggressively people were medicated, their blood sugar control still deteriorated at about the same rate.

What this tells us is that the drugs are only suppressing a symptom and that the underlying process is still at work.

What's more, metformin exposes patients to risks of its own, despite its reputation as relatively benign. For example, metformin depletes B vitamins, B12 in particular. Lowered B12 can raise homocysteine levels, which can lead to an increased risk of heart attack.

Even with all of this in the scientific literature, studies on the risks faced by diabetics are never designed to take into account the effect of the toxins we call pharmaceuticals. If you believe that it's the drugs that are making you sick, you're probably right.

The News

Kendrick, Malcolm. 2006. The Greatest Medical Scandal Ever? Red Flags. Access at http://www.redflagsdaily.com/kendrick/2006_jan27.

The Research

Bell, David. 2006. Do Sulfonylurea Drugs Increase the Risk of Cardiac Events? Canadian Medical Association Journal. January 17, 2006 (174:2): 185-6.

Inoue, Manami et al. 2006. Diabetes Mellitus and the Risk of Cancer. Archives of Internal Medicine. September 25, 2006 (166): 1871-7.

National Diabetes Center, *Coronary Heart Disease and Poor Blood Sugar Control—Cause or Effect?* Access at http://diabetes-mellitus.org/chd.htm.

Simpson, Scot. 2006. Dose-response Relation Between Sulfonylurea Drugs and Mortality in Type 2 Diabetes Mellitus. Canadian Medical Association Journal. January 17, 2006 (174:2): 169-74.

Slynkova, Katarina et al. 2006. The Role of Body Mass Index and Diabetes in the Development of Acute Organ Failure and Subsequent Mortality in an Observational Cohort. *Critical Care.* 10(5): 1-9.

Wysowski, Diane et al. 2003. Rapid Increase in the Use of Oral Antidiabetic Drugs in the United States, 1990-2001. *Diabetes Care.* June 2003 (26:6): 1852-5.

Resources

Your Own Health And Fitness, Resources on Diabetes, Insulin Resistance, Metabolic Syndrome, and Obesity. Access at http://www.yourownhealthandfitness.org/topicsDiabetes.php.

FAT AND DEATH

Katherine Flegal got into trouble. Dr. Flegal is a researcher at the Centers for Disease Control and Prevention (CDC). In April 2005 she and some colleagues published a study in which they concluded that being obese is not as dangerous as previously thought.

The Flegal study contradicted a study published a year earlier that was co-authored by her boss Julie Gerberding, director of the CDC. Dr. Flegal's findings disrupted the simple message that health officialdom wants to send about body size: excess weight is lethal. What Flegal's and other researchers' studies point to is a much more complicated relationship between fat and health.

Dr. Flegal's study looked at the relationship between body mass index (BMI) as a measure of fatness and the risk of dying. Her methods were acknowledged to be better than the methods in her boss's study, whose lead author was Ali Mokdad.

The broader Mokdad/Gerberding study estimated how Americans die, not by medical condition but by modifiable cause—what they called *actual causes of death.* Instead of heart attack and cancer, the Mokdad study counted deaths from smoking, fatness, and bullets.

The Mokdad study made headlines in March of 2004 when it concluded that fatness was right up there with smoking as a cause of death. The Flegal study moved fatness to number seven on Mokdad's list of actual causes of death—less lethal than firearms, but more lethal than sex.

Before the Flegal study was submitted for publication, it was thoroughly reviewed by the CDC. So its results were not a surprise. When the study made headlines, CDC officials at first scratched their heads. Yet within a month, Dr. Gerberding held a press conference at which she reported a reevaluation of the Flegal study. Some, but not all of the results would receive official sanction. The reevaluation put fatness back at number two on the death list.

Dr. Flegal was not invited to the press conference.

The problem was not just that the Flegal study found fatness far less lethal than the Mokdad study. The Flegal study found that people who were a little fat had a lower risk of death than people of a so-called normal weight. Dr. Flegal got off-message and so she was silenced.

What Was Missing

BMI is not an especially accurate measure of what's going on with a person's body fat. BMI is the ratio of your weight to your height (weight in kilograms divided by the square of height in centimeters or 703 times weight in pounds divided by the square of height in inches). It does not measure how much of someone's weight is fat, how the fat is distributed, nor what kind of fat it is.

The measure of fatness: Body mass index (BMI) and the corresponding weight for selected heights

Classification (BMI Range)	BMI Upper Limit	Height		
		5'0"	5'6"	6'0"
		Weight in pounds		
Underweight (less than 18.5))	18.5	95	115	136
Normal (18.5 to 25))	25	128	155	184
Overweight (25 to 30)	30	154	186	221
Mildly obese (30 to 35)	35	179	217	258
Moderately obese (35 to 40)	40	205	248	295
Severely obese (more than 40)	>40	>205	>248	>295

The principal tissues that contribute to your weight are muscle (and bone) and fat. Your body uses fat for fuel, for tissue repair and maintenance, for metabolic processes, and for insulation. You store fat in two principal locations: under your skin (subcutaneous fat) and surrounding your intestines (visceral fat).

Visceral fat is metabolically active—for example, it can produce estrogens. Subcutaneous fat is not metabolically active. So two people with the same BMI might have different health effects depending on how much of their weight is muscle, how much is fat, and how much is visceral fat.

And muscle mass by itself can have different health effects. Steven Blair, PED of the Cooper Institute has collected a vast amount of data on the relationship between physical fitness and health. In studying the relationship between fatness and health, his research (and that of others) concludes that for two people with the same BMI, the one with greater cardiorespiratory fitness has a lower risk of death, less ill health, and less visceral fat in proportion to subcutaneous fat.

So it's not just how much of your weight is fat or how much is visceral fat or how much is muscle. Whatever your degree of fatness, your health improves with cardiorespiratory fitness—that is, the fitness of your heart, blood vessels, and lungs.

Although related, cardiorespiratory fitness is not the same as physical activity. First, they differ as to how they are measured in health studies. Cardiorespiratory fitness is more accurate because it's directly measured from performing a physical task. In contrast, physical activity is typically self-reported and subject to distortion.

A more important difference is that the level of physical activity required to develop cardiorespiratory fitness differs from person to person. That is, two people with the same BMI might have the same kind and amount of physical activity, yet have different cardiorespiratory fitness.

None of this is captured by BMI.

A final factor that isn't captured by most BMI-based research is the effect of weight change on health. One study has indicated that people whose weight changes significantly are at greater risk of illness, whatever their starting BMI and regardless of whether they gained or lost weight. The greatest risk was for those who intentionally lost weight. The researchers speculate on what might cause this result—for example, that since fat sequesters toxins, burning off fat releases those toxins.

Actual Causes of Death

The Mokdad article was about more than obesity. Its treatment of actual causes of death sheds much light on the message that the CDC and with it the conventional media promote. The table below lists Mokdad's actual causes of death with the original estimates and those percentages with Flegal's revised obesity estimate.

Actual causes of death in 2000: Original Mokdad estimate with Flegal's revised estimate for obesity

	Percent of deaths	
Actual cause	Mokdad	Flegal
Tobacco	18.1%	18.1%
Poor diet and physical inactivity	16.6%	1.1%
Alcohol consumption	3.5%	3.5%
Microbial agents	3.1%	3.1%
Toxic agents	2.3%	2.3%
Motor vehicles	1.8%	1.8%
Firearms	1.2%	1.2%
Sexual behavior	0.8%	0.8%
Illicit drug use	0.7%	0.7%
Other	51.8%	67.4%

Notice that "obesity" isn't used. Instead, "poor diet and physical inactivity" is a placeholder for obesity. In the body of the Mokdad article, the connection is simply stated without reference to any research. Taking for granted that "poor diet and physical inactivity" are equivalent to obesity is an empirical leap, no matter how well-massaged it might be into our collective consciousness. In the 19th Century, it was called gluttony and sloth. Today, we don't talk of sin, but of lifestyle choices.

On closer examination, most of Mokdad's actual causes of death have the strong aroma of sin: tobacco, alcohol, firearms, sex, and drugs. In other words, it frames causes of death so that they are the result of character flaws.

But not all lethal character flaws are on Mokdad's list. Mistakes by definition are avoidable. If pharmaceutical and medical mistakes were included as an actual cause of death, they would take second place, accounting for over 10% of deaths in 2000.

The Mokdad article discusses what falls in the "Other" category—that is, over half the deaths not otherwise accounted for by Mokdad and over two-thirds if we use Flegal's obesity estimate. The article speculates that a good chunk results from socioeconomic inequity.

Socioeconomic inequity affects health in two ways. Lower status (and with it less sociopolitical power) means
• less access to health care resources and
• a greater incidence of health problems.

The greater incidence of health problems is the consequence of stress. Psychosocial stress from low status and powerlessness creates physiological stress that causes metabolic disruptions—from hormone imbalance to immune dysfunction.

Yet the official position on obesity (and the other actual causes of death) is predicated on what people choose rather than on what they endure.

Obesity as a Sign, not a Cause

The official worry is that excess weight increases health risks by causing heart attacks, strokes, diabetes, and other illnesses. Critic Paul Campos argues that this is like attributing lung cancer to the smelly clothes, yellow teeth, and bad breath caused by smoking. In other words, the obesity epidemic as an effect, not a cause.

The question is: What causes the metabolic derangement that results in obesity? We're not talking simply about endocrinology. We're talking about the many paths to excess body fat, the many actual causes of the obesity epidemic.

The official position is based on the self-limiting notion that obe-

sity has a single cause. "Inequity" is as limiting an answer as "poor diet and physical inactivity." Candidates for causing obesity include
* psychosocial stress from inequity,
* physiological stress from exposure to pollutants,
* metabolic stress from limited access to nutrient-rich foods, and
* lack of opportunities for physical activity.

Too much body fat might be bad for your health, although not as dramatically nor as universally bad as some health officials might want us to believe. Instead, excess body fat affects your health in complicated ways. How much of your weight is fat? What kind of fat is it? How is it distributed on your body? How fit are you? What weight is normal for you? What's an appropriate weight for your age? Do you have access to nutrient-rich food? Do you have opportunities for building your cardiorespiratory fitness?

The answers are about alternatives, not gluttony, sloth, or any other character flaw.

Resources

Adler, Nancy E., et al. 1999. *Socioeconomic Status and Health in Industrial Nations*. New York: New York Academy of Science.

Campos, Paul. 2005. *The Diet Myth*. New York: Gotham.

Blair, Steven N., and Tim S. Church. 2004. The Fitness, Obesity, and Health Equation: Is Physical Activity the Common Denominator? *JAMA*. September 8, 2004, 292(10): 1232-4.

Flegal, Katherine M. et al. 2005. Excess Deaths Associated With Underweight, Overweight, and Obesity. *JAMA*. April 20, 2005, 293(15): 1861-67.

Gard, Michael and Jan Wright. 2005. *The Obesity Epidemic*. New York: Routledge.

Gibbs, W. Wayt. 2005. Obesity: An Overblown Epidemic? *Scientific American*. June, 2005: 70-75.

Gregg, Edward W., et al. Secular Trends in Cardiovascular Disease Risk Factors According to Body Mass Index in US Adults. *JAMA*. April 20, 2005, 293(15): 1868-74.

Kendrick, Malcolm. 2005. Challenging the Convention on Heart Disease and Diabetes. *Your Own Health And Fitness*. Broadcast April 26, 2005.

Mokdad, Ali H. et al. 2004. Actual Causes of Death in the United States, 2000. *JAMA*. March 10, 2004, 291(10): 1238-45.

Physicians for Human Rights. 2003. *The Right to Equal Treatment*. Boston: Physicians for Human Rights.

Sørensen, TIA, et al. 2005. Intention to Lose Weight, Weight Changes, and 18-y Mortality in Overweight Individuals without Co-Morbidities. *PLoS Medicine*. June, 2005, 2(6): e171.

HEALTH INEQUITY AND TOXIC LOAD

If you want to be healthy, move to England. That was the message from a study in the May 2, 2006 issue of the Journal of the American Medical Association (*JAMA*). The motivation for doing the study as stated in the JAMA article was to see whether a society where access to medical care is universal (that is, England) has healthier people than one without universal medical care (that is, the United States).

The simple answer is yes. The English with their system of socialized medicine (much maligned in the US) have better health than Americans.

One of the authors is Michael Marmot, a leading figure in the study of the social determinants of health. The US media made sure to absolve the US medical care system from blame by attributing to Marmot the view that "Britain's universal health-care system shouldn't get credit for better health." But the best that the media could come up with as an explanation was a flaccid reference to Americans' suffering from more stress as an inherent part of our culture.

2½ Times the Cost

But let's start at the beginning. According to the Marmot study, in the United States we spend $5,274 per person per year for medical care. The English spend $2,164 per person per year. That's not half, as the US media reported, but 40%.

What Marmot and his colleagues looked at was the health of white people between 55 and 64 years old—the age when medical conditions come home to roost. The study excluded people of color so that the well-known poorer health of those populations would not affect the results. The conditions they looked at were diabetes, hypertension, all forms of heart disease, heart attack, stroke, lung disease, and cancer.

For each and every one of these conditions, people in the US were worse off than people in England. Diabetes: 75% more. Hypertension: 20% more. Heart disease: 50% more. Heart attack: 30% more. Stroke: 65% more. Lung disease: 30% more. Cancer: 75% more.

These numbers are from so-called self-reports: people in the study were asked whether a physician had ever told them they had diabetes, etc. Marmot and his colleagues acknowledged that the US medical system is diagnosis-happy. So they asked whether the difference was because we in the US suffer from overdiagnosis and overtreatment.

The people in the study were not only asked about diagnoses, but were also given a physical exam. Measurements such as blood pressure, hemoglobin A1C, C-reactive protein, and other risk markers were taken. Those measurements verified the gap.

The researchers went even further and asked whether the difference might be the result of differences in health characteristics: smoking, drinking, and body weight. When the researchers adjusted these so that the English had the same characteristics as Americans, the US statistics still came out worse than the English.

Inequality Makes You Sick

A result of the study that was ignored by the mainstream media was that in both countries your health is affected by your social class: those who are more secure have better health. With a very interesting exception: cancer. There was little difference between rich and poor in either the US or England in the incidence of cancer.

This apparent anomaly is explained by understanding that "cancer" is not a single condition such as a stroke. When the different types of cancer are examined in relation to social status, an association emerges—but it's mixed. Some cancers such as lung, cervical, and stomach cancer are more prevalent among people with low social status. Other cancers such as breast cancer and melanoma are associated with high social status.

So while some cancers have the expected association with low status, as does having a stroke, other cancers have the opposite association. People who are more likely to be healthy because of their social class are in fact more vulnerable to certain cancers.

Marmot and the commentators to his article acknowledged the negative effect on health that comes from stress due to social inequity. But Marmot was much more sophisticated in pointing to insecurity from lack of access to medical care as part of a more general insecurity, especially from the growing inequality in the distribution of income in the US as compared to England where, tattered and battered though it might be, a semblance of a social security net still exists. Commentators in the mainstream media could only talk about the stress that comes with the volatility of achieving the American Dream.

While Marmot's observation on the origins of stress is very much to the point, he ignores another source of stress: toxins in the environment. That's why the findings on cancer are so telling. That different types of cancer are associated with different social classes points to differences in both psychosocial stress and exposures to environmental toxins.

Environmental Stressors

Social insecurity is one kind of stressor. Environmental toxins are another. No study to date has brought these two exposures together to examine the relative effects of each on health.

However, over the past fifty years, the most dramatic change in exposures has been from our exposure to manufactured chemicals and emissions of ionizing and non-ionizing radiation. Although not true in every instance, Americans have been exposed to more of these toxins for a longer period of time than the English.

Our increasing environmental exposure to novel chemicals and novel electromagnetic radiation sources have been shown to be carcinogens, endocrine disruptors, neurotoxins (toxic to the nervous system), immunotoxins (toxic to the immune system), oxidative stressors, and genotoxins (toxic to DNA). For some of these exposures, the health effects are immediate and acute. For others, the health effects have long latencies and are chronic. In many cases, we know little about the long term effects.

Some of the most potent chemicals are pesticides and chlorinated organic compounds, especially PVC (polyvinyl chloride). Both pesticides and chlorinated organics have been linked not only to cancer but to neurological and endocrine disruption. These exposures begin before birth. For example, breast milk has been found to contain very high concentrations of pesticide and chlorinated organic chemical metabolites—our body turns the pesticide into another chemical that is toxic. The resulting damage to the fetus might appear as a health effect such as neurological damage at birth or it might not appear until adulthood as diabetes.

Exposures continue throughout life. For example, a study in Seattle compared children who regularly ate organic food to those who regularly ate conventional food. The researchers found that pesticide concentrations were almost ten times higher in the children who ate conventional food.

PVC is pervasive in building materials. A vast array of toxins are produced when PVC is manufactured and when it burns. PCBs (polychlorinated biphenals) are among the many byproducts. Everyone on earth has a measurable amount of PCBs, as described in the Environmental Working Group's *Body Burden* study.

Not only are the effects of many novel, manufactured chemicals unknown, the interaction between them is even more of a mystery. An article by Theo Colborn, PhD challenged current pesticide regulations by citing what we do know about multiple exposures having a synergistic effect—the toxic effect of two pesticides is more than double the effect of the individual pesticides. Dr. Colborn wrote *Our*

Stolen Future in 1996, a book that introduced the concept of endocrine disruption. The book's website now includes a broad range of information on chemical toxins.

Although less well recognized, non-ionizing radiation seems to have effects comparable to chemical toxins. The rapid increase in the use of wireless technologies such as the cellular telephone has brought considerable attention to these effects. These effects include both acute and chronic conditions, as we describe in "The WiFi Blues" on page 188 and as we've covered in several interviews, such as with Olle Johansson, PhD.

The concern with exposure to non-ionizing radiation goes even further back. Dr. Johansson and his colleague Örjan Hallberg, MSc have done several studies on the possible effect of FM broadcast signals on health, associating increased exposure to FM signals to increased incidence of colon cancer, lung cancer, breast cancer, bladder cancer, malignant melanoma, and asthma.

In a recent book, Finish journalist Gunni Nordström describes the research on the interaction between chemicals and non-ionizing radiation. The early research began in Silicon Valley when workers in computer and computer chip manufacturing plants developed sensitivities to light, skin reactions, and neurological symptoms. What researchers in this area have exposed is the possible synergistic effect of, for example, radiation from computer screens reacting with chemicals outgassed by computer equipment.

Protection

Want to be as healthy as the English? Don't move to England, minimize your exposure to environmental stressors.

In and around your home you can be exposed to chemical toxins in products you use and in the materials that make your home.

The websites for the Environmental Working Group and for Seventh Generation have resources for identifying toxins in products. These include not only obvious sources such as sprays to control ants, cockroaches, and other household pests but also scented laundry products and cosmetics. On the outside of your house or apartment building, products that control weeds and pests in the garden are also obvious toxins.

Food and water can also be sources of toxins. We've already cited the study in Seattle that showed the tenfold difference in pesticide metabolites in children who eat conventionally grown food. Concerns over water quality have led to a bottled water industry that would have seemed absurd 40 years ago. Colin Ingram's *The Drinking Water Book* provides guidance for identifying water treatment needs.

What covers the walls, ceilings, and floors of your home can be a source of toxins. Older homes might have lead-based paints. Synthetic rugs and carpets not only collect toxins brought in from the outside, they outgas toxins such as phthalates. Outside structures such as wood decks have been treated with wood preservatives that contain arsenic and outgas volatile organic compounds. The Healthy Building Network is one resource for identifying these exposures.

Most homes have an array of electrical and electronic equipment that emits electromagnetic radiation. Cell phones, cordless phones, computers, printers, fax machines, scanners, microwave ovens, refrigerators, hairdryers, and television sets are all sources of electromagnetic radiation. B. Blake Levitt's *Electromagnetic Fields* is one resource for identifying these exposures, as is our interview with her and Cindy Sage.

In addition to exposures from electrical and electronic equipment, the electrical wiring in your home might create an exposure referred to as dirty electricity. Our interview with Magda Havas, PhD is a resource for identifying this risk.

Beyond exposures that are immediate to your home are those that are brought to you—more accurately, imposed on you without your consent and often without your knowledge. For example, if you live in an area where conventional farming takes place, wind can carry pesticides and herbicides into your yard and home. In addition, antennas that broadcast signals for cell phones and wireless communication will penetrate your walls. These antennas can be on the side of buildings in plain site or hidden an architectural features such as a church steeple. Or, in the case of wireless connections, they can be in your neighbor's bedroom a short distance away.

At work and at school, all of these exposures can be present. In some case, they are exacerbated. For example, even if you use ecologically benign methods to control pests in your home, your office building or your child's school might routinely spray for pests.

While reducing exposures to toxins is important, if daunting, you can also support your body in reducing the effects of those exposures. Your liver has two basic biochemical pathways for removing toxins. Our show on "Detoxification" is one resource for supporting those pathways.

To bring this discussion full circle, the Prevention Institute has reported on how eleven communities have improved their health through activism. Our exposures to toxins are not the inevitable consequence of some natural phenomenon. They are the result of decisions by human beings with the power to expose us—and with the power to stop. Just so with Dr. Marmot's idea that less social inequity is the explanation for the better health of the English. Fighting for healthy communities is both an essential way to reduce exposures to toxins and a tonic for psychosocial stress.

The News

Johnson, Carla and Mike Stobbe. 2006. Study Shows Americans Sicker Than English. *Associated Press.* May 2, 2006.

The Research

Marmot, Michael et al. Disease and Disadvantage in the United States and in England. *Journal of the American Medical Association.* May 3, 2006 (295; 17): 2037-45.

Resources

Baillie-Hamilton, Paula. 2005. *Toxic Overload.* New York: Avery.

Cancer Prevention Coalition. Access at http://www.preventcancer.org.

Colborn, Theo. 2006. A Case for Revisiting the Safety of Pesticides: A Closer Look at Neurodevelopment. *Environmental Health Perspectives.* 114(1) January 2006: 10-7.

Colborn, Theo, et al. 1996. Our Stolen Future: Are We Threatening Our Fertility, Intelligence, and Survival? A Scientific Detective Story. New York, Dutton.

Environmental Working Group. Access at http://www.ewg.org.

Fawcett, Jeffry, 2005. Cancer by the Numbers. *Progressive Health Observer.* 8 (Fall 2005): 5,8.

Hallberg, Örjan and Olle Johansson. 2002. Cancer Trends During the 20th Century. *Journal of Australian College of Nutritional & Environmental Medicine.* 21(1) April 2002: 3-8.

Havas, Magda. 2006. Dirty Electricity and EMF Health Dangers. *Your Own Health And Fitness.* Broadcast May 30, 2006 on KPFA 94.1 FM Berkeley, CA.

Healthy Building Network. Access at http://www–.healthy–building.net.

Houlihan, Jane et al. 2003. *BodyBurden: The Pollution in People.* Oakland, CA: Environmental Working Group.

Ingram, Colin. 2006. Safe Drinking Water. *Your Own Health And Fitness.* Broadcast June 10, 1997 on KPFA 94.1 FM Berkeley, CA.

Johansson, Olle. 2006. The Science of RFR Health Risks. *Your Own Health And Fitness.* Broadcast April 25, 2006 on KPFA 94.1 FM Berkeley, CA.

Levitt, B. Blake and Cindy Sage. 2006. Where You're Exposed and What to Do: EMF and RFR. *Your Own Health And Fitness.* Broadcast March 14, 2006 on KPFA 94.1 FM Berkeley, CA.

Levitt, B. Blake. 1995. *Electromagnetic Fields: A Consumer's Guide to the Issues and How to Protect Ourselves.* New York: Harcourt.

Nordström, Gunni. 2004. *The Invisible Disease: The Dangers of Environmental Illnesses caused by Electromagnetic Fields and Chemical Emissions.* New York: O Books.

Our Stolen Future. Access at http://www.ourstolenfuture.org.

Physicians for a National Health Program. Access at http://www–.pnhp.org.

Prevention Institute. Access at http://www.preventioninstitute–.org.

Seventh Generation. Access at http://www.seventhgeneration.com.

Healing

Getting lots of rest when you're sick is a good idea. Often, your body tells you quite clearly that it needs for you to stop so it can heal.

Sometimes feeling tired is the first sign that you've caught a cold or flu. Sometimes your body insists that you rest by making you feel so exhausted that it's impossible to do anything. But sometimes rest isn't enough. Sometimes you need the help of a professional healer. Less often still, your body needs heroic intervention.

Even with professional healers—whether practicing conventional medicine, alternative medicine, or traditional medicinal arts—the starting place is how your body heals itself.

Health care institutions dominated by conventional medicine operate principally within the specific disease framework we discussed previously in "Illness" on page 259. The specific disease framework has been developed and maintained over the last century as medical science and practice have shifted from acute to chronic illness—the diagnosis and treatment of diseases people do not yet have.

The specific disease framework manifests in practice as risk factor medicine, which we discussed in "Protection and Prevention" on page 237. Although based on the idea of disease prevention, the actual practice of risk factor medicine turns risk factors into diseases as such and treats them accordingly. As we've already discussed, real prevention is based on mitigating or eliminating altogether toxic environmental exposures, both physical and social, through individual and collective action. In transforming risk factors into diseases, conventional medicine (and far too much of complementary and alternative medicine) mistakenly combats symptoms under the guise of healing.

For example, as we discussed in "Hypertension All Around" (on page 266), blood pressure outside a specified range is mistakenly diagnosed and treated as the disease hypertension. The medical practitioner subsequently intervenes on behalf of the patient to heal her. Pharmaceuticals are the principle intervention.

But are pharmaceuticals actually capable of healing risk factors recast as diseases such as hypertension, frailty, or metabolic syndrome?

The path to an answer is suggested in a study reported in *Science* that describes a method for discovering new uses for existing drugs.[1]

The method compares the so-called off-target effects of pharmaceuticals. "Off-target" is a refreshing and more accurate phrase for the more familiar "side effects." It's a recognition that drugs have biological effects, only some of which are intended.

The method that was developed by these researchers compares the chemical properties of unrelated drugs—for example, one drug used for depression and another for blood pressure. The comparison reveals unexpected target proteins—for example, proteins and cell receptors that affect heart rate. A famous example is the active ingredient for Viagra, a drug originally developed to control blood pressure. Using this method, the researchers identified 750 drug pairs out of 2,900 studied that had target protein effects not predicted from the original drugs.

The idea behind this study is quite clever: find new uses for existing drugs, products that are already on the market and have a clinical track record. This could be good news for Big Pharma. Drugs that are about to go off-patent for one use could be re-patented for another.

But let's return to the idea of off-target effects. The FDA maintains a reporting system for adverse drug effects. Drug companies are required to include this information with the drug along with information on effects uncovered by their own research. The goal of a pharmaceutical company is to get through the FDA approval process before too many negative effects show up. What the *Science* study highlights is that pharmaceuticals have additional, unexpected effects.

That this is a dangerous game is highlighted by infamous cases such as Vioxx. It passed the FDA approval process and then killed or caused harm to many people. We're further reminded of these dangers by the report of the Florida Medical Examiners Commission that in Florida in 2007 prescription drugs killed four times as many people as illegal, street drugs. [2]

Pharmaceuticals—and for that matter any biologically active substance given as a cure—invariably have both on-target and off-target effects. In either instance, drugs prevent or promote a biochemical process. The on-target effect is intended to fix biochemistry that's (allegedly) not working right.

But they don't heal.

That's what the person does. That's what his body does. It has that capacity. That's why pharmaceuticals should be the method of last resort in healing. In fact, because health is a capacity not a condition, health includes the capacity to heal. Like all other aspects of health, it's supported by how well the environments to which a person is exposed strengthen her unique biology's capacity to heal.

In 2008, the American Academy of Pediatrics recommended the use of statins in aggressively treating children with high cholesterol.[3] A member of the nutrition committee said, "The risk of giving statins at a lower age is less than the benefit you're going to get out of it." This expert went on to say that "not a whole lot" was known about the actual benefits of statins used on kids.[4]

It is some reassurance that the announcement of this policy elicited an uproar from a huge number of pediatricians. While some strongly agreed with the recommendation, others expressed dismay. One response was revealing. The pediatrician regretted the recommendation because it threatened to divert attention from the more effective solutions of diet and exercise, actions that we know can support the capacity to heal.

Magic pills. Magic procedures. Magic. And the belief in magic is on both sides of the prescription pad. Children will be given statins because the American Academy of Pediatrics, the professional organization responsible for children's health, believes it is so—even though there's "not a whole lot" known about the on-target and off-target effects on kids. However, enough is known about the effects on adults to cause alarm. But never mind. This is magic.

The fundamental point is that statins threaten to do much to children, but statins won't heal them. The drugs will suppress their cholesterol biochemistry and likely disrupt their endocrine and immune biochemistry. The drugs won't do anything about the metabolic disruptions and environmental exposures that cause their bodies to adapt by raising their cholesterol. Statins will only cure them of high cholesterol—which is not a disease. Statins will not help them heal.

This takes us back to the theme of the first article in this book, "The Placebo Effect." In the articles between there and here we've discussed some basic principles that affect healing as well as health.

- Health, and with it healing, is a capacity unique to each person's biology and how it adapts to its environment.
- Choosing and creating supportive environments that improve the capacity for health and healing: personal, natural, built, and social environments as those affect us through food, physical activity, consumption, and production.
- Doing the simplest things to support the capacity to thrive—that is, what supports health and with it the capacity to heal.

The first article in this section, "Ancient Diet Reverses Autoimmune Diseases," applies the principle of doing the simplest things first to autoimmune diseases, such as multiple chemical sensitivity. In this case, the "simplest thing" is adopting a hunter-gatherer diet—the argument being that from a biological standpoint, it's the simplest way to eat.

The second article, "What Causes a Heart Attack," debunks the conventional explanation for heart attacks and the horrifying treatments used to prevent them. Instead, we argue that it is stress—physiological and psychosocial—that causes these heart events. The simplest thing? Not stress reducing treatments, but the elimination of stress inducing environments.

In the last two articles of this section, "What's Wrong with Conventional Estrogen Therapy" and "Estrogen and Broken Hearts," we discuss the unnecessary suffering of women. The articles criticize the misinformation pandered by conventional science about hormone balance and hormone replacement. The articles go on to describe the simple actions that restore balance and health.

One of the simplest things anyone can do to support his capacity to heal is to develop the art of self-care. There are a wide range of health and healing traditions that are based on the kind of self-care we advocate. We'll mention two here.

Orthomolecular health medicine is a form of therapy that has the objective

> to restore the optimum environment of the body by correcting imbalances or deficiencies based on individual biochemistry using substances natural to the body such as vitamins, minerals, amino acids, trace elements, and essential fatty acids.[5]

Although the practice of using nutrients to support health and healing has a long history, orthomolecular medicine emerged in its current form from the work of Linus Pauling. He coined the term orthomolecular to capture the core meaning of the practice: the right molecule in the right concentration.

Work in orthomolecular medicine[6] has provided a wealth of science that enables healing based on our core principles. It has led to a popular literature that makes principles of self-care accessible to the medical civilian.[7]

Other traditions are further removed from the science that is acceptable to contemporary health care institutions. We have covered a wide variety of these on the Your Own Health And Fitness radio show.[8] We discuss one here.

In the early part of the 20th Century, Edward Bach traveled the English countryside observing the traditional use of flower essences as therapies. Using his skills as a researcher,[9] Bach developed and documented the preparation and use of these flower essences for use by the non-expert practicing self-care.[10]

The fundamental principal of Bach flower remedies is that illness comes from an emotional imbalance that has resulted from trauma. To restore health and build the capacity to heal, specific flower essences are taken to restore that balance. This is an approach shared with orthomolecular health medicine: restoring balance supports health and healing. However, the mode of action differs. Orthomolecular health medicine restores balance biochemically. Flower essence remedies affect vital forces in a way that is similar to the concept of the vital force qi in traditional Chinese medicine: imbalance results in illness; health is restored through rebalancing with practices such as acupuncture and qi gong.[11]

Bach flower essences are neither mystical nor unscientific. The remedies come from a scientific tradition referred to as empiricism.[12] This is science that is based on the careful observation of individual needs and the experience and expertise of the scientist or practitioner. Although it is a scientific method with a much longer history than currently fashionable statistical methods, it is dismissed out of hand as "unscientific." Science based on statistical analysis is not just the standard but the only method of scientific practice that is accepted by dominant institutions.

Bach flower remedies are not only based on science, they are very much based on biological science. We're just not used to thinking of emotions as biological events. However, from the research of people such as Antonio Damasio,[13] even conventional science is recognizing that our emotional and physical states are intertwined. The common sense of this science is that emotions bring the state of a person's body to his awareness and prompt him to take appropriate action. For example, we opened this article by describing how getting rest helps you recover from sickness and how your body tells you so by making you feel tired.

This is not about making emotions go away. It's about emotional and physical symptoms being two aspects of the same condition.

Conventional science attempts to heal by affecting the physical, with emotional effects seen as a side issue. Flower essence remedies and many other non-invasive therapies such as homeopathy[14] work from the other direction: treat the emotional symptoms as more fundamental but entwined with the physical symptoms.

The art of self-care is collective as well as personal. Like the art of personal self-care, the art of collective self-care works from the inside out. This is where the concepts of social capital and social networks fall short. They are empty of the felt experiences, unique needs, and local knowledge that make a living community. It is the emotional

glue of a community that enables its members to thrive, what moves
its people to create better lives.

Notes

1   Monica Campillos, et al. (2008) "Drug Target Identification Using Side-Effect Similarity."

2   Damien Cave (2008) "Legal Drugs Kill Far More Than Illegal, Florida Says" and Medical Examiners Commission (2007) *Drugs Identified in Deceased Persons by Florida Medical Examiners: 2007 Interim Report.*

3   Tara Parker-Pope (2008a) "8-Year-Olds on Statins? A New Plan Quickly Bites Back" and Stephen R. Daniels, et al. (2008) "Lipid Screening and Cardiovascular Health in Childhood."

4   Dr. Jatinder Bhatia quoted in Tara Parker-Pope (2008b) "Cholesterol Screening Is Urged for Young."

5   From the International Society for Orthomolecular Medicine, access at http://www.orthomed.org.

6   Leading professional organizations are the International Society for Orthomolecular Medicine (access at http://www.orthomed.org) and its *Journal of Orthomolecular Medicine.* Many individual countries have complementary organizations, such as the Orthomolecular Health Medicine Society (access at http://www.ohmsociety.com) in the US. Also see the Linus Pauling Institute (access at http://lpi.oregonstate.edu), Orthomolecular. Org (access at http://orthomolecular.org), and Orthomolecular Health (access at http://orthomolecularhealth.com).

7   We have interviewed some of the leading members of this movement. For example, Richard Kunin (1999) "Orthomolecular Medicine: Treating with Targeted Nutrient Therapies," Richard Kunin (2006) "Nutrient Basics," Eva Edelman (2000) "Natural Healing for Mental Disorders," and Abram Hoffer (2000) "Natural Nutrition for Children." There are also many popular writers who provide access to this knowledge, once again many of whom we have interviewed. For example, see Abram Hoffer and Andrew Saul (2008) *Orthomolecular Medicine for Everyone: Megavitamin Therapeutics for Families and Physicians,.* Jack Challem (2003) *The Inflammation Syndrome: The Complete Nutritional Program to Prevent and Reverse Heart Disease, Arthritis, Diabetes, Allergies, and Asthma* and Andrew Saul (2003) *Doctor Yourself: Natural Healing That Works.* Finally, a basic resource is the Orthomolecular Medicine News Service (access at http://www.orthomolecular.org/resources/omns/index.shtml).

8   These include well-known traditions such as homeopathy, aromatherapy, herbalism, and traditional Chinese medicine. See Your Own Health And Fitness, Resources on Homeopathy (access at http://www.yourownhealthandfitness.org/topicsHomeopathy.php) and Resources on Alternative Healing (access at http://www.yourownhealthandfitness.org/topicsAlternative.php).

9   Bach was a research bacteriologist who gained fame for many of his discoveries (Vinton McCabe (2007a) *The Healing Bouquet: Exploring Bach Flower Remedies* Chapter 1).

[10] See Bach's original writings in Edward Bach and FJ Wheeler (1997) *The Bach Flower Remedies*. Also see Vinton McCabe (2008) *"The Essence of Healing: Discovering Bach Flower Remedies."*

[11] For example, see Harriet Beinfield and Efrem Korngold (1991) *Between Heaven and Earth: A Guide to Chinese Medicine*.

[12] Kenny Ausubel ed (2004) *Ecological Medicine: Healing the Earth, Healing Ourselves*.

[13] Antonio Damasio (1994) *Descartes' Error: Emotion, Reason, and the Human Brain*, Antonio Damasio (1999) *The Feeling of What Happens: Body and Emotion in the Making of Consciousness*, Antonio Damasio (2003) *Looking for Spinoza: Joy, Sorrow, and the Feeling Brain*.

[14] See Vinton McCabe three book series that weaves together classical homeopathy, Bach flower essences, and cell salts as kindred homeopathic remedies: Vinton McCabe (2007b) *The Healing Enigma: Demystifying Homeopathy*, Vinton McCabe (2007a) The Healing Bouquet: Exploring Bach Flower Remedies, and Vinton McCabe (2009) *The Healing Echo: Discovering Homeopathic Cell Salt Remedies*. See also Vinton McCabe (2004) *Household Homeopathy: A Safe and Effective Approach to Wellness for the Whole Family* and Stephen Cummings and Dana Ullman (2004) *Everybody's Guide to Homeopathic Medicine*.

ANCIENT DIET REVERSES
AUTOIMMUNE DISEASES

I first heard it called the "caveman diet" in the offices of environmental ecologists during the 1980s.

Environmental ecologists are doctors who specialize in treating patients with environmental illness (EI) and multiple chemical sensitivities (MCS). This confluence of symptoms in people who become intolerant of modern chemical-laden environments appeared around the same time as the diagnosis of chronic fatigue syndrome (CFS).

An early arm of integrative medicine, environmental ecology combined allergy treatments with nutrient and dietary interventions designed to support an overburdened immune system.

Not Allergic, Poisoned!

For a variety of reasons, people who react to chemicals are bio-accumulating substances that other people detoxify and excrete. These "reactions" are actually poisonings. Your liver is responsible for clearing toxins from your system. Your body passes these toxins out in excrement and sweat.

The poisoning response starts with an over-exposure to pollutants and toxins, stress and trauma, and invasive medical treatments. A sluggish liver function combines with a genetic susceptibility of the immune system to overload, spilling toxins back into your tissues.

Dr. Phyllis Saifer and Dr. Nathan Becker, early pioneers in researching the etiology of EI, discovered that most of their patients had an autoimmune component to their illness stimulated by the overreaction of their sympathetic nervous system. Many of these patients had autoimmune thyroiditis (Hashimoto's) or lupus or both. The presence of autoimmune disease was thought to be a symptom of a larger failure of the immune system.

Eating Your Vitamins

The caveman or hunter-gatherer diet is based on research into pre-agricultural, Paleolithic nutrition. Physician Dr. Boyd Eaton was trained at Harvard Medical School with academic appointments in radiology and anthropology. His fascination with evolutionary medicine and Paleolithic nutrition started in the late 1970s. His many papers comparing our modern diet to that of hunter-gatherers gave rise to many popular low carbohydrate diets.

For easily 2.5 million years, humanoids ate a diet of whole foods rich in nutrients. Compared to a pre-agricultural, hunter-gatherer diet, Dr. Eaton found our modern diet lacking in the extreme. It's not surprising that our ancestors were larger and had bigger brain cases than humans who preceded the industrial revolution. Remember those tiny shoes from the Victorian era you saw in museums?

The hunter-gatherer diet is nutrient dense. You'd be surprised to see how many minerals there are in meat! Another advantage to the hunter-gatherer diet is that it's rich in natural fats. You need fat to utilize fat soluble vitamins such as A and E, both very important for healthy immune function.

Attack of the Immune System

Doctors faced with clients who fail to thrive use the hunter-gatherer diet to uncover food allergies. The rationale is common sense: reduce the load on an overburdened, misfiring immune system, symptoms abate, and healing begins. In addition, food allergies cause the mucosal barrier of the gut to become inflamed and permeable allowing tiny food particles to be released into the blood stream. This is "leaky gut." It contributes to the development of more food allergies and autoimmune reactions.

Think of it this way: when your immune system doesn't know the difference between your own tissues and something foreign, it attacks both. If it's been attacking a protein it doesn't like, it goes looking for more; if your thyroid and joints contain proteins that are similar, it attacks them. Boom! Inflammation, antibodies, and an immune system that doesn't know the difference between spinach and cancer.

This sort of dysfunction means that when *your house* is on fire, your immune system is busy watering down *the house next door*. Your resistance to allergens and viruses might be weakened, or conversely, you might have a King Kong immune system that attacks your own tissues!

In my experience, people with auto-immunity including MS, post-polio syndrome, Hashimoto's, lupus, even Crohn's and IBS benefit enormously from the immune sparing and anti-inflammatory effects of the hunter-gatherer diet. It's always the easiest and least invasive thing to try first. If it works, you eliminate the long-term damaging effects of strong immuno-suppressant drugs. Used with medication, it could certainly reduce the dose requirements.

Cavepeople Weren't Vegans

It's unfortunate that most vegetable proteins contain substances that protect them from being eaten to extinction. After all, when we eat beans, seeds, nuts, and grains we are eating the part of the plant that propagates. These contain self-protective anti-nutrients that can interfere with absorption of minerals, block the function of the thyroid gland, and make the foods harder to digest. These incomplete proteins are also more allergenic. It's hard for a vegetarian to use the hunter-gatherer diet as a tool to lower immune load and identify food allergies.

Our early ancestors ate a diet rich in animal protein and fish, foraged vegetables, fruits, nuts, and, when really lucky, a bit of honey. Their carbohydrate load was very low, and they drank lots of water. There is also evidence that they did not take animals without fat since their protein rich diet without fat made them ill. This allowed mostly older animals to be taken, sparing the young who had years of procreation left.

Where's the Hunter-gatherer Aisle?

Eating closer to our ancestors to flag food allergies can be done without a bow and arrow. With the current availability of meat, eggs, and poultry that is ethically and sustainably raised, it's possible to buy meat that is safer and more nutritious than what is industrially raised or highly processed.

When using the principles of the hunter-gatherer diet, remember that you are trying as much as possible to mimic a diet before agriculture. Avoid the use of dairy products, corn, dried beans, soy, or grains of any kind including the new alternatives to wheat. You may need to avoid alcoholic beverages since they contain not only grains but also yeasts, sulfites, and lots of histamine, all of which make allergies and autoimmune conditions worse. Watch your condiments, too: cider vinegar might be OK but not wine vinegar.

You will be concentrating on eating foods in their original, unprocessed state. But it's not necessary or even desirable to eat everything raw. Humanoids cooked food early on!

Include nuts and seeds, which you may find more digestible if you follow Sally Fallon's (*Nourishing Traditions*) suggestions of soaking them overnight in salt water, rinsing them in the morning and drying them until crisp in a low oven (150-225 degrees). This removes many of the anti-nutrients.

Animal protein contains a combination of fats including monounsaturates, the kind that is extolled in olive oil. Pork contains a whopping 60% of it. Interestingly, wild game is actually higher in saturated fat than beef or pork, so I'm mystified why both Dr. Boyd and his student Loren Cordain, PhD, who has also written about Paleolithic nutrition, stress eating only lean meats.

A Word about Fat

Long chain Omega-3 fatty acids and Omega-6s are called essential fatty acids (EFA) because your body can't make them so you must get them from food. They are necessary for proper cell function. Omega-3s are primarily in fish and flaxseed. Flax contains an oleic acid that your body has to convert to Omega-3s. This process doesn't work in some people, notably vegans and diabetics. Flax is also a potential allergen since it's a grass in the same family as linseed oil.

Hunter-gatherer diets had a much higher ratio of 3s to 6s. This is important because when the ratio is skewed favoring 6s, studies show a dramatic increase in inflammation and disease. Eliminating grains from your diet helps in the maintenance of a healthy fat ratio since grains are high in Omega-6 fats.

Another place you might be getting 6s is in nuts and vegetable oils. These oils are very fragile, they go rancid easily, and are damaged by heating. When you cook with fat, use only natural undamaged fats, never processed or trans fats. Those fats with a high saturate content aren't damaged by heating and cooking. Additionally, saturates won't affect the ratio of Omega-3s to 6s since they contain neither.

Some suggestions for cooking are coconut oil, palm oil (Spectrum Organic Shortening), ghee (clarified butter), or, if you're not allergic to dairy, butter.

Some Guidelines for Allergy Elimination

Follow this plan for at least three weeks. Allergic foods are addictive. It takes two weeks for withdrawal symptoms to abate. Cheat and back you go to day one!

Eat animal protein: fish, poultry, eggs, and red meat. Some people might find themselves allergic to eggs and beef.

Eat vegetables but not corn or dried beans. Some people have problems with onions. If you're watching your carbohydrate intake, avoid potatoes, sweet potatoes, yams, and winter squash.

Eat fresh fruits. Keep it to 2 fruits a day if you are watching your carbohydrate intake. Strawberries and citrus are allergenic for some people. Don't eat dried fruit; it's moldy and packed with concentrated sugar.

Drink lots of water, not fruit juice. And watch out for carrot, tomato, and beet juice if you are watching your carbohydrate intake.

NO alcohol.

NO grains: rice, corn, pasta, bread, tortillas, wheat including durum, semolina, kalmut, all other alternative grains, rye, oats, barley, and malt. Watch out for "thickened" soups and gravies.

Fats: have them! Use unrefined cold pressed: olive, almond or sesame oil. For cooking use clarified butter (ghee) to avoid milk solids, Spectrum's Organic Shortening (which is palm oil), or coconut oil.

Avoid legumes: soy, soy sauce and soy products such as liquid aminos and tofu, dry beans, and dry peas.

Nuts are OK unless they stimulate a strong craving response.

Avoid all sugar, honey, molasses or any other concentrated sugar. This includes sweetened fruit juice and artificial sweeteners.

Avoid all dairy, including cheese.

Watch out for ingredients in condiments. Use canola or olive oil mayonnaise. Watch out for wine vinegar. Read labels to make sure there is no corn (fructose), MSG (hydrolyzed vegetable protein), milk, whey, malt, or yeast.

Into the fourth week, if your symptoms have improved, you might want to stay the course! Although it's not part of a hunter-gatherer diet, some people can re-introduce organic milk products.

If you can't live without dairy, after the fourth week try a *single* serving of a milk product, but not cheese. Cheese contains mold which should be it's own test. Wait for 48 hours before you think you're in the clear. If you reintroduce dairy and over a week or so notice that some of your symptoms are returning, you should probably admit defeat. Some find they can reintroduce dairy if they eat it only every fourth day.

Hang onto Your Seat

Symptoms of food sensitivity and allergies include headaches, gastro-intestinal problems, brain fog, depression, anxiety, achy joints, skin problems, and sleepiness after meals.

These symptoms are masked by frequent feedings. When you eliminate and re-introduce a food you're sensitived to, symptoms may be strong.

If you have a bad reaction, you will need to de-acidify your system quickly to reduce the symptoms. A single 10,000 mg dose of buffered vitamin C works well or a half teaspoon of sodium bicarbonate (baking soda, not baking powder) in a glass of water. Keep yourself hydrated to dilute the reaction. The homeopathic remedy Histaminium in a 30C pellet held under your tongue for about ten seconds might also help, but note that the pellet is lactose (milk sugar).

My Friends Will Hate Me

With the popularity of low carb diets eating hunter-gatherer has become easier. Just tell the waiter you're on *Atkins*. It's useful to try the hunter-gatherer diet with an experimental attitude rather than asking yourself daily whether you have to deprive yourself of your favorite foods ... forever. Also remember that it's not a "diet" but a lifestyle. If it works, you will be eliminating disabling symptoms and protecting yourself from further illness by reducing the extra load on your immune system.

It may feel like you're trying to learn to walk on your hands at first because eating patterns are habituated. But soon you'll regard chocolate cake as poison.

Well, not soon, but eventually!

Resources

Audette, Ray. 2000. *NeanderThin: Eat Like a Caveman to Achieve a Lean, Strong, Healthy Body.* New York: St. Martin's.

Berman, Layna. 2004. The Hunter-Gatherer Diet. *Your Own Health And Fitness.* Broadcast March 2, 2004.

Cohen, Mark Nathan. 1996. The History of Diet. *Your Own Health And Fitness.* Broadcast January 9, 1996.

Cohen, Mark Nathan. 1991. *Health and the Rise of Civilization.* New Haven: Yale University Press.

Cordain, Loren. 2002. The Paleo Diet. *Your Own Health And Fitness.* Broadcast February 5, 2002.

Cordain, Loren. 2002. *The Paleo Diet: Lose Weight and Get Healthy by Eating the Food You Were Designed to Eat.* New York: Wiley.

Eaton, Boyd. Evolution, Diet and Health. Access at www.cast.uark.edu/local/icaes/index.html.

Enig, Mary. 2001. Dietary Fat Update. *Your Own Health And Fitness.* Broadcast July 10, 2001.

Fallon, Sally. 2001. Healthy Food Prep. *Your Own Health And Fitness.* Broadcast May 22, 2001.

Fallon, Sally. 1999. *Nourishing Traditions.* Washington, DC: New Trends Publishing.

The Paleo Diet Page. www.paleodiet.com.

WHAT CAUSES A HEART ATTACK

The official story about heart attacks is simple and it's wrong. It goes something like this:

- cholesterol accumulates on the artery walls that feed the heart;
- a chunk breaks loose and blocks blood flow to the heart (*ischemia*);
- with oxygen cut off, heart tissue dies;
- scar tissue forms over the dead (*necrotic*) area;
- the inert scar tissue disrupts the heart's electrical signals so that the heart has a seizure.

Cardiovascular disease was developed as a diagnosis to prevent heart attacks by preventing the first step: plaque build-up. A vast industry of pharmaceuticals (statins chief among them), treatments (such as for hypertension), invasive procedures (such as angioplasty), and technology (such as pacemakers) was born to treat cardiovascular disease.

Yet the rate at which people die from heart attacks has risen ever since cardiovascular disease was invented 50 years ago. Any progress in heart attack statistics is likely due to the improved methods for keeping people alive rather than any "cures" of cardiovascular disease.

It Doesn't Make Sense

Malcolm Kendrick, MD is a physician in the North of England who educates other physicians and writes regularly for the online journal Red Flags. He has for some time criticized the conventional conception of cholesterol-caused cardiovascular disease. In a recent article he called into question the entire official story as to what causes a heart attack.

Dr. Kendrick challenges the assumption that ischemia (arterial blockage) causes a heart attack. When tissue dies, your immune system causes it to disintegrate. This would create a hole in your heart and blood would spurt out. Which isn't what happens.

Dr. Kendrick also points to research showing that clots form days or weeks *before* a heart attack. In many cases there were no clots at all. In other words, a clot and its downstream effect in cutting off oxygen could not be the cause of the heart attack.

The scar tissue? Kendrick posits that it is the consequence not the cause of a heart attack. What is officially called a *myocardial infarction* ("myocardial" meaning heart, "infarction" meaning death) is actually a remodeling of heart muscle into scar tissue.

Dr. Kendrick notes that in some people certain areas of the heart can spontaneously go into a state of hibernation. Both this and the remodeling process are, he argues, "highly complex, and controlled, and active."

What causes the heart to "decide" to stop and remodel itself?

When interviewed on *Your Own Health And Fitness*, Dr. Kendrick was reluctant to speculate. But he was certain that mainstream researchers and practitioners actively avoid addressing the issues he raises. They instead cling to cholesterol lowering and the standard bag of conventional tricks to prevent heart attacks—even though they don't seem to work.

The Healthy Heart

As you grow older, your heart and cardiovascular system age: they degenerate by becoming stiff and inefficient. By holding back aging, vulnerability to heart attack can be reduced.

In conventional medicine, cardiovascular disease was invented so that heart attacks could be prevented by reducing the conditions thought to cause them—conditions such as elevated LDL cholesterol, C-reactive protein, lipoprotein(a), clotting factors, and oxidized LDL cholesterol. Each of these is connected to clotting, ischemia, and the rest of the standard story.

If Malcolm Kendrick is right, then treating conventionally conceived cardiovascular disease won't lower heart attack risk—unless the treatment coincidentally affects the underlying process that actually causes a heart attack. With the active promotion of statin drugs as the treatment of choice, the opposite is the case: conventional treatments weaken the heart and cardiovascular system.

Instead of treating people to prevent a heart attack, our current state of ignorance points to making the heart and cardiovascular system as healthy as possible. A healthy heart will better cope with the "highly complex, and controlled, and active" process that causes a heart attack. And there's a good chance that such events are less likely in a healthy heart.

A healthy heart is younger than its chronological age. The degeneration associated with an aging heart can be slowed by paying attention to five things: energy production, blood vessel stiffness, inflammation, calcium balance, and homocysteine.

Your heart has the highest concentration of mitochondria of any tissue in your body. That's because your heart consumes more energy per pound than any other tissue. Heart failure is what happens when your heart's energy production fails—the muscle can no longer work. "Healthy Mitochondria" (PHO #9) describes how to maintain energy production.

Stiffness in arteries not only makes the heart work harder it also inhibits delivery of nutrients to tissues—including the muscle tissue of the heart. Nitrogen oxide (*NO*) keeps blood vessel walls pliant. The amino acid arginine is not only a source of NO it also supports insulin sensitivity. In addition to arginine, herbal "sex tonics" such as yohimbine and ashwagandha are also good NO sources.

Arterial stiffness is affected by inflammation and calcium balance. Inflammation also affects the viscosity of blood: thicker blood makes the heart work harder. Jack Challem's *The Inflammation Syndrome* describes nutrients that protect against inflammation.

Calcification of the heart and arteries is closely associated with heart failure. Cardiovascular calcification is tied to *de*calcification of bone. Calcium is leeched from your bones and deposited in your heart muscle and artery walls.

Calcium balance is restored with adequate supplementation of vitamin D and vitamin K. Because vitamin K contributes to healthy blood clotting, conventional hypertension drugs such as warfarin (trade name Coumadin) disrupt vitamin K's role in calcium balance.

Homocysteine was originally proposed as a cause of ischemia through inflammation. But homocysteine also causes the smooth muscles of the artery walls to seize. As a result, it might play a role in the heart seizing.

Homocysteine is an intermediate product in your body's conversion of an amino acid into the antioxidant glutathione. It builds up when that process is disrupted. Typically, this is caused by a deficiency in B vitamins—B6, B12, and folic acid. You can easily restore the process with supplements.

Young hearts are less likely to suffer a heart attack. Although we might not know yet what actually causes a heart attack, you can protect yourself by keeping your heart in balance with the right nutrients.

Resources

Challem, Jack. 2003. *The Inflammation Syndrome*. New York: John Wiley and Sons.

Kendrick, Malcolm. 2005. Heart Attacks Are Not Caused by Blood Clots. *Red Flags*. Access at http://www.redflagsdaily.com.

Kendrick, Malcolm. 2007. *The Great Cholesterol Con: The Truth about What Really Causes Heart Disease and How to Avoid It*. London:John Blake.

Kendrick, Malcolm and Uffe Ravnskov. 2006. Heart Disease: What Is It Really? *Your Own Health And Fitness*. Broadcast February 28, 2006.

Ojio, Shinsuke et al. 2000. Considerable Time From the Onset of Plaque Rupture and/or Thrombi Until the Onset of Acute Myocardial Infarction in Humans. *Circulation*. October 24, 2000; 102:2063-9.

Ravnskov, Uffe. 2000. *The Cholesterol Myths*. Washington, DC: New Trends Publishing.

Rittersma, Saskia et al. 2005. Plaque Instability Frequently Occurs Days or Weeks Before Occlusive Coronary Thrombosis. *Circulation*. February 21, 2005; 111:1160-5.

The International Network of Cholesterol Skeptics. Access at http://www. thincs.org.

WHAT'S WRONG WITH CONVENTIONAL ESTROGEN THERAPY

Opening a newspaper is bad for the health of a postmenopausal woman.

In April 2004, the *Associated Press* ran an article titled "Report: Estrogen Therapy Raises Risk of Stroke, Blood Clots" which reported that "on average, the hormone (estrogen) caused 12 more strokes and 6 additional venous blood clots per 10,000 women each year."

Reading research and newspaper articles critically is a first line of defense against manipulation by market forces in the health care industry. Let's start with the numbers, 12 more strokes per 10,000, about double the number of non-lethal strokes. That's not good.

But then comes the leap of faith: taking estrogen caused this doubling of risk. The problem is that these strokes were most likely caused by estrogen that isn't balanced with progesterone and testosterone. What caused the strokes was that these women were getting the wrong treatment.

But Did They Ask the Right Question?

Before looking at the other statistics reported from the study, I'd like to discuss the study's design. This second trial by the Women's Health Initiative was conducted on 10,739 postmenopausal women aged 50-70 years with prior hysterectomy. There is no mention of whether these women had intact ovaries, smoked, were obese or diabetic, had a previous clotting incident, or a family history of CVD. These risk factors all greatly increase the risk of clots and strokes.

All women were given the same oral dose of Premarin. These women were not tested ahead to determine how much estrogen replacement they needed, or whether they needed any at all.

Premarin is extracted from pregnant mares using morally abhorrent methods. This horse estrogen includes equilin, an estrogen that is not native to humans (the three principle estrogens being estrone, estradiol, and estriol). The ratio between the estrogens in Premarin isn't the same as that produced by the human body. Since the human endocrine system depends on hormone balance, any change in the hormone ratio causes a ripple effect throughout the body.

The Importance of Estrogen

Estrogen in balance with other hormones is lifegiving. In both sexes, it is key to healthy brain function. In his book *The End of*

Stress As We Know It, Dr. Bruce McEwen describes estrogen's action.

> Estrogen stimulates neurons to form new synapses.... [I]t encourages the growth of new neurons and protects against the destructive effects of free radicals. Of all the potential benefits to the brain, the most striking is estrogen's ability to protect memory.

He goes on to discuss beta-amyloid plaques, which cause destruction of the brain in Alzheimer's disease: "Estrogen appears to protect against the destructive effects of this protein." Several studies "also found a similar reduction in the risk of Alzheimer's disease in women taking estrogen replacement therapy."

But like all hormones, estrogen depends on other hormones for its action. Without sufficient amounts of native (bio-identical) progesterone, estrogen can't do its job. Additionally, while too much estrogen can contribute to sticky or clotting blood, progesterone and testosterone both counter this effect by making the blood more fluid.

You'll Throw a Clot when You Read This!

Back to the WHI's new study using estrogen alone in women with hysterectomy. A predominant effect of hysterectomy is the drastic lowering of *all* hormones, especially testosterone!

Testosterone not only protects the heart and vascular system of both sexes, it preserves bone and muscle. As a woman ages, her testosterone lowers. She tends to gain weight as a result, with increased risk of metabolic syndrome and diabetes, further disposing her to clots and strokes.

I'm not surprised to see an increased stroke rate among these women! What does surprise me is which results were reported and which were ignored.

There was a significant reduction in the risk of hip fractures by almost half, much more impressive than the increase in strokes. Heart disease also improved, although vascular disease risk increased slightly (remember what I said about testosterone's heart protective effects).

What completely blew me away was the unreported effect on breast cancer! Unreported because it missed "statistical significance" by a hair. The rates of breast cancer in the trial group were much lower than in the controls. This is amazing since estrogen has been maligned for being provocative in breast cancer, especially when it's not balanced with progesterone. How is this NOT "statistically significant?"

Estrogen tends to be more cancer promoting when taken orally as compared to topical or trans-dermal applications. Oral estrogen takes a "first pass" through the liver, where it can be metabolized into catechol estrogen which can be oxidized by free radicals into quinone estrogen, which can damage the DNA responsible for cell replication, causing mutations and cancer.

The other missing piece is what the designers of the trial regarded as cancer. As John Lee, MD, often pointed out, breast cancer statistics include DCIS (ductal carcinoma in situ). These rarely result in malignant cancer, although they are included in breast cancer statistics. It's worth mentioning that DCIS usually disappears when estrogen is balanced with progesterone.

So What Do I Think?

This study points to the absolutely positive effects of estrogen! Here we have women taking an oral dose of horse estrogen, at a dose that probably doesn't reflect their actual needs, without the protective balancing effects of bio-identical progesterone and testosterone, and they still had reduced rates of bone loss and breast cancer!

This trial also drives home the need for hormone balancing, which would have protected these women from clotting and strokes.

And where, oh where is the trial with bio-identical progesterone? Clearly no one wants to pay for this since the sales of osteoporosis medications and anti-depressants might tank.

A few brave souls have done this research; most of it is described in *What Your Doctor May Not Tell You About Breast Cancer*. Not surprisingly, it shows bio-identical progesterone performing and synthetic progestins failing!

My advice is: first, get your hormone levels tested; then add only what you need to take care of your symptoms and maintain balance. Use only bio-identical hormones from a compounding pharmacy and use them topically. Then get ready to rock and roll!

Resources

Lee, John, MD and David Zava, PhD. 2002. *What Your Doctor May Not Tell You About Breast Cancer*. New York: Warner.

McEwen, Bruce. 2002. *The End of Stress as We Know It*. Washington, DC: Joseph Henry Press.

Women's Health Initiative Steering Committee. 2004. Effects of Conjugated Equine Estrogen in Postmenopausal Women with Hysterectomy: The Women's Health Initiative Randomized Controlled Trial. JAMA. April 13, 2004. 291(14): 1701-12.

ESTROGEN AND BROKEN HEARTS

Why is it so hard for women to get the whole story about hormone research? As a postmenopausal woman, it makes my blood... well, clot!

Two recent news items about hormone research show just how selective what gets reported is. The largest is a study reported in the February 23, 2005 issue of *JAMA* about estrogen and urinary incontinence. Another study in the February 10, 2005 issue of *The New England Journal of Medicine* reported on the effect of sudden emotional stress on the heart.

Choose the Right Form of Hormone!

The JAMA study reported that women taking oral horse estrogens and synthetic patented progestins had no improvement in vaginal dryness and incontinence. In fact, these hormones seem to have made the incontinence worse.

First of all, these hormones are not identical to those made in a woman's body, before or after menopause. You can't patent natural substances. Patenting turns substances into products and allows the company exclusive rights to the new formula. And it increases the prices the consumers pay.

Patented progestins (those that have their molecular structure altered to make them patentable) do not attach to all of the progesterone receptors, have none of the balancing effects of bioidentical progesterone, and have been shown in study after study to interfere with the healthful effects of bioidentical estrogens. They also increase uncomfortable symptoms and cancer.

Secondly, women make three different forms of estrogen. One of them does work brilliantly to restore and protect vaginal mucosa, preventing urinary incontinence, and recurrent bladder and cystitis infections. This estrogen is called estriol, abbreviated E3.

Estriol has been used in Europe for decades for postmenopausal women, intravaginally in low doses. It has never been shown to be provocative in increasing symptoms, clotting, or cancer in physiological doses.

Forty Years of Research

Dr. Henry Lemon spent forty years studying the relationship between the three estrogens and cancer risk. This research is described in *What Your Doctor May Not Tell You About Breast Cancer* by John Lee, MD and David Zava, PhD. When estriol is used intravaginally, the vaginal mucosa take up only what's needed and no more. This trans-mucosal application is the preferred route for estriol supplementation.

A 1993 Israeli study published in *The New England Journal of Medicine* followed fifty women treated with 0.5 mg of estriol every night for two weeks and then twice a week for eight months. Forty-three other women used a cream without estriol. The estriol treatment lowered the vaginal PH, which marks a rise in healthy *Lactobacilli* bacterial flora and a decrease in *E. coli*, bacteria associated with urinary infections. The incidence of urinary tract infections in the treated group decreased by 10 times.

A Swedish study published in 1994 showed equal effectiveness as opposed to women using a vaginal estradiol (E2) ring, which caused itching, urinary tract infections, *Candida* (yeast) infections, and pressure inside the vagina.

How Hard is This?

Did anyone need to do more research? Why are we seeing hormone-demonizing articles hogging the headlines, scaring women away from solutions that protect their health?

In the meantime, for urinary incontinence, vaginal dryness, or pain, try 0.5 mg of estriol (E3) by prescription from a compounding pharmacy. Use the full dose 2 to 3 days a week or half the dose intravaginally every day.

A word of caution: many women find the carrier creams used by compounders to be irritating. Your pharmacy can also formulate the prescription in a dropper bottle in oil. You then mix the dose with a lubricant of your choosing (aloe jelly works well) and apply it. Compounders will think you're going to use this under your tongue... as I wrote earlier, put this resourceful hormone into your vagina not under your tongue. Not that it will hurt you orally, it just works best intravaginal. Also, never use any form of estrogen without also using it's balancing partner, bioidentical progesterone (in a cream applied to your skin, not in your vagina).

Too Much Estradiol Will Break Your Heart

I'm sure the researchers who reported in the *New England Journal of Medicine* on the effect of sudden emotional stress didn't think they were reporting on the effects of unbalanced estradiol-to-progesterone ratio... but I do.

The article discusses a phenomenon that most of us have experienced: a tragic, stressful, or stunning emotional experience that causes heart symptoms.

What's interesting here is that when the patients were examined for the presence of a heart attack, they had experienced a reversible left ventricular dysfunction but not a heart attack. The conclusion: "Emotional stress can precipitate severe, reversible left ventricular dysfunction in patients without coronary disease." In other words, heart break!

Who's Most at Risk?

The kicker here is that the population most at risk for this complication is postmenopausal women. What do we know about these women? As the late Dr. John Lee, MD discussed in all his books, but especially in *What Your Doctor May Not Tell You About Menopause*, progesterone is the first hormone to tank at menopause. Progesterone has a quieting and sedating effect in contrast to estradiol's excitatory effect.

As women go though menopause, the balance of their hormones favors estrogen, causing them to be more *sympathetic dominant*. This refers to the part of the nervous system that is responsible for fight-or-flight.

When I see women in my practice whose progesterone levels are low, and this includes many younger women since our environment now exposes all of us to xenoestrogens, they have trouble sleeping, are irritable, and cry easily.

The progesterone dose needs vary as much as women do. Saliva testing is a great tool for checking whether you're dose is keeping you in a good ratio with estrogen. Generally, a replacement dose of progesterone is anywhere from 10 to 30 mg. For most over-the-counter progesterone creams, this would be about 1/8 teaspoon on the skin twice a day, morning and evening. Some will need more, some less. Too much causes some sleepiness or dullness, too little will cause spotting in women who are still menstruating. Certain conditions such as endometriosis will increase the dose needed.

Progesterone works best through the skin and should be stopped for two weeks each month if you're menstruating (use days 12-26 of your cycle) or just one week if you're postmenopausal.

Not Hysterical

Stress is stress. Both women and men feel better and are healthier when their sex hormones are balanced. Stress affects men by increasing cortisol levels, released during times of shock or stress. Cortisol contests and lowers testosterone. Testosterone in men (like progesterone in women) is calming, unlike synthetic testosterone, the anabolic steroids used by athletes.

Estrogen *does* seem to make women more emotive. When transsexuals change from female to male, they notice a marked decrease in their emotional volume and a smoothing out of their reactive response.

Another study published in *Nature* that hit the news was about the differences among women. The study examined women's chromosomes and found that some women are more "feminine" than others. After seeing a lot of saliva hormone results, I have to agree that there's variation there too. But mostly what I see is that women need to supplement with bioidentical, transdermal progesterone to restore their estrogen-to-progesterone ratio and their serenity... Whatever type of woman they are. *Viva le difference!*

Resources

Berman, Layna. 2005. Hormone Replacement: How, Who, and When. *Your Own Health and Fitness.* Broadcast February 1, 2005.

Berman, Layna. 2005. Hormone Intersect. *Your Own Health and Fitness.* Broadcast October 4, 2005.

Hendrix, Susan L. et al. 2005. Effects of Estrogn With and Without Progestin on Urinary Incontinence. *JAMA.* 293(8), February 23, 2005.

Lee, John 2002. What Your Doctor May Not Tell You About Menopause. *Your Own Health and Fitness.* Broadcast February 19, 2002.

Lee, John. 1996. *What Your Doctor May Not Tell You About Menopause.* New York:Warner Books.

Lee, John and David Zava. 2002. *What Your Doctor May Not Tell You About Breast Cancer.* New York:Warner Books.

Ross, Mark T. et al. 2005. The DNA Sequence of the Human X Chromosome. *Nature.* 434 (March 17, 2005): 325-37.

Wittstein, Ilan S. et al. 2005. Neurohumoral Features of Myocardial Stunning Due to Sudden Emotional Stress. *New England Journal of Medicine.* 352(6), February 10, 2005.

Health is a capacity, not a condition: it's the biological capacity to live a full, rich life. It's certainly not the absence of disease. Our work helps people build that capacity by promoting informed health decisions: in this book, on our radio show, and as health educators in private practice,

Too Much Medicine, Not Enough Health analyzes a wide range of issues. The book is intended to redirect the ideology, politics, and practice of health toward the actual lives of people and their communities. Three principles guide our work:

• each person has a unique biology and unique biological history;
• each person's body works as an ecology, with the action of each part supporting or balancing the action of other parts; and
• do the simplest things first by using the body's own capacities, what is most recognizable to it, and what is least invasive.

In our practice we often see people who have who have experienced exactly the opposite in the health care system. In this book we have described numerous instances where the aim of a health practice is to suppress symptoms instead of support a person's unique biology. We criticize this approach as failing to understand symptoms as the body's ecology working to right itself.

Along with many others, we also criticize interventionism in health and health care. This extends to prevention where a person must be turned into a patient in order to be treated for a disease he does not yet have. With an ever-widening array of preventive diagnoses and increasingly stringent criteria for risk, the net of intervention continues to expand.

Also with others, we believe that the health and health care crises arise from the juggernaut of the overdiagnosis and overtreatment that comes from symptom-centric, interventionist health practices. Our work enables escape from a system that, with increasing force, turns healthy people into patients.

Some of our work consists of revealing the media and research biases that misinform both people and practitioners. The articles in this book are demonstrations of how to work through those biases.

People are exposed most to media bias. It follows a common pattern in which journalists report the conclusions of researchers—the putative experts. The reporting is selective and is based on what is institutionally sanctioned. Overcoming media bias is made difficult by the ecclesiastical aura that surrounds "science" in our culture and what we've called the culture of expertise.

Although most people can easily grasp how media coverage is capable of bias, research bias presents a more difficult case. Contrary to the myth of scientific neutrality, sanctioned science and the researchers who practice it maintain accepted assumptions, conclusions, and methods. It is a form of science committed to a specific kind of knowledge epitomized in the sanctity of the clinical trial as the so-called gold standard. Challenges to sanctioned assumptions, conclusions, and methods are marginalized.

Practitioners of science sanctioned (and funded) by dominant health institutions have no monopoly on knowledge. Because science is the knowledge of causal relationships acquired through careful observation and reasoning, all the forms it takes should be honored.

In addition to what is culturally identified as science, whether sanctioned or not, we argue that valid knowledge is available through personal experience and local knowledge. These, too, provide an understanding of causal relationships based on careful observation and reasoning. But these are specific and concrete, not general and abstract; bottom up and not top down. These forms of knowledge do not lend themselves to—in fact resist—institutionalization and so are commonly excluded out of hand.

Environmental cues along with misinformation and bias affect health and health decisions. The media, health institutions, and commercial enterprises are obvious contributors to the information environment. But institutions also play an even larger role by shaping the personal, built, natural, and social environments that enforce people's roles and provide decision making cues—in essence by establishing what is possible and acceptable.

A more profound set of environmental factors affect health directly. In our opinion, the two most important are social inequity and toxic exposures. This is where the failure of the health and health care system is made plain. Doctors can't prescribe a social safety net. They can't prescribe that products and production processes be nontoxic. They can only prescribe pharmaceuticals, medical procedures, and perhaps recommend "lifestyle" changes.

Health and illness come from how each person's unique biology responds to exposures in her personal, built, natural, and social environments. So better health comes far more from better environments than better medical interventions. Those environmental improvements come from personal and collective action taken by people as consumers, workers, parents, children, students, neighbors, citizens, and even as patients in making environmental change that builds the capacity that is health. That is why we advocate health from the ground up.

Aarts, Henk, et al. 2008. Preparing and Motivating Behavior Outside of Awareness. *Science.* March 21, 2008. 319: 1639.

Abramson, John. 2004. *Overdosed America: The Broken Promise of American Medicine.* New York, HarperCollins.

Ackerman, Frank and Lisa Heinzerling. 2004. *Priceless: On Knowing the Price of Everything and the Value of Nothing.* New York, The New Press.

Adams, James and Charles Holloway. 2004. Pilot Study of a Moderate Dose Multivitamin/Mineral Supplement for Children with Autistic Spectrum Disorder. *Journal of Alternative and Complementary Medicine.* 10(6): 1033-9.

Adler, Nancy, et al eds. 1999. *Socioeconomic Status and Health in Industrial Nations: Social, Psychological, and Biological Pathways.* New York, New York Academy of Sciences.

AFL-CIO. 2008. *2008 Health Care for America Survey.* Washington, DC: AFL-CIO, Working America. March 2008.

Allday, Erin. 2007. Kids See Hours of Fast Food TV Ads. *San Francisco Chronicle.* March 29, 2007.

—. 2008. To Drop Pounds, Write Down Everything You Eat. *San Francisco Chronicle.* San Francisco. July 8, 2008.

Alliance for Natural Health. Access at http://www.anhcampaign.org/.

Altman, Rebecca Gasior, et al. 2008. Pollution Comes Home and Gets Personal: Women's Experience of Household Chemical Exposure. *Journal of Health and Social Behavior.* December 2008. 49(4): 417-35.

American Cancer Society, Women Skip Lifesaving Mammograms. Access at http://www.cancer.org/docroot/NWS/content/NWS_1_1x_Women_Skip_Lifesaving_Mammograms.asp.

American Public Health Association. Access at http://www.apha.org/.

Andrade, Anderson J.M., et al. 2006. A Dose–Response Study Following in Utero and Lactational Exposure to Di-(2-Ethylhexyl)-Phthalate (DEHP). *Toxicology.* October 29, 2006. 227(3): 185-92.

Angell, Marcia. 2004. *The Truth About the Drug Companies: How They Deceive Us and What to Do About It.* New York, Random House.

Animal Welfare Institute. Access at http://www.awionline.org/.

Apte, Michael, et al. 2008. Outdoor Ozone and Building-Related Symptoms in the BASE study. *Indoor Air.* April 2008. 18: 156-70.

Arbes, Samuel, et al. 2005. Prevalence of Positive Skin Test Responses to 10 Common Allergens in the US Population. *Journal of Allergy and Clinical Immunology.* 116: 377-83.

Architects / Designers / Planners for Social Responsibility Northern California Chapter. Access at http://www.adpsr-norcal.org/.

Aronowitz, Robert. 1998. *Making Sense of Illness: Science, Society, and Disease.* New York, Cambridge University Press.

Atkins, Robert. 2002. *Dr. Atkins' New Diet Revolution.* New York, Avon Books.

Audette, Ray. 2000. *Neanderthin: Eat Like a Caveman to Achieve a Lean, Strong, Healthy Body.* New York, St. Martin's.

Ausubel, Kenny ed. 2004. *Ecological Medicine: Healing the Earth, Healing Ourselves*. San Francisco, Sierra Club Books.

Bach, Edward and FJ Wheeler. 1997. *The Bach Flower Remedies*. New Canaan, Connecticutt, Keats Publishing.

Backhed, Fredrik, et al. 2005. Host-Bacterial Mutualism in the Human Intestine. *Science*. March 25, 2005. 307: 1915-20.

Badman, Michael and Jeffrey Flier. 2005. The Gut and Energy Balance: Visceral Allies in the Obesity Wars. *Science*. March 25, 2005. 307: 1909-14.

Baillie-Hamilton, Paula. 2005. *Toxic Overload*. New York, Avery Publishing Group.

Bakalar, Nicholas. 2008. Outcomes: Heeding Familiar Advice May Add Years to Your Life. *New York Times*. New York. January 22, 2008.

Balbus, John and Yewling Chee. 2004. *Dangerous Days of Summer*. Washington, DC, Environmental Defense.

Balch, Phyllis. 2002. *Prescription for Nutritional Healing: A-to-Z Guide to Supplements*. New York, Avery Publishing Group.

Banks, James, et al. 2006. Disease and Disadvantage in the United States and in England. *JAMA*. May 3, 2006. 295(17): 2037-45.

Barlett, Donald and James Steele. 2004. *Critical Condition: How Health Care in America Became Big Business and Bad Medicine*. New York, Doubleday.

Barteri, Mario, et al. 2005. Structural and Kinetic Effects of Mobile Phone Microwaves on Acetylcholinesterase Activity. *Biophysical Chemistry*. March 1, 2005. 113(3): 245-53.

Bass, Carole. 2008. Solving a Massive Worker Health Puzzle. *Scientific American*. Issue March 2008: 86-93.

Bell, David. 2006. Do Sulfonylurea Drugs Increase the Risk of Cardiac Events? *Canadian Medical Association Journal*. January 17, 2006. 174(2): 185-6.

Bennett, Gary G., et al. 2007. Safe to Walk? Neighborhood Safety and Physical Activity among Public Housing Residents. *PLoS Medicine*. October 2007. 4(10): e306.

Benyus, Janine M. 1997. *Biomimcry: Innovation Inspired by Nature*. New York, Quill.

Beral, Valerie, et al. 1999. Mortality Associated with Oral Contraceptive Use: 25 Year Follow up of Cohort of 46 000 Women from Royal College of General Practitioners' Oral Contraception Study. *BMJ*. January 9, 1999. 318.

Berkman, Lisa F. and Ichiro Kawachi eds. 2000. *Social Epidemiology*. New York, Oxford University Press

Berman, Layna. 1996. The Psychology of Exercise. *Your Own Health And Fitness*. KPFA 94.1FM. Junly 2, 1996.

—. 2001. Exercising Beyond Constraints. *Your Own Health And Fitness*. KPFA 94.1FM. April 3, 2001.

—. 2002a. Exercise: An Integrative Perspective. *Your Own Health And Fitness*. KPFA 94.1FM. January 22, 2002.

—. 2002b. The Science of Weight Training. *Your Own Health And Fitness*. KPFA 94.1FM. September 3, 2002.

—. 2003a. Exercise How-To. *Your Own Health And Fitness*. KPFA 94.1FM. Novermber 18, 2003.

—. 2003b. Insomnia. *Your Own Health And Fitness*. KPFA 94.1FM. September 23, 2003.

—. 2004a. Heart Disease: Another Perspective. *Your Own Health And Fit-

ness. KPFA 94.1FM. April 27, 2004.

—. 2004b. The Hormonal Consequences of Starch and Stress. *Your Own Health And Fitness*. KPFA 94.1FM. February 3, 2004.

—. 2004c. The Hunter-Gatherer Diet. *Your Own Health And Fitness*. KPFA 94.1FM. March 2, 2004.

—. 2005a. Allergy Alternatives. *Your Own Health And Fitness*. KPFA 94.1FM. April 19, 2005.

—. 2005b. Another Thyroid Show. *Your Own Health And Fitness*. KPFA 94.1FM. May 31, 2005.

—. 2005c. Designing a Sane Individualized Diet Plan. *Your Own Health And Fitness*. KPFA 94.1FM. January 4, 2005.

—. 2005d. Hormone Intersect. *Your Own Health And Fitness*. KPFA 94.1FM. October 4, 2005.

—. 2005e. Hormone Replacement: How, Who, and When. *Your Own Health And Fitness*. KPFA 94.1FM. February 1, 2005.

—. 2005f. Indoor Air Pollution. *Your Own Health And Fitness*. KPFA 94.1FM. March 1, 2005.

—. 2006. Detoxification. *Your Own Health And Fitness*. KPFA 94.1FM. September 19, 2006.

Berman, Layna and Jeffry Fawcett. 2005. Risk Factor Medicine. *Your Own Health And Fitness*. KPFA 94.1FM Berkeley, CA. August 30, 2005.

—. 2007a. Does Green Mean Non-Toxic? *Your Own Health And Fitness*. KPFA 94.1FM. August 28, 2007.

—. 2007b. Exercise and Disease Prevention. *Your Own Health And Fitness*. KPFA 94.1FM. July 17, 2007.

—. 2007c. Hypertension Revisited. *Your Own Health And Fitness*. KPFA 94.1FM. April 17, 2007.

—. 2007d. Overdiagnosis and Overtreatment Part 1. *Your Own Health And Fitness*. KPFA 94.1FM. January 23, 2007.

—. 2007e. Overdiagnosis and Overtreatment Part 2. *Your Own Health And Fitness*. KPFA 94.1FM. February 20, 2007.

—. 2007f. Stress Related Illness. *Your Own Health And Fitness*. KPFA 94.1FM. September 25, 2007.

—. 2008a. Aerial Spraying and Detoxification. *Your Own Health And Fitness*. KPFA 94.1FM. February 26, 2008.

—. 2008b. Doing the Simplest Things First. *Your Own Health And Fitness*. KPFA 94.1FM. June 3, 2008.

Bernstein, Richard. 1997. *Dr. Bernstein's Diabetes Solution: A Complete Guide to Achieving Normal Blood Sugars*. New York, Little, Brown & Company.

Biello, David. 2008. Smog Can Make People Sick, Even Indoors: When the Air Is Thick with Pollution, "Sick Building" Complaints Become More Common. *Scientific American*. Issue January 29, 2008.

Bioinitiative Working Group. Access at http://www.bioinitiative.org/.

Bioinitiative Working Group et al. 2007. *Bioinitiative Report: A Rationale for a Biologically-Based Public Exposure Standard for Electromagnetic Fields (ELF and RF)*. Bioinitiative Working Group. August 31, 2007.

Biomimcry Guild. Access at http://www.biomimicryguild.com/.

Biomimcry Institute. Access at http://www.biomimicryinstitute.org/.

Bjorntorp, Per ed. 1992. *Obesity.* Philadelphia, Lippincott.

—. 2001. Do Stress Reactions Cause Abdominal Obesity and Comorbidities? *Obesity Reviews.* May 2001. 2(2): 73-86.

Blair, Steven and Timothy Church. 2004. The Fitness, Obesity, and Health Equation: Is Physical Activity the Common Denominator? *JAMA.* September 8, 2004. 292(10): 1232-4.

Blanchard, Karen, et al. 2004. Mammographic Screening: Patterns of Use and Estimated Impact on Breast Carcinoma Survival. *Cancer.* August 1, 2004. 101(3): 495-507.

Blue Planet Project. Access at http://www.blueplanetproject.net/.

BN Ranch. Access at http://www.preferredmeats.com/BNranch_network.htm.

Boockvar, Kenneth and Diane Meier. 2006. Palliative Care for Frail Older Adults. *JAMA.* November 8, 2006. 296(18): 2245-53.

Bornehag, Carl-Gustav. 2004. The Association between Asthma and Allergic Symptoms in Children and Phthalates in House Dust. *Environmental Health Perspectives.* October 2004. 112(14): 1393-7.

Bower, Bruce. 2001. Youthful Nicotine Addiction May Be Growing. *Science News.* September 22, 2001. 160(12): 183.

Braungart, Michael, et al. 2007. Cradle-to-Cradle Design: Creating Healthy Emissions E a Strategy for Eco-Effective Product and System Design. *Journal of Cleaner Production.* September 2007. 15(13-14): 1337-48.

Braverman, Harry. 1974. *Labor and Monopoly Capital: The Degradation of Work in the Twentieth Century.* New York, Monthly Review Press.

Breggin, Peter. 2001. *The Anti-Depressant Fact Book: What Your Doctor Won't Tell You About Prozac, Zoloft, Paxil, Celexa, and Luvox.* Cambridge, MA, Perseus Publishing.

—. 2004. Depressing News About Antidepressants. *Your Own Health And Fitness.* KPFA 94.1FM. May 25, 2004.

Bridges, Andrew. 2007. Birth-Control Pill Halts Women's Periods. *San Francisco Chronicle.* San Francisco. May 22, 2007.

Brigham, Janet. 1998. *Dying to Quit: Why We Smoke and How We Stop.* Washington, DC, Joseph Henry Press.

Brody, Julia Green, et al. 2007. Environmental Pollutants and Breast Cancer. *Cancer.* June 15, 2007. 109(12 Suppl): 2667-711.

Brook, Robert D., et al. 2004. Air Pollution and Cardiovascular Disease: A Statement for Healthcare Professionals from the Expert Panel on Population and Prevention Science of the American Heart Association. *Circulation.* 109: 2655-71.

Buchanan, Ian, et al. 2008. Air Filter Materials, Outdoor Ozone and Building-Related Symptoms in the BASE study. *Indoor Air.* April 2008. 18: 144-55.

Buck Institute for Aging Research. Access at http://www.buckinstitute.org/.

Budnitz, Daniel S., et al. 2006. National Surveillance of Emergency Department Visits for Outpatient Adverse Drug Events. *JAMA.* October 18, 2006. 296(15): 1858-66.

Butler, Colin D. and Sharon Friel. 2006. Time to Regenerate: Ecosystems and Health Promotion. *PLoS Medicine.* October 2006. 3(10): e394.

California Alliance to Stop the Spray. Access at http://www.cassonline.org/.

California Alliance to Stop the Spray. 2008. *Light Brown Apple Moth (LBAM) Economic Impacts and Solutions.* CASS Economics Research Summary. May 5, 2008.

California Newsreel. 2008. Unnatural Causes: Is Inequality Making Us Sick?

Campbell, T. Colin and Thomas M. Campbell. 2004. *The China Study*. Dallas, Benbella Books.

Campillos, Monica, et al. 2008. Drug Target Identification Using Side-Effect Similarity. *Science*. July 11, 2008. 321(5886): 263-6.

Campos, Paul. 2004. *The Obesity Myth: Why America's Obsession with Weight Is Hazardous to Your Health*. New York, Gotham.

Cancer Prevention Coalition. Access at http://www.preventcancer.org/.

Caress, Stanley and Anne Steinemann. 2009. Prevalence of Frangrance Sensitivity in the American Population. *journal of Environmental Health*. March 2009. 71(7): 46-50.

Carey, Benedict. 2008. More Expensive Placebos Bring More Relief. *New York Times*. New York. March 5, 2008.

Carlo, George and Martin Schram. 2001. *Cell Phone: Invisible Hazards in the Wireless Age: An Insider's Alarming Discoveries About Cancer and Genetic Damage*. New York, Carroll & Graf.

Caruso, Claire C, et al. 2004. *Overtime and Extended Work Shifts: Recent Findings on Illnesses, Injuries, and Health Behaviors*. Cindinnati, OH:National Institute for Occupational Safety and Health. 2004-143. April 2004.

Caruso, Denise. 2007. A Challenge to Gene Theory, a Tougher Look at Biotech. *New York Times*. New York. July 1, 2007.

Cave, Damien. 2008. Legal Drugs Kill Far More Than Illegal, Florida Says. *New York Times*. New York. June 14, 2008.

Centers for Disease Control and Prevention. 2003. *Second National Report on Human Exposure to Environmental Chemicals*. National Center for Environmental Health. NCEH Pub. No. 02-0716.

—. 2005. Increase in Poisoning Deaths Caused by Non-Illicit Drugs - Utah, 1991-2003. *MMWR Morb Mortal Wkly Rep*. January 21, 2005. 54(2): 33-6.

—. 2007. Unintentional Poisoning Deaths - United States, 1999-2004. *MMWR Morb Mortal Wkly Rep*. February 9, 2007. 56(5): 93-6.

Challem, Jack. 2003. *The Inflammation Syndrome: The Complete Nutritional Program to Prevent and Reverse Heart Disease, Arthritis, Diabetes, Allergies, and Asthma*. New York, John Wiley and Sons.

—. 2004. Inflammation and Chronic Disease. *Your Own Health And Fitness*. KPFA 94.1FM. July 13, 2004.

—. 2005a. *Feed Your Genes Right*. Hoboken, NJ, Wiley & Sons.

—. 2005b. Feed Your Genes Right. *Your Own Health And Fitness*. KPFA 94.1FM. March 15, 2005.

Chang, Alicia. 2007. Study: Obesity Is 'Socially Contagious'. *San Francisco Chronicle*. San Francisco. July 25, 2007.

Chao, H. Jasmine, et al. 2003. The Work Environment and Workers' Health in Four Large Office Buildings. *Environmental Health Perspectives*. July 2003. 111(9): 1242-8.

Cheng, Maria. 2008. Healthy Habits Can Mean 14 Extra Years. *San Francisco Chronicle*. San Francisco. January 8, 2008.

ChildTrauma Academy. Access at http://childtraumaacademy.org/.

Christakis, Nicholas A. and James H. Fowler. 2007. The Spread of Obesity in a Large Social Network over 32 Years. *N Engl J Med*. 357(4): 370-9.

Citizens for Health. Access at http://www.citizens.org/.

Clapp, Richard W., et al. 2007. *Environmental and Occupational Causes of Cancer: New Evidence, 2005–2007.* Lowell, Massachusetts: Lowell Center for Sustainable Production, University of Massachusetts. October 2007.

Coghlan, Andy. 2006. Diabetes Spotlight Falls onto Fish. *New Scientist.* Issue September 30, 2006.

—. 2007. Genetic Testing: Informed Choice or Waste of Money? *New Scientist.* Issue October 3, 2007.

Cohen, Mark Nathan. 1991. *Health and the Rise of Civilization.* New Haven, Yale University Press.

—. 1996. The History of Diet. *Your Own Health And Fitness.* KPFA 94.1FM. January 9, 1996.

Colborn, Theo. 2006. A Case for Revisiting the Safety of Pesticides: A Closer Look at Neurodevelopment. *Environmental Health Perspectives.* January 2006. 114(1): 10-7.

Collaborative on Health and the Environment. Access at http://www.healthandenvironment.org/.

Commoner, Barry. 1971. *The Closing Circle: Nature, Man, and Technology.* New York, Random House.

Community Food Security Coalition. Access at http://www.foodsecurity.org/.

Community Supported Agriculture. Access at http://www.nal.usda.gov/afsic/pubs/csa/csa.shtml.

Cone, Maria. 2007. Common Chemicals Are Linked to Breast Cancer. *Los Angeles Times.* Los Angeles. May 14, 2007.

Consonni, Dario, et al. 2008. Mortality in a Population Exposed to Dioxin after the Seveso, Italy, Accident in 1976: 25 Years of Follow-Up. *Am J Epidemiol.* April 1, 2008. 167(7): 847-58.

Cordain, Loren. 2002a. The Paleo Diet. *Your Own Health And Fitness.* KPFA 94.1FM. February 5, 2002.

—. 2002b. *The Paleo Diet: Lose Weight and Get Healthy by Eating the Food You Were Designed to Eat.* New York, John Wiley and Sons.

Coren, Stanley. 1997. *Sleep Thieves.* New York, Free Press.

Cummings, Stephen and Dana Ullman. 2004. *Everybody's Guide to Homeopathic Medicine.* New York, Penguin.

Cummins, Joe and Sam Burcher. 2008. Sex Hormones and City Life. *Institute of Science in Society.* May 16, 2088.

Dadd, Debra Lynn. 2005. *Home Safe Home: Creating a Healthy Home Environment by Reducing Exposure to Toxic Household Products.* New York, Jeremy P. Tarcher/Penguin.

Dallman, Mary F., et al. 2003. Chronic Stress and Obesity: A New View of "Comfort Food". *Proceedings of the National Academy of Science.* September 30, 2003. 100(20): 11696-701.

Damasio, Antonio. 1994. *Descartes' Error: Emotion, Reason, and the Human Brain.* New York, GP Putnam's Sons.

—. 1999. *The Feeling of What Happens: Body and Emotion in the Making of Consciousness.* New York, Harcourt.

—. 2003. *Looking for Spinoza: Joy, Sorrow, and the Feeling Brain.* New York, Harcourt.

Danese, Andrea, et al. 2007. Childhood Maltreatment Predicts Adult Inflammation in a Life-Course Study. *Proceedings of the National Academy of Science.* January 23, 2007. 104(4): 1319-24.

Daniels, Stephen R., et al. 2008. Lipid Screening and Cardiovascular Health in Childhood. *Pediatrics.* July 2008. 122(1): 198-208.

Danthanarayana, Wijesiri. 1983. Population Ecology of the Light Brown Apple Moth, Epiphyas Postvittana (Lepidoptera: Tortricidae). *The Journal of Animal Ecology.* February 1983. 52(1): 1-33.

Darmon, Nicole and Adam Drewnowski. 2008. Does Social Class Predict Diet Quality? *Am J Clin Nutr.* May 2008. 87(5): 1107-17.

DataCenter. Access at http://www.datacenter.org/.

Daughton, Christian. 2003. Cradle-to-Cradle Stewardship of Drugs for Minimizing Their Environmental Disposition While Promoting Human Health. *Environmental Health Perspectives.* May 2003. 111(5): 757-74.

—. 2004. Non-Regulated Water Contaminants: Emerging Research. *Environmental Impact Assessment Review.* 24: 711-32.

Davis, Aaron C. 2008. Moth-Spraying PR Deal Suspended Amid Questions. *San Francisco Chronicle.* San Francisco. March 13, 2008.

Davis, Devra. 2007. *The Secret History of the War on Cancer.* New York, Basic Books.

de Gelder, Beatrice. 2006a. Toward a Biological Theory of Emotional Body Language. *Biological Theory.* Spring 2006. 1(2): 130-2.

—. 2006b. Towards the Neurobiology of Emotional Body Language. *Nature Reviews Neuroscience.* March 2006. 7: 242-9.

Debra Lynn Dadd Website. Access at http://www.dld123.com/.

Dembe, Allard E., et al. 2007. Associations between Employees' Work Schedules and the Vocational Consequences of Workplace Injuries. *J Occup Rehabil.* October 12, 2007. 17: 641-51.

Dembner, Alice. 2006. Science Gaining on Elders' Frailty. *Boston Globe.* Boston. September 3, 2006.

Dement, William. 1999. *The Promise of Sleep.* New York, Delacorte Press.

—. 2001. Sleep. *Your Own Health And Fitness.* KPFA 94.1FM. December 4, 2001.

Diabetes Prevention Program Research Group. 2002. Reduction in the Incidence of Type 2 Diabetes with Lifestyle Intervention or Metformin. *N Engl J Med.* February 7. 346(6): 393-403.

Diem, Elisabeth, et al. 2005. Non-Thermal DNA Breakage by Mobile-Phone Radiation (1800mhz) in Human Fibroblasts and in Transformed Gfsh-R17 Rat Granulosa Cells in Vitro. *Mutat Res.* 583: 178-83.

Dietary Guidelines Advisory Committee. 2005. *The Report of the Dietary Guidelines Advisory Committee on Dietary Guidelines for Americans, 2005.* Washington, DC:USDA and US Department of Health and Human Services,.

Doubeni, Chyke A., et al. 2008. Perceived Accessibility as a Predictor of Youth Smoking. *Ann Fam Med.* July/August 2008. 6(4): 323-30.

Duncan, Glen, et al. 2004. Prevalence and Trends of a Metabolic Syndrome Phenotype among US Adolescents, 1999–2000. *Diabetes Care.* October 2004. 27(10): 2438-43.

Eaton, S. Boyd and Stanley B. Eaton. 2003. An Evolutionary Perspective on Human Physical Activity: Implications for Health. *Comparative Biochemistry and Physiology Part A.* September 2003. 136: 153-9.

Eaton, S. Boyd, et al. 2002. Evolution, Diet, and Health. In *Human Diet: Its Origin and Evolution*. Ungar, Peter S. and Mark F. Teaford eds. Westport, CT, Bergin & Garvey: 7-18.

Eckburg, Paul B., et al. 2005. Diversity of the Human Intestinal Microbial Flora. *Science*. June 10, 2005. 308: 1635-8.

Ecological Options Network. Access at http://www.eon3.net/.

Ecological Options Network. 2008. Stop Them before They Spray Again: Reports from the LBAM Front Lines.

Edelman, Eva. 1998. *Natural Healing for Schizophrenia and Other Common Mental Disorders, 2nd Edition*. Eugene, Oregon, Borage Books.

—. 2000. Natural Healing for Mental Disorders. *Your Own Health And Fitness*. KPFA 94.1FM. November 7, 2000.

Edible Schoolyard. Access at http://www.edibleschoolyard.org/.

Elliott, David, et al. 2007. Helminths as Governors of Immune-Mediated Inflammation. *Int J Parasit*. 37: 457-64.

ENCODE Project Consortium. 2007. Identification and Analysis of Functional Elements in 1% of the Human Genome by the ENCODE Pilot Project. *Nature*. June 14, 2007. 447: 799-816.

Enig, Mary. 2000. *Know Your Fats: The Complete Primer for Understanding the Nutrition of Fats, Oils, and Cholesterol*. Silver Spring, MD, Bethesda Press.

—. 2001. Dietary Fat Update. *Your Own Health And Fitness*. KPFA 94.1FM. July 10, 2001.

—. 2004. Dietary Fats: Myths and Science. *Your Own Health And Fitness*. KPFA 94.1FM. January 13, 2004.

Environmental Working Group. Access at http://www.ewg.org/.

Environmental Working Group, National Tap Water Quality Database. Access at http://www.ewg.org/sites/tapwater/.

Environmental Working Group, Skin Deep Cosmetic Safety Database. Access at http://www.cosmeticsdatabase.com/.

Epstein, Samuel. 1998. *The Politics of Cancer Revisited*. Fremont Center, NY, East Ridge Press.

Epstein, Samuel, et al. 2001. Dangers and Unreliability of Mammography: Breast Examina-Tion Is a Safe, Effective, and Practical Alternative. *International Journal of Health Services*. 31(3): 605-15.

Evans, Lynette. 2008. Forget the Fragrance. *San Francisco Chronicle*. San Francisco. August 2, 2008: F3.

Fagerlund, Richard. 2008. Moth Spraying Likely to Harm More Than Help. *San Francisco Chronicle*. San Francisco. February 23, 2008.

Fagin, Dan, et al. 1996. *Toxic Deception: How the Chemical Industry Manipulates Science, Bends the Law, and Endangers Your Health*. Secaucus, NJ, Birch Lane Press.

Fallon, Sally. 2001. Healthy Food Prep. *Your Own Health And Fitness*. KPFA 94.1FM. May 22, 2001.

—. 2004. Fake Foods. *Your Own Health And Fitness*. KPFA 94.1FM. February 24, 2004.

Fallon, Sally and Mary Enig. 1999. *Nourishing Traditions: The Cookbook That Challenges Politically Correct Nutrition and the Diet Dictocrats*. Washington, DC, New Trends.

—. 2003. *Comments to the 2005 Dietary Guidelines Advisory Committee.* December 18, 2003.

Farm to School. Access at http://www.farmtoschool.org/.

Farmer, Paul, et al. 2006. Structural Violence and Clinical Medicine. *PLoS Medicine.* October 2006. 3(10): e449.

Fawcett, Jeffry. 2005c. Antioxidant Follies. *Progressive Health Observer.* December 2004/January 2005. 4: 1ff.

—. 2005d. Cancer by the Numbers. *Progressive Health Observer.* Fall 2005. 8: 5ff.

—. 2006a. Healthy Mitochondria. *Progressive Health Observer.* Winter 2006. 9: 2ff.

FDA, Cell Phone Facts: Consumer Information on Wireless Phones. Access at http://www.fda.gov/cdrh/wireless/braincancer040606.html.

FDA, Cell Phone Facts: Do Wireless Phones Pose a Health Hazard? Access at http://www.fda.gov/cellphones/qa.html#22.

Fergusson, Dean, et al. 2005. Association between Suicide Attempts and Selective Serotonin Reuptake Inhibitors: Systematic Review of Randomised Controlled Trials. *BMJ.* 330: 396-403.

Fernández-Armesto, Felipe. 2002. *Near a Thousand Tables: A History of Food.* New York, Free Press.

Fine, Ben. 1998. *The Political Economy of Diet, Health and Food Policy.* New York, Routledge

—. 2000. *Social Capital Versus Social Theory: Political Economy and Social Science at the Turn of the Millennium.* New York, Routledge.

—. 2002. *The World of Consumption: The Material and the Cultural Revisited.* New York, Routledge.

Fischer, Douglas. 2007. Scientists Expose Body Toxin Risks: Synthetic Chemicals May Affect Two Generations' Ability to Have Children. *Oakland Tribune.* February 2, 2007.

Fischer, Frank. 1990. *Technocracy and the Politics of Expertise.* Newbury Park, CA, Sage Publications.

—. 2000. *Citizens, Experts, and the Environment: The Politics of Local Knowledge.* Durham, Duke University Press.

Fisk, Donald M. 2001. American Labor in the 20th Century. *Compensation and Working Conditions.* Fall 2001. 3-8.

Flegal, Katherine M., et al. 2005. Excess Deaths Associated with Underweight, Overweight, and Obesity. *JAMA.* April 20, 2005. 293(15): 1861-7.

Ford, Earl S., et al. 2004. Increasing Prevalence of the Metabolic Syndrome among US Adults. *JAMA.* October 2004. 27(10): 2444-9.

Forster, Sophie and Nilli Lavie. 2007. High Perceptual Load Makes Everybody Equal: Eliminating Individual Differences in Distractibility with Load. *Psychological Science.* 18(5): 377-81.

Fostering Sustainable Behavior. Access at http://www.cbsm.com/public/world.lasso.

Frank, Lawrence D., et al. 2003. *Health and Community Design: The Impact of the Built Environment on Physical Activity.* Washington, DC, Island Press.

Fried, Linda, et al. 2001. Frailty in Older Adults: Evidence for a Phenotype. *The Journal of Gerontology.* 56: M146-57.

Frumkin, Howard. 2001. Beyond Toxicity: Human Health and the Natural Environment. *Am J Prev Med.* 20(3): 234-40.

—. 2003. Healthy Places: Exploring the Evidence. *Am J Public Health.* September 2003. 93(9): 1451-6.

Gandhi, Gursatej. 2005. Genetic Damage in Mobile Phone Users: Some Preliminary Finding. *Ind J Hum Genet.* 11(2): 99-104.

Gangi, Shabnam and Olle Johansson. 2000. A Theoretical Model Based Upon Mast Cells and Histamine to Explain the Recently Proclaimed Sensitivity to Electric and/or Magnetic Fields in Humans. *Medical Hypothesis.* 54(4): 663-71.

Gant, Charles. 2004. End Addictions with Nutrient Therapy. *Your Own Health And Fitness.* KPFA 94.1FM. February 10, 2004.

Gant, Charles and Greg Lewis. 2002. *End Your Addiction Now.* New York, Warner Books.

Gantz, Walter. 2007. *Food for Thought: Television Food Advertising to Children in the United States,* Kaiser Family Foundation Report.

Gard, Michael and Jan Wright. 2005. *The Obesity Epidemic: Science, Morality, and Ideology* New York, Routledge.

Gauderman, W. James, et al. 2004. The Effect of Air Pollution on Lung Development from 10 to 18 Years of Age. *N Engl J Med.* September 9, 2004. 351(11): 1057-67.

Gellene, Denice. 2006. Benefits from Vitamins Are Few. *Los Angeles Times.* Los Angeles. May 18, 2006.

—. 2007. Obesity Is 'Contagious,' Study Finds. *Los Angeles Times.* Los Angeles. July 26, 2007.

Gibbs, W. Wayt. 2005. Obesity: An Overblown Epidemic? *Scientific American.* June 2005. 70-5.

Gigerenzer, Gerd. 2000. *Adaptive Thinking: Rationality in the Real World.* New York, Oxford University Press.

—. 2007. *Gut Feelings: The Intelligence of the Unconscious.* New York, Viking.

Gigerenzer, Gerd and Reinhard Selten eds. 2001. *Bounded Rationality: The Adaptive Toolbox.* Cambridge, MA, MIT Press.

Gilbert, Scott F. 2005. Mechanisms for the Environmental Regulation of Gene Expression: Ecological Aspects of Animal Development. *Journal of Bioscience.* February 2005. 30(1): 65-74.

Gladwell, Malcolm. 2005. *Blink: The Power of Thinking without Thinking.* New York, Little, Brown & Company.

Glantz, Stanton A. 2006. Smoking: The Truth. *Your Own Health And Fitness.* KPFA 94.1FM. February 21, 2006.

Glantz, Stanton A. and Edith D. Balbach. 2000. *Tobacco War: Inside the California Battles.* Berkeley, University of California Press.

Glaser, Ronald and Janet Kiecolt-Glaser. 2005. Stress-Induced Immune Dysfunction: Implications for Health. *Nature Reviews Immunology.* March 2005. 5: 243-51.

Goines, Lisa and Louis Hagler. 2007. Noise Pollution: A Modern Plague. *Southern Medical Journal.* March 2007. 100(3): 287-94.

Goodman, Steven N. 2002. The Mammography Dilemma: A Crisis for Evidence-Based Medicine? *Ann Intern Med.* September 3, 2002. 157(5): 363-4.

Gordon, Rachel. 2008. SF Traffic Noise Risks Health of 1 in 6. *San Francisco Chronicle.* San Francisco. October 8, 2008.

Grant, Bridget F., et al. 2004. Nicotine Dependence and Psychiatric Disorders in the United States. *Arch Gen Psychiatry.* November 2004. 61(11): 1107-15.

Graveline, Duane. 2004. *Lipitor, Thief of Memory: Statin Drugs and the Misguided War on Cholesterol.* West Conshohocken, PA, Infinity Publishing.

Greenpeace, Greenwashing. Access at http://stopgreenwash.org/.

Gregg, Edward W., et al. 2005. Secular Trends in Cardiovascular Disease Risk Factors According to Body Mass Index in US Adults. *JAMA.* April 20, 2005. 293(15): 1868-74.

Hadley, Caroline. 2004. Should Auld Acquaintance Be Forgot... *EMBO Reports.* 5. 12. Issue December 2004: 1122-4.

Hallberg, Örjan and Olle Johansson. 2002a. Cancer Trends During the 20th Century. *Journal of the Autralasian College of Nutrition and Environmental Medicine.* 21(1): 3-8.

—. 2002b. Melanoma Incidence and Frequency Modulation (FM) Broadcasting. *Archives of Environmental Health.* 57(1): 32-40.

—. 2005. FM Broadcasting Exposure Time and Malignant Melanoma Incidence. *Electromagnetic Biology and Medicine.* 24: 1-8.

Hamilton, Donald. 1999. *Homeopathic Care for Cats and Dogs.* Berkeley, CA, North Atlantic Books.

Hamilton, Garry. 2005. Filthy Friends and the Rise of Allergies. *New Scientist.* 2495. Issue: April 16, 2005.

Hardell, Lennart, et al. 2006. Pooled Analysis of Two Case-Control Studies on Use of Cellular and Cordless Telephones and the Risk of Malignant Brain Tumours Diagnosed in 1997-2003. *Int J Oncol.* 28(2): 502-18.

Harrington, J Malcolm. 2001. Health Effects of Shift Work and Extended Hours of Work. *Occupational and Environmental Medicine.* January 2001. 58(1): 68ff.

Hartig, Terry, et al. 1991. Restorative Effects of Natural Environment Experiences. *Environment and Behavior.* January 1991. 23(1): 3-26.

Hauser, Russ, et al. 2004. Medications as a Source of Human Exposure to Phthalates. *Environmental Health Perspectives.* May 2004. 112(6): 751-3.

Havas, Magda. 2006. Dirty Electricity and EMF Health Dangers. *Your Own Health And Fitness.* KPFA 94.1FM. May 30, 2006.

Hawkin, Paul, et al. 1999. *Natural Capitalism: Creating the Next Industrial Revolution.* New York, Little, Brown & Company.

Hawthorne, Michael and Darnell Little. 2008. Chicago's Toxic Air. *Chicago Tribune.* Chicago. September 28, 2008.

Health Care for All. Access at http://www.healthcareforall.org/.

Health Care Without Harm. Access at http://www.noharm.org/.

Health Protection Agency. Mobile Telephony and Health: Health Protection Advice. Access at http://www.hpa.org.uk/radiation/understand/information_sheets/mobile_telephony/health_advice.htm.

Healthy Building Network. Access at http://www.healthybuilding.net/.

Hemminger, Pat. 2005. Damming the Flow of Drugs into Drinking Water. *Environmental Health Perspectives.* October 2005. 113(10): A679-81.

Henderson, Diedtra. 2004. Nicotine Research Points to Key Molecule. *Washington Post.* Washington, DC. November 4, 2004.

Hendrix, Susan L., et al. 2005. Effects of Estrogen with and without Progestin on Urinary Incontinence. *JAMA.* 293(8): 935-48.

Higdon, Jane. 2003. *An Evidence-Based Approach to Vitamins and Minerals: Health Benefits and Intake Recommendations.* New York, Thieme.

Hitchcock, Christine L. and Jerilynn C. Prior. 2004. Evidence About Extending the Duration of Oral Contraceptive Use to Suppress Menstruation.

Women's Health Issues. November-December 2004. 14(6): 201-11.

Hodgson, Michael. 2002. Indoor Environmental Exposures and Symptoms. *Environmental Health Perspectives.* August 2002. 110(Supplement 4): 663-7.

Hoffer, Abram. 1999. *Dr. Hoffer's ABC of Natural Nutrition for Children with Learning Disabilities, Behavioral Disorders, and Mental State Disorders.* Kingston, Ontarios, Quarry Health Books.

——. 2000. Natural Nutrition for Children. *Your Own Health And Fitness.* KPFA 94.1FM. May 16, 2000.

Hoffer, Abram and Andrew Saul. 2008. *Orthomolecular Medicine for Everyone: Megavitamin Therapeutics for Families and Physicians.* Laguna Beach, CA, Basic Health.

Hofrichter, Richard ed. 2003. *Health and Social Justice: Politics, Ideology, and Inequity in the Distribution of Disease.* San Francisco, Jossey-Bass.

Hollis, Jack F., et al. 2008. Weight Loss During the Intensive Intervention Phase of the Weight-Loss Maintenance Trial. *Am J Prev Med.* August 2008. 35(2): 118-26.

Holtz, Timothy, et al. 2006. Health Is Still Social. *PLoS Medicine.* October 2006. 3(10): e419.

Hooper, Rowan. 2006. Men Inherit Hidden Cost of Dad's Vices. *New Scientist.* Issue January 7, 2006: 10.

Houlihan, Jane, et al. 2003. *BodyBurden: The Pollution in People.* Washington, DC, Environmental Working Group.

How Clean Is Your Air? Access at http://www.chicagotribune.com/news/local/rsei-database,0,3220483.htmlstory.

Hu, Gang, et al. 2004. Prevalence of the Metabolic Syndrome and Its Relation to All-Cause and Cardiovascular Mortality in Nondiabetic European Men and Women. *Arch Intern Med.* May 24, 2004. 164: 1066-76.

Huang, Han-Yao, et al. 2006. *Multivitamin/Mineral Supplements and Prevention of Chronic Disease.* AHRQ. AHRQ Publication No. 06-E012.

Humane Farm Animal Care. Access at http://www.certifiedhumane.com/.

Hunter, Lori M. 2007. Climate Change, Rural Vulnerabilities, and Migration. *Population Reference Bureau.* June 2007.

Hurley, Susan. 2005. Social Heuristics That Make Us Smarter. *Philosophical Psychology.* October 2005. 18(5): 585-612.

Idaghdour, Youssef, et al. 2008. A Genome-Wide Gene Expression Signature of Environmental Geography in Leukocytes of Moroccan Amazighs. *PLoS Genetics.* April 2008. 4(4): e1000052.

Independent Expert Group on Mobile Phones. 2000. *Mobile Phones and Health.* Chilton, Oxfordshire, UK, NRPB.

Independent Vitamin Safety Review Panel. 2006. Report of the Independent Vitamin Safety Review Panel. *Orthomolecular Medicine News Service.* May 23, 2006.

Ingram, Colin. 2006a. Safe Drinking Water. *Your Own Health And Fitness.* KPFA 94.1FM. October 3, 2006.

——. 2006b. *The Drinking Water Book.* Berkeley, CA, Celestial Arts.

Inoue, Manami, et al. 2006. Diabetes Mellitus and the Risk of Cancer. *Arch Intern Med.* September 25, 2006. 166: 1871-7.

International Association of Fire Fighters. 2005. *Position on the Health Effects from Radio Frequency/Microwave (RF/MW) Radiation in Fire Department Facilities from Base Stations for Antennas and Towers for the Conduction of Cell Phone Transmissions,* International Association of

Fire Fighters, Division of Occupational Health, Safety and Medicine. International Network of Cholesterol Skeptics. Access at http://www.thincs.org/.

International Society for Orthomolecular Medicine. Access at http://www. orthomed.org/.

Jackson, Peter, et al. 2006. Mobilising the Commodity Chain Concept in the Politics of Food and Farming. *Journal of Rural Studies.* April 2006. 22(2): 129-41.

Jacobs, Jane. 1993. *The Death and Life of Great American Cities.* New York, Modern Library.

Johansson, Olle. 2004. Screen Dermatitis and Electrosensitivity: Preliminary Observations in the Human Skin. In *Electromagnetic Environments and Health in Buildings.* Clements-Croome, Derek ed. New York, Spon Press: 377-90.

—. 2006. The Science of RFR Health Risks. *Your Own Health And Fitness.* KPFA 94.1FM. April 25, 2006.

Johansson, Olle, et al. 1999. A Case of Extreme and General Cutaneous Light Sensitivity in Combination with So-Called 'Screen Dermatitis' and 'Electrosensitivity' - a Successful Rehabilitation after Vitamin a Treatment - a Case Report. *Journal of the Autralasian College of Nutrition and Environmental Medicine.* April 1999. 18(1): 13-6.

Johansson, Olle and Doug Loranger. 2005. Electrosmog. *Your Own Health And Fitness.* KPFA 94.1FM. November 29, 2005.

Johnson, Carla and Mike Stobbe. 2006. Study Shows Americans Sicker Than English. *Washington Post.* Washington, DC. May 2, 2006.

Johnson, Eric J. and Daniel Goldstein. 2003. Do Defaults Save Lives? *Science.* November 21, 2003. 302: 1338-9.

Joy, Janet E., et al eds. 2005. *Saving Women's Lives: Strategies for Improving Breast Cancer Detection and Diagnosis.* Washington, DC, National Academies Press.

Katzmarzyk, Pete T., et al. 2005. Metabolic Syndrome, Obesity, and Mortality: Impact of Cardiorespiratory Fitness. *Diabetes Care.* February 2005. 28(2): 391-7.

Kawachi, Ichiro. 2006. Commentary: Social Capital and Health: Making the Connections One Step at a Time. *International Journal of Epidemiology.* July 26, 2006. 35(4): 989-93.

Kawachi, Ichiro, et al eds. 1999. *The Society and Population Health Reader: Income Inequality and Health.* New York, The New Press.

Kay, Jane. 2006. Toxic Toys: San Francisco Prepares to Ban Certain Chemicals in Products for Kids, but Enforcement Will Be Tough -- and Toymakers Question Necessity. *San Francisco Chronicle.* November 19, 2006.

—. 2008. Experts Question Plan to Spray to Fight Moths. *San Francisco Chronicle.* San Francisco. March 6, 2008.

Kellart, Stephen R. and Edward O. Wilson eds. 1993. *The Biophilia Hypothesis.* Washington, DC, Island Press.

Kendrick, Malcolm. 2003. High Blood Pressure: It's a Symptom, Not a Disease, Stupid! *Red Flags Daily.* January 9, 2003. Access at http://www. thincs.org/Malcolm.index.htm.

—. 2005a. Challenging the Convention on Heart Disease and Diabetes. *Your Own Health And Fitness.* KPFA 94.1FM. April 26, 2005.

—. 2005b. Heart Attacks Are Not Caused by Blood Clots. *Red Flags Daily.* September 12, 2005. Access at http://www.thincs.org/Malcolm.index.htm.

—. 2006. The Greatest Medical Scandal Ever? *Red Flags Daily.* January 27,

2006. Access at http://www.thincs.org/Malcolm.index.htm.

—. 2007. *The Great Cholesterol Con: The Truth About What Really Causes Heart Disease and How to Avoid It.* London, John Blake.

Kendrick, Malcolm and Uffe Ravnskov. 2006. Heart Disease: What Is It Really? *Your Own Health And Fitness.* KPFA 94.1FM. February 28, 2006.

Khamsi, Roxanne. 2006. The Dirty Truth About Allergies. *New Scientist.* 18. 26. Issue June 16, 2006.

Khaw, Kay-Tee, et al. 2008. Combined Impact of Health Behaviours and Mortality in Men and Women: The EPIC-Norfolk Prospective Population Study. *PLoS Medicine.* 5(1): e12.

Klein, Gary. 1998. *Sources of Power: How People Make Decisions.* Cambridge, MA, MIT.

Klein, Hilary Dole and Adrian M. Wenner. 2001. *Tiny Game Hunting: Environmentally Healthy Ways to Trap and Kill the Pests in Your House and Garden.* Berkeley, University of California Press.

Kolata, Gina. 2006. If You've Got a Pulse, You're Sick. *New York Times.* New York. May 21, 2007.

—. 2007. Find Yourself Packing It On? Blame Friends. *New York Times.* New York. July 26, 2007.

Kovner, Guy. 2007. Working out Reverses Aging, Novato Researchers Find. *Santa Rosa Press Democrat.* Santa Rosa. May 23, 2007.

Kregel, Kevin and Hannah Zhang. 2007. An Integrated View of Oxidative Stress in Aging: Basic Mechanisms, Functional Effects, and Pathological Considerations. *American Journal of Physiology - Regulatory, Integrative and Comparative Physiology.* January 2007. 292: R18-36.

Kuffel, Frances. 2004a. Passing for Thin. *Your Own Health And Fitness.* KPFA 94.1FM. June 8, 2004.

—. 2004b. *Passing for Thin: Losing Half My Weight and Finding My Self.* New York, Broadway Books.

Kunin, Richard. 1999. Orthomolecular Medicine: Treating with Targeted Nutrient Therapies. *Your Own Health And Fitness.* KPFA 94.1FM. September 14, 1999.

—. 2006. Nutrient Basics. *Your Own Health And Fitness.* KPFA 94.1FM. January 31, 2006.

Laaksonen, David E., et al. 2005. Physical Activity in the Prevention of Type 2 Diabetes. *Diabetes.* January 2005. 51: 158-65.

LaDou, Joseph. 2006a. Occupational and Environmental Medicine in the United States: A Proposal to Abolish Workers' Compensation and Reestablish the Public Health Model. *Int J Occup Environ Health.* April/June 2006. 12(2): 154-68.

—. 2006b. Occupational Health in the Semiconductor Industry. In *Challenging the Chip: Labor Rights and Environmental Justice in the Global Electronics Industry.* Smith, Ted, et al eds. Philadelphia, Temple University Press.

Lai, Henry. 2005. Biological Effects of Radiofrequency Electromagnetic Fields. In *Encyclopedia of Biomaterials and Biomedical Engineering.* Bowlin, Gary L. and Gary E. Wnek eds. New York, Marcel Dekker: 1-8.

Lai, Henry and Narendra Pal Singh. 1995. Acute Low-Intensity Microwave Exposure Increases DNA Single-Strand Breaks in Rat Brain Cells. *Bioelectromagnetics.* 16: 95-104.

—. 1996. Single- and Double-Strand DNA Breaks in Rat Brain Cells after

325

Acute Exposure to Low-Level Radiofrequency Electromagnetic Radiation. *Int J Radiat Biol.* 69: 513-21.

Lakoff, George. 1996. *Moral Politics: What Conservatives Know That Liberals Don't.* Chicago, University of Chicago Press.

—. 2008. *The Political Mind: Why You Can't Understand 21st-Century American Politics with an 18th-Century Brain.* New York, Viking.

Lakoff, George and Mark Johnson. 1999. *Philosophy in the Flesh: The Embodied Mind and Its Challenge to Western Thought.* New York, Basic Books.

Langer, Peter, et al. 2005. Hands-Free Mobile Phone Conversation Impairs the Peripheral Visual System to an Extent Comparable to an Alcohol Level of 4-5 G 100 Ml. *Hum Psychopharmacol Clin Exp.* 20: 65-6.

Langsjoen, Peter 2003. Discussions: Jan 2003 About Hypertension. *The International Network of Cholesterol Science.* January 3, 2003.

Larson, Magali Sarfatti. 1977. *The Rise of Professionalism: A Sociological Analysis.* Berkeley, University of California Press.

Lawlor, Debbie. 2004. Those Confounded Vitamins: What Can We Learn from the Difference between Observational Versus Randomized Trial Evidence? *The Lancet.* May 22, 2004. 363: 1724-7.

Layton, Lyndsey. 2009. No Bpa for Baby Bottles in U.S. *Washington Post.* Washington, DC. March 6, 2009.

Lazarus, David. 2007. How Water Bottlers Tap into All Sorts of Sources. *San Francisco Chronicle.* San Francisco. January 19, 2007: C1ff.

Lean, Geoffrey. 2007. EU Watchdog Calls for Urgent Action on Wi-Fi Radiation. *The Independent.* London. September 16, 2007.

Lee, Duk-Hee, et al. 2007a. Association of Serum Concentrations of Persistent Organic Pollutants with the Prevalence of Learning Disability and Attention Deficit Disorder. *J Epidemiol Community Health.* 61: 591-6.

—. 2007b. Association between Serum Concentrations of Persistent Organic Pollutants and Insulin Resistance among Nondiabetic Adults. *Diabetes Care.* June 2007. 30(3): 622-8.

—. 2006. A Strong Dose-Response Relation between Serum Concentrations of Persistent Organic Pollutants and Diabetes. *Diabetes Care.* 29(7): 1638-44.

—. 2007c. Extended Analyses of the Association between Serum Concentrations of Persistent Organic Pollutions and Diabetes. *Diabetes Care.* June 2007. 30(3): 1596-8.

Lee, John. 1996. *What Your Doctor May Not Tell You About Menopause.* New York, Warner.

—. 1999. *What Your Doctor May Not Tell You About Premenopause.* New York, Warner.

—. 2002. What Your Doctor May Not Tell You About Menopause. *Your Own Health And Fitness.* KPFA 94.1FM. February 19, 2002.

—. 2003. *Hormone Balance for Men.* Phoenix, AZ, Hormones Etc.

Lee, John and David Zava. 2002. *What Your Doctor May Not Tell You About Breast Cancer.* New York, Warner.

Lee, SoJung, et al. 2005. Cardiorespiratory Fitness Attenuates Metabolic Syndrome Risk Independent of Abdominal Subcutaneous and Visceral Fat in Men. *Diabetes Care.* April 2005. 28(4): 895-91.

Leonhardt, David. 2007. What's a Pound of Prevention Really Worth? *New York Times.* New York. January 24, 2007.

Lerner, Maura and Josephine Marcotty. 2007. No-Period Pill: Is It Meddling, or Convenience. *Minneapolis-St. Paul Star Tribune*. Minneapolis-St. Paul. May 28, 2007.

Levitt, B. Blake. 2007. *Electromagnetic Fields: A Consumer's Guide to the Issues and How to Protect Ourselves*. New York, Authors Guild.

—. 2008. Safe Cell Tower Siting. *Your Own Health And Fitness*. KPFA 94.1FM. March 11, 2008.

Levitt, B. Blake and Janet Newton. 2006. Wireless Public Health Crisis. *Your Own Health And Fitness*. KPFA 94.1FM. February 7, 2006.

Levitt, B. Blake and Cindy Sage. 2006. Where You're Exposed and What to Do: EMF and RFR. *Your Own Health And Fitness*. KPFA 94.1FM. March 14, 2005.

Ley, Ruth, et al. 2005. Obesity Alters Gut Microbial Ecology. *Proceedings of the National Academy of Science*. August 2, 2005. 102(31): 11070-5.

Linus Pauling Institute. Access at http://lpi.oregonstate.edu/.

Lipski, Elizabeth. 2004. *Digestive Wellness*. New York, McGraw-Hill.

Liu, Simin, et al. 1999. Whole-Grain Consumption and Risk of Coronary Heart Disease: Results from the Nurses' Health Study. *Am J Clin Nutr*. September 1999. 70: 412-9.

Lu, Chensheng, et al. 2008. Dietary Intake and Its Contribution to Longitudinal Organophosphorus Pesticide Exposure in Urban/Suburban Children. *Environmental Health Perspectives*. April 2008. 116(4): 537-42.

Lunder, Sonya. 2004. Toxic Cosmetics. *Your Own Health And Fitness*. KPFA 94.1FM. August 17, 2004.

Lynch, John, et al. 1997. Why Do Poor People Behave Poorly? Variation in Adult Health Behaviours and Psychosocial Characteristics by Stages of the Socioeconomic Lifecourse. *Soc Sci Med*. 44(6): 809-19.

Lynch, John and George Kaplan. 2000. Socioeconomic Position. In *Social Epidemiology*. Berkman, Lisa F. and Ichiro Kawachi eds. Oxford, Oxford University Press: 13-35.

MacDonald, Thomas and Giovanni Monteleone. 2005. Immunity, Inflammation, and Allergy in the Gut. *Science*. March 25, 2005. 307: 1920-5.

Macpherson, Andrew J., et al. 2005. Immune Responses That Adapt the Intestinal Mucosa to Commensal Intestinal Bacteria. *Immunology*. June 2005. 115(2): 153-62.

Markowitz, Gerald and David Rosner. 2002. *Deceit and Denial: The Deadly Politics of Industrial Pollution*. Berkeley, University of California Press.

Marks, Robert. 2002. *The Origins of the Modern World: A Global and Ecological Narrative*. New York, Rowman and Littlefield.

Marmot, Michael and Richard G. Wilkinson eds. 2006. *Social Determinants of Health*. New York, Oxford University Press.

Marohn, Stephanie. 2003. *The Natural Medicine Guide to Depression*. Charlottesville, VA, Hampton Roads Publishing Company.

Marois, Rene and Jason Ivanoff. 2005. Capacity Limits of Information Processing in the Brain. *Trends in Cognitive Sciences*. June 2005. 9(6): 296-305.

McCabe, Vinton. 2004. *Household Homeopathy: A Safe and Effective Approach to Wellness for the Whole Family*. Laguna Beach, CA, Basic Health.

—. 2007a. *The Healing Bouquet: Exploring Bach Flower Remedies*. Laguna Beach, CA, Basic Health.

—. 2007b. *The Healing Enigma: Demystifying Homeopathy*. Laguna Beach, CA, Basic Health.

—. 2008. The Essence of Healing: Discovering Bach Flower Remedies. *Your*

Own Health And Fitness. KPFA 94.1FM. September 23, 2008.

—. 2009. *The Healing Echo: Discovering Homeopathic Cell Salt Remedies.* Laguna Beach, CA, Basic Health.

McDonough, William and Michael Braungart. 2002. *Cradle to Cradle: Remaking the Way We Make Things.* New York, North Point Press.

McEwen, Bruce. 2004. Understanding Stress. *Your Own Health And Fitness.* KPFA 94.1FM. January 20, 2004.

—. 2008. Central Effects of Stress Hormones in Health and Disease: Understanding the Protective and Damaging Effects of Stress and Stress Mediators. *Eur J Pharm.* 583: 174-85.

McEwen, Bruce and Elizabeth Norton Lasley. 2002. *The End of Stress as We Know It.* Washington, DC, Joseph Henry Press.

McKenzie-Mohr, Doug and William Smith. 1999. *Fostering Sustainable Behavior: An Introduction to Community-Based Social Marketing.* Gabriola Island, British Columbia, New Society Publishers.

McKinley, Jesse. 2008. California Holds Off on Crop-Spraying Plan. *New York Times.* New York. April 25, 2008.

McPherson, Marianne and Lauren Korfine. 2004. Menstruation across Time: Menarche, Menstrual Attitudes, Experiences, and Behaviors. *Women's Health Issues.* November-December 2004. 14(6): 193-200.

McPherson, Ruth. 2007. A Common Allele on Chromosome 9 Associated with Coronary Heart Disease. *Sciencexpress.* May 3, 2007.

Medical Examiners Commission. 2007. *Drugs Identified in Deceased Persons by Florida Medical Examiners: 2007 Interim Report.* Tallahassee, FL: Florida Department of Law Enforcement. December 2007.

Melov, Simon, et al. 2007. Resistance Exercise Reverses Aging in Human Skeletal Muscle. *PLoS ONE.* 2(5): e465.

Melton, Lisa. 2006. The Antioxidant Myth. *New Scientist.* Issue August 5, 2006.

Microwave News. Access at http://www.microwavenews.com/.

Miller, Edgar R., et al. 2005. Meta-Analysis: High-Dosage Vitamin E Supplementation May Increase All-Cause Mortality. *Ann Intern Med.* January 4, 2005. 142(1): 37-46.

Minkler, Meredith ed. 2002. *Community Organizing and Community Building for Health.* New Brunswick, NJ, Rutgers University Press

Mokdad, Ali H., et al. 2004. Actual Causes of Death in the United States, 2000. *JAMA.* March 10, 2004. 291(10): 1238-45.

Moore, Elizabeth. 2006. *It's Child's Play: Advergaming and the Online Marketing of Food to Children,* Kaiser Family Foundation Report.

Motluk, Alison. 2007. How Many Things Can You Do at Once? *New Scientist.* Issue April 7, 2007: 28-31.

Murray, Christopher J.L., et al. 2006. Eight Americas: Investigating Mortality Disparities across Race, Counties, and Race-Counties in the United States. *PLoS Medicine.* September 2006. 3(9): e260.

MyPyramid.gov. Access at http://www.mypyramid.gov/.

Nagourney, Eric. 2008. Safety: Nonstandard Work Shifts May Hinder Recovery. *New York Times.* New York. January 29, 2008.

National Association of County and City Health Officials. Access at http://www.naccho.org/.

National Campaign to Control Hypertension. Access at http://www.controlhypertension.org/.

National Center for Health Statistics. 2004. *Health, United States, 2004, with Chartbook on Trends in the Health of Americans.* Hyattsville, Maryland:US Department of Health and Human Services. 2004-1232. September 2004.

National Diabetes Center, Coronary Heart Disease and Poor Blood Sugar Control. Access at http://diabetes-mellitus.org/chd.htm.

National Radiological Protection Board. 2004. *Mobile Phones and Health 2004.* Chilton, Oxfordshire, UK, NRPB.

National Sleep Foundation. 2000. *Adolescent Sleep Needs and Patterns.* Washington, DC:

—. 2005. *2005 Sleep in America Poll.* Washington, DC:

Natural Building Network. Access at http://www.naturalbuildingnetwork.org/.

Navarro, Vicente ed. 2002. *The Political Economy of Social Inequalities: Consequences for Health and Quality of Life.* Amityville, NY, Baywood Publishing Company.

Navarro, Vicente, et al. 2006. Politics and Health Outcomes. *The Lancet.* September 16, 2006. 368(9540): 1033-7.

Nazaroff, William W, et al. 2006. *Indoor Air Chemistry: Cleaning Agents, Ozone and Toxic Air Contaminants.* Sacramento:California Air Resources Board. April 2006.

Nebeker, Jonathan R., et al. 2005. High Rates of Adverse Drug Events in a Highly Computerized Hospital. *Arch Intern Med.* May 23, 2005. 165(10): 1111-6.

Nestle, Marion. 2002. *Food Politics: How the Food Industry Influences Nutrition and Health.* Berkeley, University of California Press.

NIH State-of-the-Science Panel. 2006. National Institutes of Health State-of-the-Science Conference Statement: Multivitamin/Mineral Supplements and Chronic Disease Prevention. *Ann Intern Med.* September 5, 2006. 145(5): 364-71.

Nordstron, Gunni. 2004. *The Invisible Disease: The Dangers of Environmental Illnesses Caused by Electromagnetic Fields and Chemical Emissions.* New York, O Books.

O'Brien, Mary. 2000. *Making Better Environmental Decisions: An Alternative to Risk Assessment.* Cambridge, MA, MIT.

Ojio, Shinsuke, et al. 2000. Considerable Time from the Onset of Plaque Rupture and/or Thrombi until the Onset of Acute Myocardial Infarction in Humans. *Circulation.* October 24, 2000. 102: 2063-9.

Olsen, Ole and Peter C. Gøtzsche. 2001a. Cochrane Review of Screening for Breast Cancer with Mammography. *The Lancet.* October 20, 2001. 358(9290): 1340-2.

—. 2001b. Cochrane Review on Screening for Breast Cancer with Mammography [Letter]. *The Lancet.* 358: 1340-2.

—. 2001c. Screening for Breast Cancer with Mammography. *Cochrane Database of Systematic Reviews.* 4: CD001877.

Organic Consumers Association. Access at http://www.organicconsumers.org/.

Organic Prairie. Access at http://www.organicprairie.com/.

Ornish, Dean. 2007. *The Spectrum: A Scientifically Proven Program to Feel Better, Live Longer, Lose Weight, and Gain Health.* New York, Ballantine.

Orthomolecular Health. Access at http://orthomolecularhealth.com/.

Orthomolecular Health Medicine Society. Access at http://www.ohmsociety.com/.

Orthomolecular Medicine News Service. Access at http://www.orthomolecular. org/resources/omns/index.shtml.

Orthomolecular.Org. Access at http://orthomolecular.org/.

Our Stolen Future. Access at http://www.ourstolenfuture.org/.

Packer, Lester and Carol Colman. 1999. *The Antioxidant Miracle*. New York, John Wiley and Sons.

Paleolithic Diet Page. Access at http://www.paleodiet.com/.

Pall, Martin. 2007. *Explaining Unexplained Illness*. Binghamton, NY, Harrington Park Press.

Pappas, Gregory. 2006. Geographic Data on Health Inequities. *PLoS Medicine*. September 2006. 3(9): e357.

Parker-Pope, Tara. 2008a. 8-Year-Olds on Statins? A New Plan Quickly Bites Back. *New York Times*. New York. July 8, 2008.

—. 2008b. Cholesterol Screening Is Urged for Young. *New York Times*. New York. July 7, 2008.

Pearson, Aria. 2007. Obesity's Helper in Triggering Diabetes. *New Scientist*. Issue April 14, 2007.

Physicians for a National Health Program. Access at http://www.pnhp.org/.

Physicians for Human Rights. 2003. *The Right to Equal Treatment*. Boston, Physicians for Human Rights.

Prentice, Jessica. 2006. *Full Moon Feast: Food and the Hunger for Connection*. White River Junction, VT, Chelsea Green.

Prevention Institute. Access at http://www.preventioninstitute.org/.

Prochaska, James, et al. 1995. *Changing for Good: A Revolutionary Six-Stage Program for Overcoming Bad Habits and Moving Your Life Positively Forward*. New York, Avon Books.

Pugh, Tony. 2007. US Economy Leaving Record Numbers in Severe Poverty. *McClatchy Newspapers*. February 23, 2007.

Putnam, Robert D. 2000. *Bowling Alone: The Collapse and Revival of American Community*. New York, Simon and Schuster.

Putnam, Robert D., et al. 2003. *Better Together: Restoring the American Community*. New York, Simon and Schuster.

Raloff, Janet. 2006. How Advertising Is Becoming Child's Play. *Science News*. 170. 5. Issue July 29, 2006.

Rampton, Sheldon and John Stauber. 2001. *Trust Us, We're Experts! How Industry Manipulates Science and Gambles with Your Future*. New York, Jeremy P. Tarcher/Putnam.

Ratneshwar, S., et al eds. 2000. *The Why of Consumption: Contemporary Perspectives on Consumer Motives, Goals, and Desires*. New York, Routledge.

Ravnskov, Uffe. 2000. *The Cholesterol Myths: Exposing the Fallacy That Cholesterol and Saturated Fat Cause Heart Disease*. Washington, DC, New Trends.

Real, Terrence. 1997. Male Depression. *Your Own Health And Fitness*. KPFA 94.1FM. July 15, 1997.

—. 1998. *I Don't Want to Talk About It*. New York, Fireside.

Reznik, Oleg. 2005. *The Secrets of Medical Decision Making: How to Avoid Becoming a Victim of the Health Care Machine*. Ann Arbor, Michigan, Loving Healing Press.

Riley, James C. 2001. *Rising Life Expectancy: A Global History*. New York, Cambridge University Press.

Risk-Screening Environmental Indicators (RSEI). Access at http://www.epa.gov/oppt/rsei/.

Rittersma, Saskia, et al. 2005. Plaque Instability Frequently Occurs Days or Weeks before Occlusive Coronary Thrombosis. *Circulation*. February 21, 2005. 111: 1160-5.

Robbins, John. 2007. *Healthy at 100*. New York, Ballantine.

Rosch, Paul J. 2003. The Emperor's New Clothes: Aggressive New Guidelines for "Prehypertension." *The Weston A. Price Foundation*. November 23, 2005.

Rose, Geoffrey. 1992. *The Strategy of Preventive Medicine*. Oxford, Oxford University Press

Rosen, George. 1993. *A History of Public Health*. Baltimore, Johns Hopkins University Press

Ross, Gilbert. 2007. SF Should Drop Ban on Certain Toys. *San Francisco Chronicle*. January 7, 2007.

Ross, Mark T., et al. 2005. The DNA Sequence of the Human X Chromosome. *Nature*. March 17, 2005. 434: 325-37.

Royte, Elizabeth. 2006. Drugging the Waters. *OnEarth*. Fall 2006: 26-31.

Rudel, Ruthann A., et al. 2007. Chemicals Causing Mammary Gland Tumors in Animals Signal New Directions for Epidemiology, Chemicals Testing, and Risk Assessment for Breast Cancer Prevention. *Cancer*. June 15, 2007. 109(12 Suppl): 2635-66.

Ruff, Christopher. 2000. Body Mass Prediction from Skeletal Frame Size in Elite Athletes. *American Journal of Physical Anthropology*. December 2000. 113(4): 507-17.

Ruff, Christopher, et al. 1993. Postcranial Robusticity in Homo. I: Temporal Trends and Mechanical Interpretation. *American Journal of Physical Anthropology*. May 1993. 91(1): 21-53.

Sage, Cindy. 2009. Regulating Wireless Radiation. *Your Own Health And Fitness*. KPFA 94.1FM. March 17, 2009.

Sage, Cindy. 2005. Smart Exposures: Understanding Risks from EMF and RFR. *Your Own Health And Fitness*. KPFA 94.1FM. July 19, 2005.

Sage, Cindy and David O. Carpenter. 2007. Bioinitiative: Standards for Electrosmog. *Your Own Health And Fitness*. KPFA 94.1FM. November 11, 2007.

Sahlins, Marshall. 2004. *Stone Age Economics*. New York, Routledge.

San Francisco Techconnect. Access at http://www.sfgov.org/techconnect/.

Sapolsky, Robert M. 1994. *Why Zebra's Don't Get Ulcers: A Guide to Stress, Stress-Related Diseases, and Coping*. New York, WH Freeman and Company.

—. 2001. The Biological Consequences of Stress. *Your Own Health And Fitness*. KPFA 94.1FM. September 25, 2001.

Saul, Andrew. 2003. *Doctor Yourself: Natural Healing That Works*. Long Beach, California, Basic Health Publications.

Schapiro, Mark. 2007. *Exposed: The Toxic Chemistry of Everyday Products and What's at Stake for American Power*. White River Jct, Vermont, Chelsea Green Publishing.

—. 2008. Why the US Is Importing Toxic Products. *Your Own Health And Fitness*. KPFA 94.1FM. June 17, 2007.

Schlosser, Eric. 2001. *Fast Food Nation: The Dark Side of the All-American Meal*. New York, Houghton Mifflin.

Schoenthaler, Stephen and Ian Bier. 2000. The Effect of Vitamin-Mineral Supplementation on Juvenile Delinquency among American Schoolchildren: A Randomized, Double-Blind Placebo-Controlled Trial. *J Altern Complement Med*. 6(1): 7-17.

Schoenthaler, Stephen, et al. 2000. The Effect of Vitamin-Mineral Supplementation on the Intelligence of American Schoolchildren: A Randomized, Double-Blind Placebo-Controlled Trial. *J Altern Complement Med*. 6(1): 19-29.

Schulze, Matthias B., et al. 2004. Sugar-Sweetened Beverages, Weight Gain, and Incidence of Type 2 Diabetes in Young and Middle-Aged Women. *JAMA*. 292(8): 927-34.

Science and Environmental Health Network. Access at http://www.sehn.org/.

Scuteri, Angelo, et al. 2005. The Metabolic Syndrome in Older Individuals. *Diabetes Care.* April 2005. 28(4): 882-8.

Severson, Kim. 2008. Los Angeles Stages a Fast Food Intervention. *New York Times.* New York. August 13, 2008.

Shabecoff, Philip and Alice Shabecoff. 2008. *Poisoned Profits: The Toxic Assault on Our Children.* New York, Random House.

Shin, Annys. 2008. Toxin Found in 'Natural,' 'Organic' Items. *Washington Post.* Washington, DC. March 15, 2008.

Sigman, Mariano and Stanislas Dehaene. 2006. Dynamics of the Central Bottleneck: Dual-Task and Task Uncertainty. *PLoS Biology.* July 2006. 4(7): e220.

Silent Spring Institute. Access at http://www.silentspring.org/.

Simpson, Scot. 2006. Dose-Response Relation between Sulfonylurea Drugs and Mortality in Type 2 Diabetes Mellitus. *Canadian Medical Association Journal.* January 17, 2006. 174(2): 169-74.

Singer, Natasha. 2007. Natural, Organic Beauty. *New York Times.* New York. November 1, 2007.

Slater, Arthur. 2005. Controlling Pests without Toxins. *Your Own Health And Fitness.* KPFA 94.1FM. May 3, 2005.

Slesin, Louis. 2005. When Enough Is Never Enough: A Reproducible EMF Effect at 12 Mg. *Microwave News.* 25(2): 1-2.

—. 2006. EMF Health News. *Your Own Health And Fitness.* KPFA 94.1FM. July 11, 2006.

Slynkova, Katarina, et al. 2006. The Role of Body Mass Index and Diabetes in the Development of Acute Organ Failure and Subsequent Mortality in an Observational Cohort. *Critical Care.* 10(5): 1-9.

Smink, Agnes, et al. 2008. Exposure to Hexachlorobenzene During Pregnancy Increases the Risk of Overweight in Children Aged 6 Years. *Acta Paediatrica.* July 2008. 97(10): 1465-9.

Smith, Melissa Diane. 2002. *Going against the Grain: How Reducing and Avoiding Grains Can Revitalize Your Health.* New York, Contemporary Books.

Solomon, Gina. 2003. Asthma and the Environment. *The Collaborative on Health and the Environment.* April 2003.

Sørensen, Thorkild I.A., et al. 2005. Intention to Lose Weight, Weight Changes, and 18-Y Mortality in Overweight Individuals without Co-Morbidities. *PLoS Medicine.* June 2005. 2(6): e171.

Sperber, Dan and Deirdre Wilson. 2002. Pragmatics, Modularity and Mind-Reading. *Mind and Language.* February/April 2002. 17(1/2): 3-23.

Squires, Sally. 2006. Panel Finds Conflicting Data on Multivitamin Benefit. *Washington Post.* Washington, DC. May 18, 2006: A15.

Srinivasan, U. Thara, et al. 2008. The Debt of Nations and the Distribution of Ecological Impacts from Human Activities. *Proceedings of the National Academy of Science.* February 5, 2008. 105(5): 1768-73.

Stansfeld, Stephen A and Mark P Matheson. 2003. Noise Pollution: Non-Auditory Effects on Health. *British Medical Bulletin.* December 2003. 68(1): 243-57.

Starr, Paul. 1982. *The Social Transformation of American Medicine.* New York, Basic Books.

Stein, Rob. 2007. Pill That Suppresses Periods Ok'd. *Washington Post.* Washington, DC. May 23, 2007.

Steinemann, Anne. 2008a. Foul Fragrance. *Your Own Health And Fitness.* KPFA 94.1FM. September 9, 2008.

—. 2008b. Fragranced Consumer Products and Undisclosed Ingredients. *Environmental Impact Assessment Review.* January 2009. 29(1): 32-8.

Steiner, Frederick. 2002. *Human Ecology: Following Nature's Lead.* Washington, DC, Island Press.

Stiglitz, Joseph E. 1987. The Causes and Consequences of the Dependence of Quality on Price. *Journal of Economic Literature.* March 1987. 25: 1-48.

Stop the Spray. Access at http://www.stopthespray.org/.

Story, Louise. 2008. Ftc Asks If Carbon-Offset Money Is Well Spent. *New York Times.* New York. January 9, 2008.

Strayer, David L., et al. 2006. A Comparison of the Cell Phone Driver and the Drunk Driver. *Human Factors.* Summer 2006. 48(2): 381-91.

Sturm, R. and D.A. Cohen. 2004. Suburban Sprawl and Physical and Mental Health. *Public Health.* 118: 488-96.

Susan G. Komen for the Cure. Access at http://cms.komen.org/komen/index.htm.

Sustainable Health Institute. Access at http://www.sustainablehealthinstitute.org/.

Svoboda, Elizabeth. 2008. The Worms Crawl In. *New York Times.* New York. July 1, 2008.

Swedish Association for the Electrosensitive. Access at http://www.feb.se/index_int.htm.

Szasz, Andrew. 2007. *Shopping Our Way to Safety: How We Changed from Protecting the Environment to Protecting Ourselves.* Minneapolis, University of Minnesota Press.

—. 2008. Shopping Our Way to Safety. *Your Own Health And Fitness.* KPFA 94.1FM. April 8, 2008.

Szreter, Simon and Michael Woolcock. 2004. Health by Association? Social Capital, Social Theory, and the Political Economy of Public Health. *International Journal of Epidemiology.* July 28, 2004. 33(4): 650-67.

Tapper, Andrew R., et al. 2004. Nicotine Activiation of α4* Receptors: Sufficient for Reward, Tolerance, and Sensitization. *Science.* November 5, 2004. 306: 1029-32.

Tarkan, Laurie. 2008. Doctors Say Medication Is Overused in Dementia. *New York Times.* New York. June 24, 2008.

Tarlov, Alvin R. and Robert F. St. Peter eds. 2000. *The Society and Population Health Reader: A State and Community Perspective.* New York, The New Press.

Tennessen, Carolyn M. and Bernadine Cimprich. 1995. Views to Nature: Effects on Attention. *Journal of Environmental Psychology.* March 1995. 15(1): 77-85.

Thayer, Robert. 2003. *Calm Energy: How People Regulate Mood with Food and Exercise.* New York, Oxford University Press.

Thun, Michael J., et al. 2008. Risky Business: Tools to Improve Risk Communication in a Doctor's Office. *JNCI.* June 19, 2008. 100(12): 830-1.

Tomlinson, Mark. 2003. Lifestyle and Social Class. *European Sociological Review.* February 2003. 19(1): 97-111.

Tuomilehto, Jaakko. 2007. Counterpoint: Evidence-Based Prevention of Type 2 Diabetes: The Power of Lifestyle Management. *Diabetes Care.* February 2007. 30(2): 435-8.

Tzoulas, Konstantinos, et al. 2007. Promoting Ecosystem and Human Health in Urban Areas Using Green Infrastructure: A Literature Review. *Landscape and Urban Planning.* 81: 167-78.

Ulrich, Roger S. 1984. View through a Window May Influence Recovery from Surgery. *Science.* April 27, 1984. 224: 420-1.

—. 1993. Biophilia, Biophobia, and Natural Landscapes. In *The Biophilia Hypothesis.* Kellart, Stephen R. and Edward O. Wilson eds. Washington, DC, Island Press: 73-137.

US Department of Health and Human Services and US Department of Agriculture. 2005. *Dietary Guidelines for Americans, 2005.* Washington, DC: US Government Printing Office. January 2005.

Velasquez-Manoff, Moises. 2008. The Worm Turns. *New York Times.* New York. June 29, 2008.

Verkerk, Robert. 2006. Protecting Access to Natural Products. *Your Own Health And Fitness.* KPFA 94.1FM. June 20, 2006.

vom Saal, Frederick and Claude Hughes. 2005. An Extensive New Literature Concerning Low-Dose Effects of Bisphenol A Shows the Need for a New Risk Assessment. *Environmental Health Perspectives.* August 2005. 113(8): 926-33.

Waber, Rebecca L., et al. 2008. Commercial Features of Placebo and Therapeutic Efficacy. *JAMA.* March 5, 2008. 299(9): 1016-7.

Wade, Nicholas. 2007. Gene Identified as Risk Factor for Heart Ills. *New York Times.* New York. May 4, 2007.

Walsh, William. 2005. Reducing Violent Behavior and Depression with Nutrients. *Your Own Health And Fitness.* KPFA 94.1FM. January 11, 2005.

Walton, Douglas. 1997. *Appeal to Expert Opinion: Arguments from Authority.* University Park, PA, Pennsylvania State University Press.

Weaver, Ian CG, et al. 2004. Epigenetic Programming by Maternal Behavior. *Nature Neuroscience.* 7: 847-54.

Weiss, Bernard and David C. Bellinger. 2006. Social Ecology of Children's Vulnerability to Environmental Pollutants. *Environmental Health Perspectives.* October 2006. 114(10): 1476-85.

Welch, H. Gilbert. 2004. *Should I Be Tested for Cancer? Maybe Not and Here's Why.* Berkeley, University of California Press.

—. 2008. Campaign Myth: Prevention as Cure-All. *New York Times.* New York. October 7, 2008.

Welch, H. Gilbert, et al. 2007. What's Making Us Sick Is an Epidemic of Diagnoses. *New York Times.* New York. January 2, 2007.

Welch, John S. 2003. Ritual in Western Medicine and Its Role in Placebo Healing. *Journal of Religion and Health.* Spring 2003. 42(1): 21-33.

Welfare State Growing Despite Overhauls. 2007. *New York Times.* New York. February 26, 2007.

Wen, Ming, et al. 2007. Neighbourhood Deprivation, Social Capital and Regular Exercise During Adulthood: A Multilevel Study in Chicago. *Urban Studies.* December 2007. 44(13): 2651-71.

Werner, Inge, et al. 2007. *Toxicity of Checkmate® LBAM-F and Epiphyas Postvittana Pheromone to Ceriodaphnia Dubia and Fathead Minnow (Pimephales Promelas) Larvae.* Davis, CA:University of California Davis, School of Veterinary Medicine. November 28, 2007.

Weston A. Price Foundation. Access at http://www.westonaprice.org/.

Wilson, Edward O. 1986. *Biophilia*. Boston, Harvard University Press.

Wireless Philadelphia. Access at http://www.wirelessphiladelphia.org/.

Wittstein, Ilan S., et al. 2005. Neurohumoral Features of Myocardial Stunning Due to Sudden Emotional Stress. *N Engl J Med*. 352(6): 539-48.

Woloshin, Steven, et al. 2008a. The Risk of Death by Age, Sex, and Smoking Status in the United States: Putting Health Risks in Context. *JNCI*. June 19, 2008. 100(12): 845-53.

—. 2008b. *Know Your Chances: Understanding Health Statistics*. Berkeley, University of California Press.

Women's Health Initiative Steering Committee. 2004. Effects of Conjugated Equine Estrogen in Postmenopausal Women with Hysterectomy: The Women's Health Initiative Randomized Controlled Trial. *JAMA*. April 13, 2004. 291(14): 1701-12.

Woolf, Steven. 2006. The Rising Prevalence of Severe Poverty in America. *Am J Prev Med*. 31(4): 332-41.

Wysowski, Diane, et al. 2003. Rapid Increase in the Use of Oral Antidiabetic Drugs in the United States, 1990-2001. *Diabetes Care*. 26(6): 1852-5.

Xu, Shujun, et al. 2006. Chronic Exposure to GSM 1800-Mhz Microwaves Reduces Excitatory Synaptic Activity in Cultured Hippocampal Neurons. *Neuroscience Letters*. May 8, 2006. 398(3): 253-7.

Yasko, Amy and Garry Gordon. 2006. Nutrigenomic Testing and the Methylation Pathway. *Townsend Letter*. January 2006: 69-73.

Your Own Health And Fitness. Access at http://www.yourownhealthandfitness.org/.

Zand, Janet, et al. 1999. *Smart Medicine for Healthier Living: A Practical A-to-Z Reference to Natural and Conventional Treatments for Adults*. Garden City Park, New York, Avery Publishing Group.

Zava, David, et al. 2007. Menstrual Suppression Cautions. *Your Own Health And Fitness*. KPFA 94.1FM. May 29, 2007.

ZRT Laboratory. Access at http://www.zrtlab.com/.

LaVergne, TN USA
27 December 2010
210215LV00004BA/8/P